NEUROLOGY
IN PRIMARY CARE

NEUROLOGY
IN PRIMARY CARE

Andrea C. Adams, MD
Consultant, Department of Neurology,
Mayo Clinic and Mayo Foundation;
Assistant Professor of Neurology,
Mayo Medical School; Rochester, Minnesota

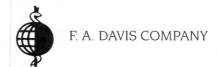

F. A. DAVIS COMPANY

As new scientific information becomes available through basic and clinical research, recommended treatments and drug therapies undergo changes. The author and publisher have done everything possible to make this book accurate, up to date, and in accord with accepted standards at the time of publication. The author, editors, and publisher are not responsible for errors or omissions or for consequences from application of the book, and make no warranty, expressed or implied, with regard to the contents of the book. Any practice described in this book should be applied by the reader in accordance with professional standards of care used with regard to the unique circumstances that may apply in each situation. The reader is advised always to check product information (package inserts) for changes and new information regarding dose and contraindications before administering any drug. Caution is especially urged when using new or infrequently ordered drugs. Nothing in this publication implies that Mayo Foundation endorses the products or equipment mentioned in this book.

Library of Congress Cataloging-in-Publication Data
Adams, Andrea C., 1955–
   Neurology in primary care / Andrea C. Adams.
     p. ; cm.
   Includes bibliographical references and index.
   ISBN 0-8036-0538-2 (alk. paper)
   1. Neurology—Handbooks, manuals, etc.   2. Nervous
system—Diseases—Handbooks, manuals, etc.   3. Primary care
(Medicine)—Handbooks, manuals, etc.
   [DNLM: 1. Nervous System Diseases—Handbooks.   3. Primary Health Care—Handbooks
WL 39 A211 2000]   I. Title.
   RC355 .A33 2000
   616.8—dc21

                                   00-031824

Dedicated to
Gene
and in memory of
Brunhilda

PREFACE

Neurology in Primary Care is intended to provide succinct and essential neurologic information for busy practicing primary care clinicians. Time is a rare commodity for these professionals, and the text, tables, and illustrations have been designed to provide quick and concise information.

Neurology is a rapidly changing specialty, with more therapeutic options available to treat neurologic disease. Neurologic symptoms such as headache, backache, and dizziness are frequent complaints that cause patients to seek medical care. *Neurology in Primary Care* was designed to give clinicians the necessary neurologic information for the diagnosis and management of these common neurologic problems.

This book will also be useful to medical students, neurology and medicine residents, and paramedical personnel who need a concise source of information on outpatient neurologic practice.

I want to thank Robert C. Benassi, emeritus Chair of the Section of Visual Information, and M. Alice McKinney, Section of Visual Information, for their expert help with the illustrations. I also thank O. Eugene Millhouse, PhD, Roberta J. Schwartz, Virginia Dunt, and Mary Schwager of the Section of Scientific Publications for their conscientious help in editing and preparing the manuscript for publication. I also thank Robert D. Brown, Jr., MD, for many of the radiographs. Finally, it is a pleasure to thank Jasper R. Daube, MD, and all my colleagues in the Department of Neurology at Mayo Cinic for their support and collegiality.

CONTENTS

PART I. EXAMINATION AND TESTING

1

THE NEUROLOGIC EXAMINATION 3
Gait Examination 4
Speech 5
Mental Status Examination 6
Cranial Nerves 6
   Olfactory Nerve, CN I 7
   Optic Nerve, CN II 7
   Oculomotor Nerve, CN III 10
   Trochlear Nerve, CN IV 11
   Trigeminal Nerve, CN V 11
   Abducens Nerve, CN VI 12
   Facial Nerve, CN VII 12
   Vestibulocochlear Nerve, CN VIII 13
   Glossopharyngeal Nerve, CN IX 14
   Vagus Nerve, CN X 14
   Spinal Accessory Nerve, CN XI 14
   Hypoglossal Nerve, CN XII 14
Motor Examination 14
Sensory Examination 16
Reflex Examination 19
Coordination Examination 23
Pediatric Examination 24
Geriatric Examination 24

2

DIAGNOSTIC TESTS 27
Cerebrospinal Fluid Analysis and Lumbar Puncture 28

ix

Indications   28
Contraindications   28
Procedure   28
Electroencephalography   30
Evoked Potentials   32
Nerve Conduction Studies and Electromyography   33
Nerve Conduction Studies   33
Muscle Studies   34
Neuroimaging   34
Computed Tomography   34
Magnetic Resonance Imaging   35
Angiography   37
Myelography   37

PART II. NEUROLOGIC SYMPTOMS

3

HEADACHE   41
Headache Red Flags   42
Diagnostic Testing   44
Neuroimaging   45
Electroencephalography   45
Lumbar Puncture   45
Other Tests   45
Classification   45
Principles of Therapy   46
Migraine Headache   48
Phases of Migraine   48
Types of Migraine   49
Associations of Migraine   50
Medications   52
Tension-Type Headache   57
Tension-Type Headache and Migraine   57
Treatment   58
Chronic Daily Headache   58
Cluster Headache   58
Treatment   59
Headaches of Short Duration   59
Post-Traumatic Headache   61
Temporal Arteritis   62
Facial Pain   63
Trigeminal Neuralgia   63
Glossopharyngeal Neuralgia   64
Occipital Neuralgia   64
Atypical Facial Pain   65

Herpes Zoster and Postherpetic Neuralgia   **65**
Temporomandibular Joint Dysfunction   **66**

4   SPINE AND LIMB PAIN   **69**
Spinal Anatomy   **71**
Evaluation of Spine Pain   **71**
Diagnostic Tests   **76**
Radiculopathy   **77**
Spinal Stenosis   **78**
Cervical Spondylosis   **80**
Whiplash   **82**
Spinal Surgery   **83**
Plexopathy   **85**

5   DIZZINESS   **89**
Diagnostic Approach   **90**
Vertigo   **94**
   Peripheral Causes   **96**
   Central Causes   **97**
Presyncope   **99**
Disequilibrium   **100**
Ill-Defined Dizziness   **102**

6   SENSORY LOSS AND PARESTHESIAS   **103**
Diagnostic Approach   **104**
Diabetic Neuropathy   **109**
   Generalized Sensorimotor Polyneuropathy   **110**
   Diabetic Autonomic Neuropathy   **111**
   Diabetic Polyradiculoneuropathy   **112**
   Truncal Neuropathy   **112**
   Mononeuropathy   **112**
Neuropathy of Other Endocrine Disorders   **113**
Metabolic Neuropathies   **113**
   Nutritional Disorders   **113**
   Chronic Renal Failure   **114**
   Porphyria   **114**
   Critical Illness   **114**
Toxic Neuropathies   **114**
Connective Tissue Disease   **114**
Dysproteinemic Polyneuropathy   **115**
Infectious Neuropathy   **116**
Inflammatory Neuropathies   **116**
   Acute Inflammatory Demyelinating Polyneuropathy   **116**
   Chronic Inflammatory Demyelinating
      Polyradiculoneuropathy   **118**
Focal Neuropathies   **118**

Carpal Tunnel Syndrome | 118
Other Compression Neuropathies | 119

7

WEAKNESS | **123**
Diagnostic Approach | 124
  Family History | 124
  Motor Examination | 125
  EMG | 125
  Muscle Biopsy | 125
Inherited Myopathies | 126
  Muscular Dystrophies | 126
  Myotonic Dystrophy | 126
Inflammatory Myopathies | 127
  Dermatomyositis | 127
  Polymyositis | 127
  Inclusion Body Myositis | 127
  Associated Conditions and Findings | 127
  Treatment | 128
Myopathies Associated with Drugs and Toxins | 128
Endocrine Myopathies | 128
Disorders of the Neuromuscular Junction | 130
  Myasthenia Gravis | 130
    Diagnostic Tests | 130
    Treatment | 131
    Factors That Exacerbate Myasthenia Gravis | 131
  Lambert-Eaton Syndrome | 132
  Botulism | 132
Motor Neuron Disease | 132
  Poliomyelitis | 134
  Cramps and Fasciculations | 134

8

MEMORY LOSS | **135**
Diagnostic Approach | 136
  History | 136
  Neurologic Examination | 139
  Mental Status Examination | 139
  Laboratory Investigation | 141
Forms of Dementia | 143
  Alzheimer Dementia | 143
  Dementia With Lewy Bodies | 147
  Vascular Dementia | 147
  Normal-Pressure Hydrocephalus | 149
  Frontotemporal Dementia | 150

9

SPELLS, SEIZURES, AND SLEEP DISORDERS | **153**
Spells | 154
Seizures | 155

Diagnostic Approach to a First Seizure 155
Treatment of Seizure Disorder 160
Epilepsy in Women 164
Sleep Disorders 165
Excessive Daytime Somnolence 166
Insomnia 167
Parasomnias 168

10 PAIN 171
General Management Principles 173
Diagnostic Approach 173
Treatment 174
Painful Polyneuropathy 178
Complex Regional Pain Syndromes 179
Postherpetic Neuralgia 179
Central Pain 180
Neuropathic Cancer Pain 180
Mental Disorders and Pain 181

PART III. COMMON NEUROLOGIC DISEASES

11 CEREBROVASCULAR DISEASE 185
Diagnostic Approach 186
Is It a Vascular Event? 187
Is Hospitalization Required? 188
Is the Event Hemorrhagic or Ischemic? 188
Does the Event Localize to the Anterior or Posterior
Circulation? 189
What Is the Mechanism? 190
Prevention of a First Stroke 192
Strategies 192
Modifiable Risk Factors 192
Hypertension 193
Myocardial Infarction 193
Atrial Fibrillation 194
Diabetes Mellitus 194
Carotid Artery Stenosis 194
Cigarette Smoking 195
Alcohol Consumption 195
Physical Activity 195
Dietary Factors 195
Other Factors 195
Symptomatic Carotid Artery Stenosis 196
Stroke in Young Adults 198
Migrainous Stroke 199
Arterial Dissection 199

Illicit Drug Use   **199**
Hematologic Disorders   **200**
Cardiac Causes   **200**
Treatment of Acute Stroke: Thrombolytic Therapy   **200**
Hemorrhagic Stroke   **201**

12   **MOVEMENT DISORDERS**   **203**
Classifying Movement Disorders   **204**
Diagnostic Approach to Movement Disorders   **204**
Parkinsonism   **207**
Features of Parkinsonism   **208**
Tremor   **208**
Bradykinesia   **208**
Rigidity   **208**
Postural Instability   **209**
Other Manifestations   **209**
Differential Diagnosis   **210**
Medical Treatment of Parkinson Disease   **210**
Managing Late Complications of Parkinson Disease   **213**
Motor Fluctuations   **213**
Dyskinesias   **215**
Other Late Complications   **215**
Surgical Therapy for Parkinson Disease   **215**
Tremor   **216**
Definition   **216**
Types   **216**
Dystonia   **219**
Definition and Types   **219**
Treatment   **220**
Tics and Tourette Syndrome   **220**
Definition and Types   **221**
Treatment   **221**
Tardive Syndromes   **221**
Diagnosis   **221**
Treatment   **222**

13   **IMMUNE AND INFECTIOUS DISEASES**   **225**
Multiple Sclerosis   **226**
Features and Types   **227**
Diagnostic Approach   **228**
Diagnostic Laboratory Support   **230**
Differential Diagnosis   **233**
Epidemiology   **233**
Prognosis   **234**
Pregnancy   **234**
Disease-Modifying Therapy   **235**
Symptomatic Therapy   **236**

Optic Neuritis   **237**
Connective Tissue Diseases and the Vasculitides   **237**
Infectious Diseases of the Nervous System   **238**
   HIV Infection   **238**
   Lyme Disease   **242**

14   **NEURO-ONCOLOGY**   **245**
Primary Brain Tumors   **246**
   Diagnostic Approach   **246**
   Management   **248**
Spinal Cord Tumors   **250**
Neurologic Complications of Systemic Disease   **251**
   Metastases   **251**
     Diagnosis   **252**
     Treatment   **252**
   Epidural Spinal Cord Compression   **252**
   Meningeal Carcinoma   **253**
   Neurologic Complications of Therapy   **253**
   Paraneoplastic Syndromes   **254**
     Definition, Description, and Diagnosis **254**
     Treatment   **256**

INDEX   **259**

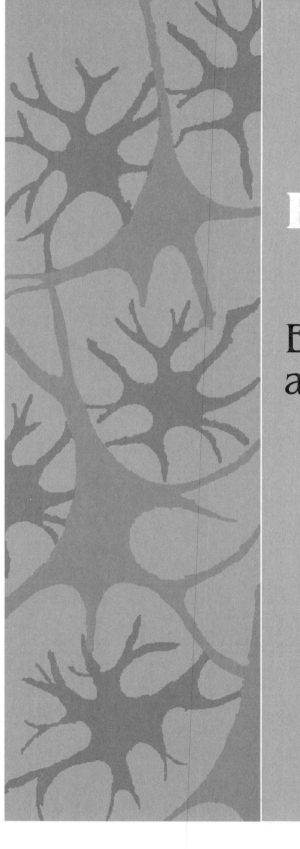

PART I

Examination and Testing

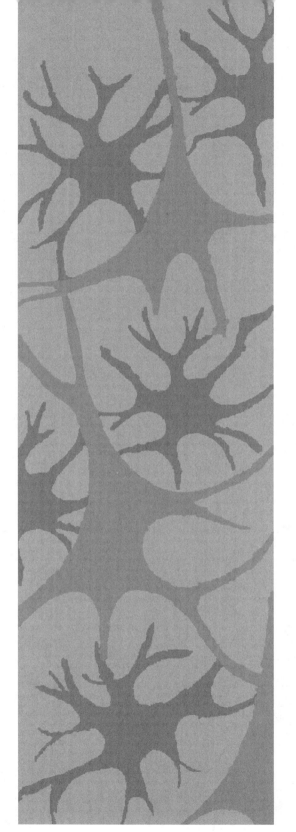

CHAPTER 1

The Neurologic Examination

CHAPTER OUTLINE

Gait Examination
Speech
Mental Status Examination
Cranial Nerves
    Olfactory Nerve, CN I
    Optic Nerve, CN II
    Oculomotor Nerve, CN III
    Trochlear Nerve, CN IV
    Trigeminal Nerve, CN V
    Abducens Nerve, CN VI
    Facial Nerve, CN VII
    Vestibulocochlear Nerve, CN VIII
    Glossopharyngeal Nerve, CN IX
    Vagus Nerve, CN X
    Spinal Accessory Nerve, CN XI
    Hypoglossal Nerve, CN XII
Motor Examination
Sensory Examination
Reflex Examination
Coordination Examination
Pediatric Examination
Geriatric Examination

The neurologic examination is the most important part of the evaluation of a patient with neurologic symptoms or disease. Most neurologists schedule 1 hour for the evaluation of a new patient; this is considerable compared with the 15 to 30 minutes scheduled by primary care physicians for a new patient. Therefore, it is imperative for primary care providers to maximize the limited time available for the examination.

The neurologic history usually provides all the information needed to understand the disease process. The temporal profile of symptoms is critical. The sudden onset of symptoms suggests a vascular cause of the illness. In contrast, slowly progressive symptoms suggest a degenerative or neoplastic process. Infections and inflammatory processes are often subacute, and a fluctuating course may indicate demyelinating disease. For example, the sudden onset of severe headache suggests subarachnoid hemorrhage instead of a brain tumor, which is associated with progressive headache of several months' duration.

The results of a neurologic examination help to localize the problem in the nervous system. A relatively complete neurologic examination can be performed in a limited time by attending to the patient's gait, speech, and mental status. The often-reported "grossly intact" or "CN II-XII intact" conveys little useful information. A description of the patient's gait as he or she walks from the waiting room to the examining room and a description of the speech and use of language during the history taking often cover many of the important features of a neurologic examination. For example, the report that a patient walks with a shuffling gait and has microphonic speech and memory difficulty or that the patient has a wide-based staggering gait, slurred (dysarthric) speech, and poor attention provides meaningful neurologic data.

GAIT EXAMINATION

Watch the patient walk. Normal walking depends on several factors that reflect function at every level of the nervous system: motor, sensory, balance, and reflex systems. Gait changes with age and is sensitive to diseases of the nervous system. Gait disorders are common in elderly persons and frequently contribute to the risk of falling.

Normal walking requires equilibrium and locomotion. Equilibrium involves the ability to assume an upright posture and to maintain balance. Locomotion is the ability to initiate and maintain rhythmic stepping. Both components involve sensory input from the vestibular, proprioceptive, tactile, and visual systems and proper function of motor and reflex systems.

Nonneurologic factors that affect gait include the musculoskeletal and cardiovascular systems. Familiar examples are the slow exercise-intolerant gait of a patient with congestive heart failure and the limp of a patient with degenerative joint disease. Gaits and their typical features and associated diseases are summarized in Table 1–1. The similarities between various gait disorders reflect the limited ways patients adjust to deteriorating performance.

The neurologic examination begins with how the patient is sitting in the waiting room chair. Secondary gain may be suggested when a patient with work-related low back pain sits comfortably, with legs crossed and reading a magazine, and then walks painfully into the examination room. A patient with proximal muscle weakness needs to push off with the hands to become upright, and a patient with parkinsonism has to make several rocking attempts before being able to stand.

Note how the patient stands. The posture, the position of the extremities, and the position of the head provide important diagnostic information. Watch how the patient initiates movement. Patients with parkinsonism or certain degenerative disorders have trouble starting (called "ignition failure"). Does the patient require gait aids such as a cane or a companion's arm? Is the stance wide-based, as in cerebellar disorders? Is the head held perfectly still, as in vestibular disorders? Watch the symmetry of associated movements, such

TABLE 1–1. GAIT TYPES: CHARACTERISTICS AND ASSOCIATED DISEASES

Gait Type	Characteristics	Associated Diseases
Antalgic	Painful, flexed, slow	Low back pain, arthritis
Hemiplegic or hemiparetic	Flexed arm, extended leg with circumduction	Stroke
Myopathic	Waddle, proximal muscle weakness of hip girdle with excess pelvic rotation	Polymyositis, muscular dystrophies
Spastic, diplegic	Stiff, bouncy, circumduction of legs, scissors-like gait	Cervical myelopathy, vitamin B_{12} deficiency, multiple sclerosis, cerebral palsy
Sensory ataxia	Footdrop, high steppage gait	Peripheral neuropathy, peroneal palsy, L5 radiculopathy, multiple sensory deficits
Vestibular ataxia	Wide-based, head held still, cautious gait	Benign positional vertigo, ototoxic drugs (aminoglycoside antibiotics)
Parkinsonian or extrapyramidal	Flexed posture, small steps, shuffling, turn en bloc, trouble initiating movement, festinating	Parkinson disease, drug-induced parkinsonism (phenothiazines)
Cerebellar ataxia	Wide-based, lateral instability, erratic foot placement	Alcoholism, phenytoin toxicity, multiple sclerosis
Psychogenic, astasia-abasia	Odd gyrations, near falling, fluctuating movement	Conversion disorder
Orthopedic	Similar to antalgic and myopathic	Prosthetic joints
Frontal gait, gait apraxia, "lower body parkinsonism"	Wide-based, short stride, trouble with starts and turns, feet glued to ground	Normal pressure hydrocephalus, small vessel disease, multiple strokes

as arm swing. A useful exercise for improving the power of observation is to watch the gait of people in a public place.

SPEECH

Speech is an integral part of the neurologic examination and can be evaluated while the medical history is being taken. Evaluation of a patient's speech and the usual examination of the head, eyes, ears, nose, and throat (HEENT examination) include examining cranial nerves (CNs) II through XII. The primary lower motor neurons for speech include the trigeminal (CN V), facial (CN VII), vagus (CN X), and hypoglossal (CN XII) cranial nerves. The glossopharyngeal (CN IX) and accessory (CN XI) nerves may also be involved. The phrenic nerve from the fourth cervical segment (C4) of the spinal cord innervates the diaphragm, and the spinal intercostal nerves innervate the thoracic intercostal muscles.

Understanding the different types of dysarthria is essential for evaluating speech. *Dysarthria* is a term for a group of motor speech disorders caused by dysfunction of the peripheral or central nervous system. Dysarthria is the imperfect articulation of speech, and abnormalities are apparent in the speed, strength, range, and timing of speech or in the accuracy of speech movements. The different types of dysarthria are listed in Table

1–2 and include flaccid, spastic, ataxic, hypo-kinetic, hyperkinetic, and mixed.

MENTAL STATUS EXAMINATION

Most of the mental status examination can be performed while the history is being taken. However, when the patient or the patient's family complains of memory or cognitive difficulty, further evaluation is recommended. Often, formal testing is not done because of lack of time. Short standardized screening tests such as the Mini-Mental State Examination (MMSE) and the short test of mental status, which is used at the Mayo Clinic, are useful screening devices for dementia. They also are time-consuming, and the results often are not sensitive enough for recognizing early cognitive decline. The tests are valuable as screening tools for elderly patients, because they establish baseline function, can be used for longitudinal monitoring, and suggest whether further testing or referral is needed. Paramedical personnel can perform the test-

ing. Testing is recommended for elderly patients before elective hospitalization, because dementia is a major risk factor for delirium in a hospital setting.

Areas of cognitive function that need to be tested include attention, recent and remote memory, language, praxis, visual-spatial relationships, judgment, and calculations. Specific testing is recommended because mildly demented patients with preserved social skills are able to converse superficially and their cognitive deficits can be easily missed. Factors that must be considered in the interpretation of the results include the patient's age, educational level, ethnicity, and primary language (if other than English). Table 1–3 summarizes how specific cognitive function is tested and provides anatomical and clinical correlation. Mental status testing is discussed in more detail in Chapter 8.

CRANIAL NERVES

Together, the HEENT and speech examinations provide a rapid and relatively compre-

TABLE 1–2. TYPES OF DYSARTHRIA: CHARACTERISTICS, LOCALIZATION OF LESION, ASSOCIATED DISEASES

Type (Deficit)	Characteristics	Localization of Lesion	Associated Diseases
Flaccid (weakness)	Hypernasal, breathy, audible inspiration (stridor)	Lower motor neuron	Amyotrophic lateral sclerosis, lower motor neuron disease
Spastic or pseudobulbar palsy (spasticity)	Slow rate, strained, reduced variability of pitch and loudness	Bilateral upper motor neuron	Multiple strokes
Ataxic (incoordination)	Irregular, scanning	Cerebellum	Cerebellar degenerative disease
Hypokinetic (rigidity and reduced range of movement)	Rapid rate	Basal ganglia	Parkinson disease
Hyperkinetic (involuntary movement)	Variable rate, loudness, distorted vowels	Basal ganglia	Huntington disease
Mixed	Spastic-flaccid Spastic-ataxic		Amyotrophic lateral sclerosis, lower motor neuron disease, multiple sclerosis

TABLE 1–3. TESTS OF COGNITIVE FUNCTION, WITH ANATOMICAL AND CLINICAL CORRELATION

Cognitive Function	Mental Status Test	Pathophysiology or Anatomy	Associated Disease or Feature
Attention	Digit span	Toxic-metabolic, diffuse, multifocal	Acute confusional syndrome
Memory	Recall	Medial temporal lobe, association cortex	Alzheimer disease
Language	Name objects, repeat phrase, follow commands	Left (dominant) hemisphere	Aphasia
Praxis	Show how to use a hammer	Left (dominant) frontal or parietal lobe	Apraxia
Calculation	Arithmetic	Left parietal lobe	Acalculia
Visual-spatial	Draw a cube or clock	Right hemisphere	Neglect
Executive function, judgment	Abstractions, proverbs	Frontal lobes	Behavioral changes

hensive evaluation of the cranial nerves. However, if the patient's primary complaint involves the cranial nerves, a more thorough evaluation is needed.

OLFACTORY NERVE, CN I

Olfactory sense is not routinely tested, but the absence of smell (anosmia) can be a complaint that warrants further investigation. Each nostril is tested with a nonirritating aroma to avoid stimulation of the trigeminal nerve. Common testing agents used are mint and coffee. The common causes of anosmia are nasal or paranasal disease and viral infections. Trauma is another frequent cause of anosmia. Hyposmia, or decreased olfactory sensation, is associated with several degenerative disorders, including Parkinson disease, Alzheimer disease, and human immunodeficiency virus (HIV)–dementia complex. Frequently, medications and environmental agents cause decreased olfaction. The perversion of smell (parosmia) and unpleasant odors (cacosmia) occur in psychiatric disease and develop after head trauma. Hyperosmia, or increased olfactory sensation, may occur with migraine headache. Olfactory hallucinations are often an aura in temporal lobe seizures.

OPTIC NERVE, CN II

The optic nerve and visual pathway encompass a major portion of the central nervous system; thus, evaluation of this system provides considerable information. The pertinent structures are the retina, optic nerve, optic chiasm, optic tract, and optic radiations in the temporal and parietal lobes, and the primary visual cortex in the occipital lobe. Visual testing should include assessing central and peripheral vision and the pupillary light reflex (Fig. 1–1) and performing a funduscopic examination. Test visual acuity in each eye with correction (glasses on), and test visual fields with glasses off, so the frames do not obstruct vision.

The pupillary light reflex consists of input (CN II, afferent limb), output (CN III, efferent limb), and an intermediary station (midbrain, or interneuron). If pupil abnormalities are found on examination, the next step is to determine which arm of the reflex is affected. Most often, anisocoria (unequal pupils) is a normal variation, but the asymmetry is slight and both pupils react to light and accommodation. Common pupil abnormalities and associated clinical conditions are summarized in Figure 1–2. A small pupil (miosis) associated with ptosis (droopy eyelid) and anhidrosis (absence of sweating) is called

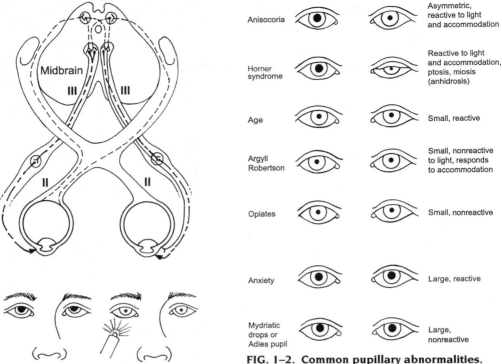

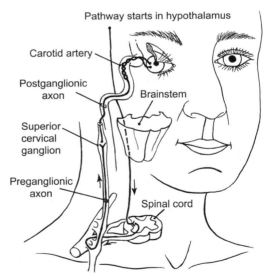

Afferent limb = CN II   – – – –
Interneuron = midbrain
Efferent limb = CN III   — – – —

FIG. 1–1. Pathway of pupillary light reflex. CN, cranial nerve.

FIG. 1–2. Common pupillary abnormalities.

Horner syndrome and results from sympathetic dysfunction. The sympathetic system can be affected in several places along its extended course (Fig. 1–3). A central autonomic tract, which controls the sympathetic system, descends from the hypothalamus through the lateral part of the brainstem. Horner syndrome frequently occurs with a lateral brainstem infarct, such as that associated with the lateral medullary (or Wallenberg) syndrome. This descending tract ends in the intermediolateral cell column of the upper thoracic cord, from which sympathetic fibers (preganglionic) leave the spinal cord and ascend in the sympathetic chain. Tumors at the apex of the lung (Pancoast tumor), thyroid tumors, or any cervical abnormality can cause Horner syndrome by interfering with these sympathetic fibers. The preganglionic

FIG. 1–3. Pathway for sympathetic control of the pupil. Interruption of this pathway results in Horner syndrome. (Modified from Patten, J: Neurological Differential Diagnosis. Springer-Verlag, New York, 1977, p 7, with permission.)

sympathetic fibers end in the superior cervical ganglion, from which postganglionic sympathetic fibers leave and join the carotid artery and travel with it to CN III.

Visual loss caused by optic neuropathy is characterized by decreased visual acuity, abnormal color vision (dyschromatopsia), an afferent pupillary defect, nerve fiber-type visual field defect (e.g., altitudinal visual field defect), and swelling or atrophy of the optic nerve (Fig. 1–4). Optic neuritis is the most common cause of optic neuropathy in young adults and presents with acute visual loss. Anterior ischemic optic neuropathy is the most common optic neuropathy in middle-aged and older adults. An altitudinal visual field defect (e.g., visual loss in the lower half of the visual field in one eye) often occurs in anterior optic neuropathy, with swelling of the optic disk from nonembolic occlusion of one of the posterior ciliary arteries. Further

evaluation or referral is recommended for patients with any visual field defect that suggests optic neuropathy.

Lack of time is often given as a reason for not performing visual field testing; however, confrontation testing can be done relatively quickly and can provide valuable information. Patients do not complain of visual field loss, and clinically silent lesions may be detected. It is best to test each eye separately and to ask the patient to look straight at the examiner's eye. Bring the target object (e.g., finger, pen) in from the periphery of each quadrant of the eye. Record the visual fields as seen by the patient. Monocular visual field loss indicates a lesion of the optic nerve. A bilateral temporal field deficit indicates a pituitary lesion or optic chiasm lesion. Homonymous hemianopia (visual loss on the same side in each eye) indicates a lesion of the optic radiations on the side of

FIG. 1–4. Funduscopic examination. Top, Appearance of normal fundus. **Bottom,** Comparison of normal optic disk and optic disk in papilledema and optic atrophy. In papilledema, the margins of the disk are blurred; also note the fullness of the veins. In optic atrophy, the disk is pale and has sharp margins. (**Top** modified from Liu, GT: Disorders of the eyes and eyelids. In Samuels, MA, and Feske, S (eds): Office Practice of Neurology. Churchill Livingstone, New York, 1996, pp 40–74, with permission. **Bottom** modified from Patten, J: Neurological Differential Diagnosis. Springer-Verlag, New York, 1977, p 27, with permission.)

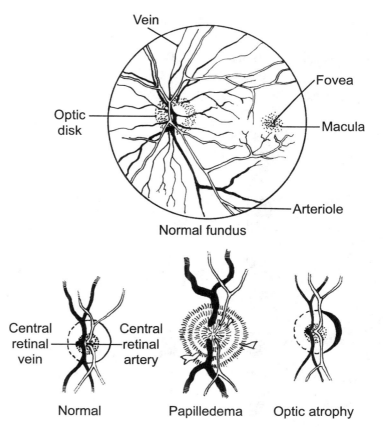

the brain opposite that of the patient's deficit (i.e., right visual field loss indicates left brain lesion). Visual field loss involving the upper quadrant of each eye ("pie in the sky") indicates a temporal lobe lesion and a "pie in the floor," a parietal lobe problem (Fig. 1–5).

OCULOMOTOR NERVE, CN III

The oculomotor nerve supplies the levator palpebra superioris, medial rectus, superior rectus, inferior rectus, and inferior oblique muscles of the eye. It also is the efferent limb of the pupillary light reflex. A patient

FIG. 1–5. Visual field defects.

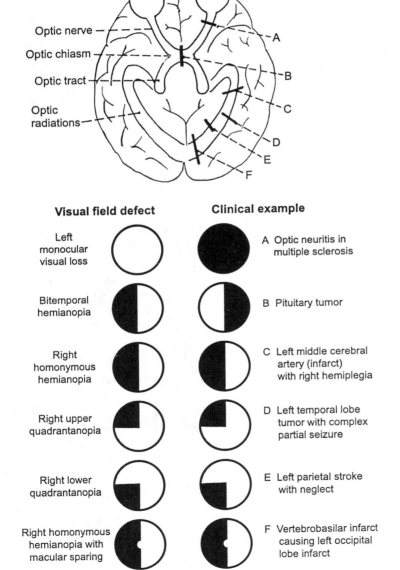

Visual field defect   **Clinical example**

Left monocular visual loss

A Optic neuritis in multiple sclerosis

Bitemporal hemianopia

B Pituitary tumor

Right homonymous hemianopia

C Left middle cerebral artery (infarct) with right hemiplegia

Right upper quadrantanopia

D Left temporal lobe tumor with complex partial seizure

Right lower quadrantanopia

E Left parietal stroke with neglect

Right homonymous hemianopia with macular sparing

F Vertebrobasilar infarct causing left occipital lobe infarct with an eye movement problem may complain of double vision (diplopia), blurry vision, and even dizziness, described as disequilibrium. CN III palsy is often due to a vascular problem from diabetes mellitus, hypertension, or atherosclerosis. A patient with paralysis of CN III has ptosis, and the eye is positioned down and out (Fig. 1–6). If both pupils are equal and reactive to light (pupil sparing), the paralysis is less likely caused by a compressive lesion. Further evaluation or referral is warranted.

Test CN III, IV, and VI by having the patient follow your finger or a light to the right, left, up, down, and diagonally in both directions. Figure 1–6 indicates which muscle is tested and gives examples of how dysfunction of CN III, IV, and VI would appear and be recorded. Both eyes are tested together, but if weakness is noted or the patient complains of double vision, then each eye should be tested separately.

TROCHLEAR NERVE, CN IV

The trochlear nerve supplies the superior oblique muscle that moves the eye down toward the nose. An isolated CN IV palsy is often due to trauma. Patients most often complain of vertical diplopia and have a tendency to keep their head tilted away from the affected side to reduce double vision.

TRIGEMINAL NERVE, CN V

The trigeminal nerve, the largest cranial nerve, is the primary sensory nerve of the face and head. The motor component innervates the muscles of mastication (masseter, temporal, and pterygoid muscles). Test these muscles by having the patient clench the jaw while you palpate the masseter and temporal muscles on each side and watch the jaw open. Deviation of the jaw indicates

FIG. 1–6. Extraocular muscle dysfunction. Extraocular muscles: **IO,** inferior oblique; **IR,** inferior rectus; **LR,** lateral rectus; **MR,** medial rectus; **SO,** superior oblique; **SR,** superior rectus. 0 = normal, −1 = weak, −2 = very weak, −3 = severe weakness, −4 = complete paralysis.

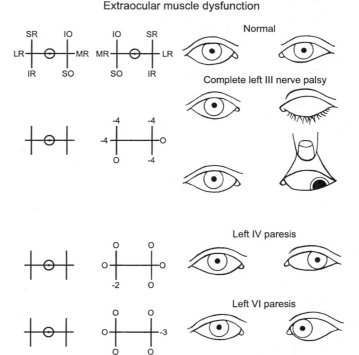

muscle weakness; the deviation is toward the side of the involved nerve.

The sensory distribution of the three branches of the trigeminal nerve is shown in Figure 1–7. This anatomical information is helpful in understanding a patient's complaint of facial pain or numbness. A quick screen of facial sensation is to touch each side of the forehead, cheek, and chin and ask if the sensation is "about the same" on both sides. The ophthalmic branch supplies the upper part of the face, including the cornea, as far as the vertex of the head. This branch is the afferent limb of the corneal reflex (stimulation of the cornea of one eye produces blinking and tearing in both eyes). This reflex is useful in evaluating a comatose patient because it allows you to examine CN V, the pons, and CN VII (the efferent limb of the corneal reflex). In an awake patient, testing the corneal reflex provides objective in-

formation about the patient's complaint of facial numbness. With the patient looking to one side (to avoid blinking due to visual threat), lightly touch the edge of the cornea with a corner of a piece of tissue that has been twisted to a point.

The most common clinical syndrome associated with the trigeminal nerve is trigeminal neuralgia, discussed in Chapter 3.

ABDUCENS NERVE, CN VI

The abducens nerve innervates the lateral rectus muscle, which moves the eye laterally. Patients complain of horizontal double vision that is most prominent when they look to a particular side, which is the side of the deficit. To compensate, patients turn their head toward the side of the lesion. CN VI nerve palsies are more frequent than CN III or IV nerve palsies. Neoplasm is a frequent cause of CN VI nerve palsy.

FACIAL NERVE, CN VII

The facial nerve innervates the muscles of facial expression and contains parasympathetic axons that innervate the salivary and lacrimal glands. Its sensory axons innervate taste buds on the anterior two-thirds of the tongue. Test the nerve by telling patients to "Wrinkle your forehead," "Close your eyes," and "Show me your teeth." Note the symmetry of movements.

In a patient with a facial nerve palsy, involvement of the forehead and eye indicates a peripheral nerve lesion (distal to the internal auditory meatus, Fig. 1–8). The phrase "tear, ear, taste, and face" describes the end points of the branches of the nerve to the lacrimal gland, stapedius muscle, taste buds on the anterior two-thirds of the tongue, and facial muscles. The most common cause of a peripheral facial palsy, often called "Bell palsy," is idiopathic. Approximately 85% of people with this condition recover over a 2- to 3-week period. Most patients require reassurance that they have not had a stroke. The dry cornea needs to be protected from abrasion. Frequently, eye patching is ineffective

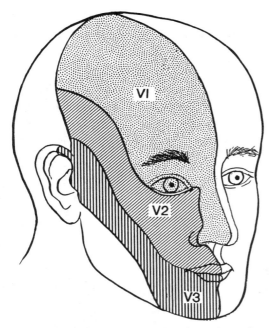

FIG. 1–7. Distribution of the three branches (V1, V2, and V3) of the trigeminal nerve. V1, Ophthalmic branch; **V2,** maxillary branch; **V3,** mandibular branch. (Modified from Patten, J: Neurological Differential Diagnosis. Springer-Verlag, New York, 1977, p 41, with permission.)

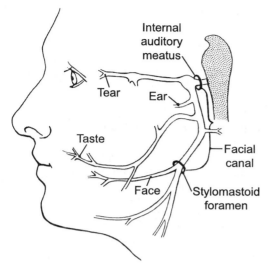

FIG. 1–8. Peripheral distribution of the facial nerve.

because the eye is often open under the patch. Artificial tears help lubricate the eye during the day, and ocular ointments can be used at night, with patching or taping.

The evaluation of facial paralysis often puts primary care providers in a difficult position. The most likely diagnosis is idiopathic facial palsy, which will resolve spontaneously without unnecessary and expensive testing. However, there is the risk of delaying prompt intervention for less common causes of facial paralysis such as tumors, infection, and systemic illness. Unless there are atypical features or evidence to suggest systemic illness, it is reasonable to allow 2 to 3 weeks for spontaneous recovery.

The proper treatment of idiopathic facial palsy is under debate. Corticosteroids are often used to speed recovery and to avoid complete paralysis. If used, these agents should be started early. A suggested dose is 1 mg/kg per day for 7 days, then tapered to zero over the next 10 days. Treatment with acyclovir (or famciclovir) is supported by studies that suggest idiopathic facial palsy is caused by a herpes simplex or varicella-zoster virus infection. Studies have shown better outcome for patients with Ramsay Hunt syndrome (varicella-zoster infection with facial paralysis and herpetic eruption in

the ear) treated with prednisone and acyclovir at 800 mg 5 times a day for 7 days.

VESTIBULOCOCHLEAR NERVE, CN VIII

The vestibulocochlear nerve transmits information from the vestibular apparatus (for balance) and cochlea (for hearing) to the brain. The vestibular portion of the nerve is not routinely tested in the office. Caloric testing is a useful test for vestibular function. Vestibular deficits that are seen on the neurologic exam include problems with gait and balance and nystagmus. Vestibular function is considered in Chapter 5.

Auditory acuity can be assessed during the interview by noting the patient's response to softly spoken words. Some examiners hold up a watch and measure the distance from which the patient is able to hear it. If a more detailed evaluation is needed, audiology referral is recommended.

A tuning fork can be used to distinguish between hearing loss due to middle ear disease (conductive loss) and that due to sensorineural injury (perceptive loss). In the Rinne test, a vibrating tuning fork is placed on the patient's mastoid process until the patient reports not being able to hear the vibrations, after which the tuning fork is held near the ear. Normally, and in patients with sensorineural hearing loss, the vibrations are still audible when the tuning fork is held by the ear because air conduction is better than bone conduction. This is not the case in conduction loss (i.e., bone conduction is better than air conduction). The Rinne test is used in conjunction with the Weber test, in which the tuning fork is held on the vertex of the head. If the patient has either normal hearing or conductive deficits, the tuning fork vibrations should be heard equally in both ears. However, in sensorineural hearing loss, the sound will appear to be diminished in the affected ear.

Trouble hearing and noise in the ear (tinnitus) are the most frequent complaints that indicate involvement of the cochlear portion of CN VIII. Common causes of hearing loss include age (presbycusis) and exposure to noise. Anything that affects hearing can cause tinnitus. Ototoxic drugs that should be familiar to primary care providers include aminoglycoside antibiotics, antineoplastic drugs, anti-inflammatory medicines, diuretics, and antimalarial drugs.

GLOSSOPHARYNGEAL NERVE, CN IX

The gag reflex is used to test the glossopharyngeal nerve (and the vagus nerve, CN X) clinically. A tongue depressor applied to the posterior pharynx causes the pharyngeal muscles to contract, with or without gagging. This test is unpleasant for patients, and only exceptionally does it provide information that cannot be obtained by assessing the patient's speech and watching the patient swallow spontaneously.

Glossopharyngeal neuralgia is an uncommon disorder characterized by paroxysms of lancinating pain in the structures the nerve innervates: the ear, base of the tongue, lower jaw, and tonsillar fossa. Occasionally, syncope occurs as part of glossopharyngeal neuralgia because CN IX innervates the carotid sinus.

VAGUS NERVE, CN X

The gag reflex is also used to test the vagus nerve. The motor component of this nerve supplies the muscles of the pharynx and larynx. Although the vagus nerve is the most important of the parasympathetic nerves, it is difficult to assess clinically. This nerve is involved in many reflexes, including cough, vomiting, and swallowing reflexes. Dysphagia and dysarthria are the most common clinical features of vagal dysfunction, because of weakness of the muscles of the pharynx and larynx.

SPINAL ACCESSORY NERVE, CN XI

The spinal accessory nerve innervates the trapezius and sternocleidomastoid muscles. Test this nerve by having the patient turn his or her head, and then assess the strength of each sternocleidomastoid muscle against resistance. To test the trapezius, that is, to assess muscle strength and symmetry, ask the patient to shrug the shoulders. The nerve can be injured by intracranial or cervical trauma. The clinical presentation may include shoulder pain, winging of the scapula, and weak elevation of the shoulder.

HYPOGLOSSAL NERVE, CN XII

The hypoglossal nerve innervates the tongue. To test this nerve, have the patient stick the tongue out and move it from side to side. Look for weakness, atrophy, fasciculations, and abnormal movements. Unilateral weakness causes the tongue to deviate to the side of the lesion. Hypoglossal dysfunction results in dysarthria. It is important to inspect the tongue for fasciculations if motor neuron disease is suspected. A note of caution: familiarize yourself with how a normal tongue looks before ascribing fasciculations to what may be normal quivering of the tongue. The tongue can also be valuable in "above the neck" assessment of rapid alternating movements when testing coordination.

MOTOR EXAMINATION

Watching the patient stand and walk is a major portion of the motor examination. If an ambulatory patient is able to walk on the toes and heels, to hop, and to squat, lower extremity strength is well within normal limits and individual muscle testing may not be needed. Evaluation of the motor system involves assessing the symmetry of muscle strength, bulk, and tone. Abnormal muscle movement like fasciculations should be noted. All the major muscle groups can be tested with the patient seated. For easy comparison of the left and right sides, test both sides simultaneously. Simultaneous testing (done quickly and with encouragement) may also reduce give-way weakness in a patient who wants to exaggerate symptoms.

Test the proximal and distal muscles of all four extremities. The deltoid (arms abducted against resistance), biceps, and triceps muscles are good proximal upper extremity muscles to test. Grip strength is a good measure of distal upper extremity strength. If proximal muscle weakness is suspected, test neck flexion. Normally, the examiner should not be able to overcome the powerful neck muscles. Test for drift by asking the patient to hold both arms straight out in front, with the palms up. This is useful for detecting subtle weakness of the upper extremity, which is expressed as pronation and lowering of the weak arm.

Patients often complain of "weakness," a term they use to imply illness. How the weakness limits their ability to perform normal daily activities will reveal more about the complaint of weakness. For example, proximal muscle weakness is suggested when patients report difficulty walking up stairs or keeping their arms raised when fixing their hair. Fatigable weakness or weakness that is more prominent at the end of the day may suggest myasthenia gravis. If the patient has a history of fatigable weakness, repetitive muscle strength should be tested.

The anatomy of the motor system, important in understanding the physical findings found on motor examination, is sketched in Figure 1–9. The major tract of the motor system is the corticospinal, or pyramidal, tract, which originates in the precentral gyrus (primary motor cortex) of the frontal lobe. The areas of the body are represented systematically along the precentral gyrus. The leg is represented on the medial surface and the face, arm, and hand, on the lateral surface. At the junction between the medulla and spinal cord, the corticospinal tract crosses the midline (pyramidal decussation). Because of this decussation, the right cerebral hemisphere controls the muscles on the left side of the body and the left hemisphere controls those on the right side. The origin, course, and termination of the corticospinal tract constitute the *upper motor neuron*. The clinical features of an upper motor neuron problem include weakness, spasticity, hyperreflexia, and extensor plantar reflex, or Babinski sign ("up-going toe").

The lower motor neuron consists of the motor nerve cell (anterior horn cell) in the spinal cord or brainstem and its axon, which courses through a peripheral nerve to end in a muscle. The lower motor neuron is also called the "final common pathway." Clinical features of a lower motor neuron lesion in-

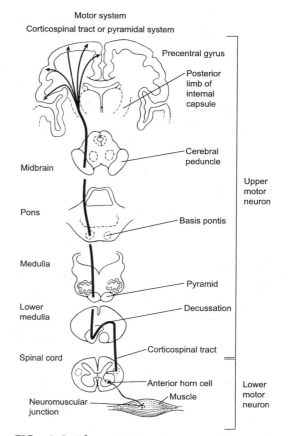

FIG. 1–9. The motor system: corticospinal tract, or pyramidal system, and lower motor neuron (anterior horn cell).

clude weakness, decreased deep tendon reflexes, muscle loss or atrophy, and fasciculations. Upper and lower motor neuron dysfunctions are compared in Table 1–4. Other components of the motor system, including the basal ganglia ("extrapyramidal system") and cerebellum, are discussed in Chapter 12.

The pattern of weakness and the associated neurologic findings help to localize the lesion in the nervous system. Figure 1–10, from the Mayo neurology examination form, lists the major muscles that are tested in a comprehensive neurologic examination, with the nerve that innervates the muscle in parentheses and the associated nerve root. Proximal muscle weakness indicates a myopathy, whereas distal muscle weakness may indicate a peripheral neuropathy, especially if there are associated sensory findings.

TABLE 1–4. COMPARISON OF UPPER MOTOR NEURON AND LOWER MOTOR NEURON DYSFUNCTION

Clinical Feature	Upper Motor Neuron	Lower Motor Neuron
Weakness	Yes	Yes
Muscle tone	Increased (spasticity)	Decreased
Muscle stretch reflexes	Increased	Decreased
Muscle bulk	Normal (disuse atrophy)	Atrophy
Fasciculations	No	Yes
Babinski sign	Yes	No

Fascicul.	Size	Strength	R	L	Strength	Size	Fascicul.
			Temporal-Masseter	V			
			Pterygoid	V			
			Forehead	VII			
			Orbic. oculi	VII			
			Mouth (retraction)	VII			
			Palate-Pharynx	X			
			Sternomastoid	XI			
			Trapezius	XI			
			Tongue	XII			
			Neck flexors	C 1-6			
			Neck extensors	C 1-T1			
			Muscle Bulk Uppers	nl abn			
			Ext. rotat. (suprascap.)	C 56			
			Pector. maj. (pector.)	C5-T1			
			Deltoid (axill.)	C 56			
			Biceps (musculocut.)	C 56			
			Brachioradialis (radial)	C 56			
			Supinator (radial)	C 56			
			Pronator teres (median)	C 67			
			Triceps (radial)	C 678			
			Wrist ext. (radial)	C 678			
			Wrist flex. (med. & uln.)	C 678 T1			
			Digit ext. (radial)	C 78			
			Digit flex. (med. & uln.)	C 78 T1			
			Thenar (med.)	C 8 T 1			
			Hypothenar (uln.)	C 8 T1			
			Interossei (uln.)	C 8 T1			
			Abdomen	T6 - L1			
			Rectal sphinct.	S 34			
			Muscle Bulk Lowers	nl abn			
			Iliopsoas (femor.)	L 234			
			Adduct. thigh (obtur.)	L 234			
			Abduct. thigh (sup. glut.)	L 45 S1			
			Gluteus max. (inf. glut.)	L 5 S12			
			Quadriceps (femor.)	L 234			
			Hamstrings (sciat.)	L 45 S1			
			Anter. tibial (peron.)	L 45			
			Toe ext. (peron.)	L 45 S1			
			Ext. hal. long. (peron.)	L 5 S1			
			Peronei (peron.)	L 5 S1			
			Post. tibial (tib.)	L 5 S1			
			Toe flex. (tib.)	L 5 S1			
			Gastroc. Soleus (tib.)	L 5 S12			

FIG. 1–10. The major muscles tested in a comprehensive neurologic examination (part of the Mayo neurology examination form).

Weakness of a specific muscle suggests a problem with the nerve that innervates the muscle. For example, a patient with footdrop who has normal strength in the posterior tibial muscle (foot inversion) is more likely to have a peroneal nerve palsy than a radiculopathy of the fifth lumbar root. A patient with footdrop and entirely normal findings on the sensory examination may have motor neuron disease. The patterns of weakness seen at different levels of the nervous system are summarized in Table 1–5.

SENSORY EXAMINATION

The frequency of sensory complaints—pain, numbness, and tingling—encountered in clinical practice emphasizes the importance of the sensory examination. However, the responses to sensory testing are subjective, and some patients provide misleading or exaggerated responses that complicate the interpretation of the findings. Therefore, it is important to be familiar with the essential anatomy of the sensory system and to correlate the sensory findings with more objective information obtained from the motor and reflex examinations.

The major types of somatic sensation are exteroceptive sense, including pain and temperature sensation, and proprioceptive sense, including position and vibratory sensation. Pain and temperature sensation are conveyed via the spinothalamic tract and vibration and position sense, via the dorsal column–lemniscal pathway. Both tracts also convey the sensation of touch. A clinically relevant point about the spinothalamic tract

TABLE 1–5. PATTERNS OF WEAKNESS BY ANATOMICAL DIVISION

Division (Disease)	Clinical Example	Examination Findings		Other Clinical Features
		Motor	Sensory	
Muscle (myopathy)	Polymyositis	Proximal weakness	Normal	Diffuse myalgias
Neuromuscular junction	Myasthenia gravis	Fatigable weakness	Normal	Diplopia, ptosis
Peripheral nerve (neuropathy)	Peroneal palsy	Weak peroneal-innervated muscles	Peroneal nerve distribution	Injury at knee
Nerve root (radiculopathy)	L5 radiculopathy	All the above findings plus weakness of other L5-innervated muscles (posterior tibial, foot inversion)	Sensory loss in dermatomal distribution	Back pain
Anterior horn cell (motor neuron disease)	Amyotrophic lateral sclerosis	Lower motor neuron and upper motor neuron muscle weakness	Normal	Atrophy, fasciculations
Spinal cord (myelopathy)	Cervical spondylosis	Upper motor neuron weakness	Sensory level	Babinski sign
Brainstem	Brainstem glioma	Upper motor neuron weakness	Variable	Cranial nerve involvement
Cerebral cortex	Cortical infarction	Upper motor neuron weakness	Cortical sensation (discriminative sensation, joint position sense, 2-point discrimination, graphesthesia)	Language impairment (if dominant hemisphere), visuospatial problems

(pain and temperature) is that the axons cross the midline near their origin in the spinal cord and ascend laterally in the cord. The dermatomes of the body are represented in a systematic fashion in the tract, with the sacral dermatomes laterally (near the surface of the cord) and the cervical segments medially (near the gray matter). The axons forming the dorsal columns do not cross in the spinal cord; instead, they end on neurons in the medulla, whose axons immediately cross the midline to form the medial lemniscus. Thus, in the spinal cord and medulla, the spinothalamic and dorsal column lemniscal tracts are separated, but they come together at the level of mid pons. Because of this arrangement, pain and temperature sensation may be lost over part of the body, while vibratory sensation and position sense are spared. This sensory dissociation can occur with lesions only in the spinal cord, medulla, or lower pons. In contrast, all sensory modalities are represented together at the level of the thalamus. This explains why the thalamic

TABLE 1–6. COMMON PATTERNS OF SENSORY DEFICIT

Anatomy	Clinical Example	Sensory Loss: Pain/ Temperature or Vibratory/Joint Position	Distribution of Sensory Abnormality	Associated Features
Peripheral nerve (mononeuropathy)	Carpal tunnel syndrome	Both	Precisely in the distribution of median nerve	Weakness of muscles of median nerve, wrist pain
Nerve root (radiculopathy)	L5 radiculopathy	Both	Dermatomal distribution	Weakness of L5-innervated muscles, back pain
Peripheral nerve (peripheral neuropathy or polyneuropathy)	Diabetic neuropathy	Both	Stocking-glove pattern	Painful paresthesias, autonomic neuropathy
Spinal cord				
Commissural syndrome	Syringomyelia	Pain/temperature	Band-like or cape-like pattern	Arnold-Chiari malformation
Brown-Séquard syndrome	Trauma	Both	Ipsilateral pain/temp, contralateral vibratory/joint position	Ipsilateral motor deficit
Dorsal cord syndrome	Subacute combined degeneration (vitamin B_{12} deficiency)	Vibration/joint position	Area distal to level of lesion	Babinski sign
Brainstem	Brainstem infarction	For mid pons or rostral: both	Ipsilateral face and contralateral body	Cranial nerve involvement depending on level of brainstem involvement
		For medial medulla: vibratory/joint position	Contralateral body	
		For lateral medulla: pain/ temperature	Ipsilateral face and contralateral body	
Thalamus	Thalamic infarction	Both	Dense contralateral face and body	Thalamic pain syndrome
Cerebral cortex	Middle cerebral artery infarction	Discriminative sensation, joint position sense, 2-point discrimination, graphesthesia	Contralateral face and limbs	Hemiparesis, aphasia (if dominant hemisphere)

syndrome is characterized by dense sensory loss of all modalities over an entire half of the body and face. Lesions of the postcentral gyrus, or primary somesthetic cortex, are associated with loss of discriminative sensation: joint position, two-point discrimination, stereognosis (the appreciation of the form of an object by touch), and graphesthesia (the ability to recognize figures written on the skin). Only a minimal deficit of touch, pain, temperature, and vibratory sensation may be noted with cortical lesions. The sensory pattern typical of lesions at various levels of the nervous system is summarized in Table 1–6 and Figure 1–11.

In neurologic practice, the minimal sensory examination includes testing pain and/or temperature sensation and joint position and/or vibration sensation in all four extremities. In primary care practice, it may not be necessary to perform a sensory examination unless the patient has a sensory complaint or abnormal gait. While testing a patient's gait and station, determine whether the patient can stand with the feet close together and with the eyes open. If the patient is able to do this, ask him or her to close the eyes (Romberg test); this test assesses proprioceptive function. A normal person may sway slightly, but marked swaying or falling indicates proprioceptive deficit (Romberg sign). Patients with a Romberg sign may report difficulty walking to the bathroom in the dark or have trouble maintaining their balance while in the shower (because of reduced visual input). In comparison, patients with cerebellar dysfunction sway with their eyes open. Patients with conversion disorder or another factitious illness tend to sway from the hips rather than the ankles and, despite a wide sway arc, maintain their balance. Asking the patient to perform the finger-to-nose test during this examination is a useful distraction.

If there is a sensory complaint, it is useful for the patient to outline the area of deficit, so you can examine that area more closely. Diagrams of dermatomes and areas supplied by individual peripheral nerves are useful in localizing a specific sensory complaint (Fig. 1–12). To test spinothalamic function, use a disposable straight pin or safety pin. Tell the patient you are going to touch him or her lightly with a pin (it is not necessary to penetrate the skin) and demonstrate what you are going to do before you start. Ask the patient to call the sensation "sharp" when touched with the point of the pin and "dull" when touched with your finger or the head of the pin. Testing at the base of the nail bed avoids most calluses on the fingers. Assessing whether the patient can distinguish sharp from dull before asking him or her to compare the sensation on the two sides of the body often avoids any tendency the pa-

tient may have to exaggerate the sensory signs. Asking the question "Is it about the same?" helps the patient avoid over-interpretation of minimal differences in stimulation. Whether it is necessary to test more than the hands and feet depends on the patient's presenting complaint. If there is a history of spine symptoms, it may be necessary to test several dermatomes or to look for a sensory level. It is usually more convenient to check for sharp versus dull sensation than to test temperature sensation. Temperature sensation can be tested by using a cold tuning fork or reflex hammer; however, it is more difficult for patients to compare temperature sensation on the two sides of the body than to compare sharp or dull sensation.

Proprioception can be tested by the Romberg test or by testing vibratory sensation or joint position sense. Vibratory sensation is often quicker to test than joint position sense, but it requires a tuning fork. Use a large tuning fork (128 Hz), especially when testing elderly patients, in whom testing with a small tuning fork may falsely indicate proprioceptive deficit. Hold the tuning fork on the nail bed of a finger and the great toe and ask if the person can appreciate the "buzz." Most adults can appreciate vibratory sensation at the toes. If vibration is not appreciated, move the tuning fork proximally to a bony prominence, for example, the lateral malleolus, tibia, or knee. Test both sides. If asymmetry is noted in a patient prone to exaggerate, hold the tuning fork on the side of diminished sensation and ask the patient to report when the buzz is no longer felt; this may minimize the perceived deficit.

Testing joint position sense is useful in assessing cortical sensory loss. First, demonstrate the test. Hold one of the patient's distal phalanges laterally, and move the joint up or down a few millimeters. Ask the patient to report, without looking, the direction relative to the last position. Coordination tests like the finger-to-nose test, which the patient is asked to perform with eyes closed, also assess motion and position sense.

REFLEX EXAMINATION

The examination of reflexes provides the most objective information obtained with

FIG. 1–11. Patterns of sensory deficit.

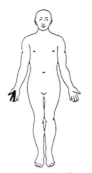

Mononeuropathy
right median nerve
(carpal tunnel)

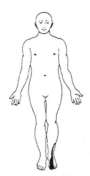

Radiculopathy
Left L5

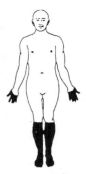

Peripheral
neuropathy
(polyneuropathy)

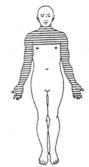

Commissural syndrome
C2-T2 syringomyelia
(pain and temperature only)

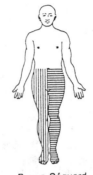

Brown-Séquard
R hemisection at T10
vibration/joint position
pain and temperature

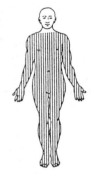

Dorsal column
subacute combined
degeneration

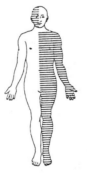

R lateral brainstem
infarct

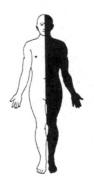

R thalamic infarct

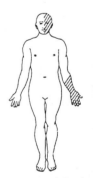

R cortical infarct

≡ Pain and temperature

||| Vibration and joint position

■ Combined

/// Joint position, graphesthesia
discriminative sensation

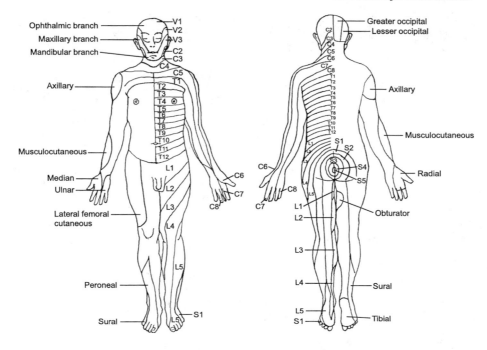

FIG. 1–12. Dermatomes (C2-S5) and area of distribution of peripheral nerves.

the neurologic examination. Although reflexes can be reinforced or decreased, they are involuntary motor responses to sensory stimuli and do not depend on voluntary control. Importantly, reflex tests can be performed in a patient who is confused or in a coma. Reflex abnormalities may be the first indication of neurologic disease.

The major reflexes are muscle stretch (or deep tendon) reflexes, superficial reflexes, and pathologic reflexes, specifically the plantar (or Babinski) reflex. The muscle stretch reflexes that are routinely tested in neurologic practice are the biceps, brachioradialis, triceps, quadriceps, and gastrocnemius-soleus reflexes, named for the muscle tested. The afferent limb of the reflex arc is a sensory nerve root (Table 1–7). The interneuron is in the spinal cord, and the efferent limb is the motor nerve to the muscle. Any process that affects any component of the reflex arc will alter the reflex. For example, the ankle, or gastrocnemius-soleus, reflex may be absent in a patient with diabetic

neuropathy or with a herniated disk affecting the first sacral (S1) nerve root. Upper motor neuron lesions that reduce inhibition (producing hyperreflexia) or cerebellar or brainstem lesions that reduce facilitation (producing hyporeflexia) can affect this reflex arc. Drugs and metabolic factors also can affect reflexes; for example, hyperreflexia occurs with hyperthyroidism and central nervous system stimulants, and hyporeflexia occurs with hypothyroidism.

Several techniques can be used to elicit muscle stretch reflexes. All major muscle stretch reflexes can be tested with the patient seated and the arms resting in the lap. This position allows rapid comparison of the right to left sides and limits the patient's movement. Testing from side to side can be repeated quickly if there is a question about the symmetry of the reflex. Because it is essential for the patient to be relaxed, talk to the patient during this portion of the examination to divert his or her attention. If the patient remains tense, ask him or her to look

TABLE 1–7. DEEP TENDON REFLEXES AND CORRESPONDING NERVE ROOT, NERVE, AND MUSCLES SUPPLIED BY NERVE AND ROOT

Reflex	Root	Nerve	Muscles Supplied by Nerve Only	Other Muscles Supplied by Same Root but Different Nerve
Biceps	C6	Musculocutaneous	Biceps	Pronator teres (median)
Brachioradialis	C5-C6	Radial	Brachioradialis, triceps	External rotator–infraspinatus (suprascapular)
Triceps	C7	Radial	Triceps, wrist extensors	Pronator teres (median), wrist flexors (median and ulnar)
Quadriceps	L3-L4	Femoral	Quadriceps, iliopsoas	Adductors of thigh (obturator)
Gastrocnemius-soleus	S1	Tibial	Gastrocnemius-soleus, posterior tibial	Gluteus maximus (inferior gluteal)

up, to bite down, or to interlock the fingers and pull the hands apart (Jendrassik method) as you tap the tendon with the reflex hammer. The Achilles tendon (gastrocnemius-soleus muscles) reflex, or ankle jerk, can easily be elicited by having the patient kneel on a chair while you put minimal pressure with one hand on the ball of the patient's foot and then tap the tendon with the reflex hammer.

How the findings are interpreted depends on the results of other portions of the neurologic examination. For example, both the biceps and brachioradialis reflexes test the C5-C6 root, but the biceps muscle is innervated by the musculocutaneous nerve and the brachioradialis muscle by the radial nerve. Thus, if one reflex is abnormal but not the other, the lesion is likely to be along a peripheral nerve and not the C5–C6 root. Information from the reflex examination in conjunction with the results of the motor and sensory examinations is used to localize a problem with the nerve root, plexus, peripheral nerve, and so forth (Table 1–7, Fig. 1–12). Symmetric hyperreflexia in conjunction with flexor plantar reflexes may be a normal finding in an anxious patient. However, in an elderly patient, hyperreflexia may represent cervical spondylosis. Diffuse hyporeflexia can be a normal finding if there is

no other abnormality. Ankle jerks that are reduced or absent are common in peripheral neuropathy.

Other muscle stretch reflexes can be tested to aid in the interpretation of the neurologic findings, such as the jaw, internal hamstring, and Hoffman (finger flexor) reflexes. The internal hamstring reflex tests the L5 nerve root. If the reflex is asymmetric, suspect an L5 radiculopathy. However, the value of this reflex may be theoretical because of the difficulty in eliciting it. The jaw and finger flexor reflexes typically reflect hyperreflexia.

Superficial reflexes are elicited by stimulating the skin or mucous membranes. These reflexes include the corneal, pharyngeal, abdominal, cremasteric, anal, and bulbocavernosus reflexes. The corneal and pharyngeal (gag) reflexes have already been discussed in relation to cranial nerves. Although the other reflexes are not routinely tested, they can provide valuable information.

The afferent and efferent pathways of the abdominal reflexes are the intercostal nerves at T6-T9 for the epigastric region and T11-L1 for the hypogastric region. The absence of abdominal reflexes suggests corticospinal tract, or upper motor neuron, injury. Abdominal reflexes are tested with the patient supine and the arms at the sides. Stroke, or gently scratch with a blunt object, the four quadrants around the umbilicus, Normally, the umbilicus moves toward the stimulus. The reflex may not be present if the patient is obese or multiparous, has had an abdominal operation, or is tense. Unilateral loss of these reflexes indicates a unilateral corticospinal tract lesion and may be an important clinical clue to early multiple sclerosis. The unilateral absence of abdominal reflexes is sometimes considered a reason to perform magnetic resonance imaging in patients with idiopathic scoliosis, to rule out syringomyelia.

The cremasteric reflex tests the L1-L2 nerve roots. Stimulation of the inner aspect of the thigh, as in abdominal reflex testing, causes elevation of the testicle. Loss of this reflex may indicate an upper motor neuron lesion or lesion of cord segment L1 or L2.

The anal reflex tests segments S2-S4. It is useful in evaluating patients with suspected injury of the sacral spinal cord (conus medullaris or cauda equina). Gently scratch the skin around the patient's anus to produce contraction of the anal ring, which can be detected or palpated with a gloved fingertip.

The plantar reflex is evoked by stroking the bottom of the foot from the heel forward with the end of a reflex hammer or wooden applicator. After age 1 year, the normal response is flexion of the toes. The stimulus should be applied as lightly as possible to elicit the normal flexor response. Use a stronger stimulus if there is no response. A painful stimulus or one that tickles may elicit a withdrawal response. The abnormal response, called the "Babinski sign," is extension of the great toe and associated fanning of the other toes (extensor plantar reflex). This sign indicates a corticospinal tract lesion (see Fig. 1–9).

The plantar reflex has to be tested carefully to avoid misinterpretation of the results. If there is question about the response, stroke the foot with the leg extended (having the patient extend the leg while seated can be used as a modified straight leg test for eliciting back or root pain). To reduce the problem of withdrawal, divert the patient's attention by discussing unrelated matters. If excessive withdrawal is encountered, stroke the lateral aspect of the sole (Chaddock) or run two knuckles down both sides of the tibia (Oppenheim). The latter is very uncomfortable for the patient and should be reserved for equivocal results.

COORDINATION EXAMINATION

Cerebellar function is assessed by testing coordination and rapid alternating movements, and the results can serve as a crosscheck for other parts of the neurologic examination. However, this testing may not be needed if the patient has a normal gait and speech pattern and no complaints about coordination.

The finger-to-nose test is a convenient test of coordination. Ask the patient to extend both arms out in front of the body (observe for static tremor) and to touch the nose with an index finger, first with the right hand and then with the left, and to repeat the action. Abnormalities in rate, range, direction, and force of movement indicate incoordination. The movement should be symmetric. Next, ask the patient to continue the activity with the eyes closed (this also tests position sense). Apraxia may become apparent in a patient with dementia. A comparable test for the lower extremities is to have the patient place the heel on the opposite knee and run the heel down the shin as smoothly as possible.

Rapid alternating movements of the tongue (wiggling the tongue from side to side), hands (turning the hand palm up, palm down, palm up, and so on), fingers (tapping the index finger against the thumb), and feet (tapping the foot) also test coordination. Evaluate the rate and range of the movement. Movement on the two sides should be symmetric; this is not dependent on hand dominance. The sound the movement makes (e.g., shoe tap on the floor or hand pat on the knee) is often helpful in detecting an abnormality, a "syncopated rhythm," which may be missed by observation alone. Although movement may be slowed by weakness, the rate of movement should be regular. Unilateral abnormalities are consistent with ipsilateral cerebellar lesions. Patients with Parkinson disease may demonstrate a decreased *range* of movement but an increased *rate* of movement.

PEDIATRIC EXAMINATION

The pediatric neurologic examination needs to be adapted to the age, temperament, and comfort of the child. Generally, observing the child is essential: watch how the child moves and plays while you take the medical history. Playing with the child and making a game of the examination (e.g., touching the penlight turns the light on) can provide the necessary information and make the encounter a pleasant experience for the child. Finger puppets and other toys are extremely helpful in getting the child's attention and cooperation. The sequence of the examination has to be flexible. Begin the examination with a fun activity like running down the hallway, and reserve the less pleasant parts (measuring head circumference) for the end, after rapport has been achieved. Consult developmental tables for normal motor, language, adaptive, and social behaviors appropriate for age (Table 1–8).

GERIATRIC EXAMINATION

Many abnormalities seen in elderly patients on the neurologic examination are attributed to age. The problem is that many of these abnormalities should be attributed to diseases that are common in the elderly. To avoid overlooking findings that indicate neurologic disease, you should not expect to find any abnormality on neurologic examination of the elderly. Do not be cavalier in attributing abnormal results to "aging" or "disease of aging." The clinical relevance of physical findings is important to consider. Primitive reflexes such as the snout or suck reflex and gait difficulties are common in the elderly. However, functional implications such as falling are much more important to the patient than the presence or absence of a snout reflex. Examining performance-oriented measures of posture and balance is important in the elderly. These include assessing the patient's ability to stand up from

---

TABLE 1–8. LANDMARKS FOR NORMAL DEVELOPMENT OF MOTOR, LANGUAGE, AND SOCIAL SKILLS: 2 TO 48 MONTHS

2 Months

Lifts head up several seconds while
   prone
Startle reaction to loud noise
Smiles responsively
Begins to vocalize single sounds

6 Months

Lifts head while supine
Sits with support
Babbles
Rolls from prone to supine

12 Months

Walks with assistance
Uses 2 to 4 words with meaning
Uses pincer grasp
Understands a few simple
   commands

18 Months
Throws ball
Feeds self
Uses many intelligible words
Climbs stairs with assistance

24 Months

Runs
Speaks in 2- to 3-word sentences
Kicks ball
Uses pronouns ("you," "me," "I")

36 Months

Rides tricycle
Copies a circle
Repeats 3 numbers or a sentence
   of 6 syllables
Plays simple games

48 Months

Hops on one foot, throws ball
   overhand
Identifies the longer of two lines,
   draws a man with 2 to 4 parts
Tells a story
Plays with children, with social
   interaction

TABLE 1–9. GERIATRIC NEUROLOGIC EXAMINATION

Examination	Age-Associated Changes	Common Diseases
Mental status	Reduced visual perception Reduced constructional ability	Dementia, depression
Cranial nerves	Decreased olfaction Decreased pupillary size and reactivity, presbyopia Decreased smooth pursuit movements Limited upward gaze and convergence Presbycusis	Glaucoma, macular degeneration, cataracts Environmental noise damage Positional vertigo from cupulolithiasis
Motor	No age-related weakness	Parkinsonism Stroke Arthritis Reduced cardiovascular fitness
Sensory	Reduced vibratory sensation in lower extremities	Peripheral neuropathy Medication effect Diabetes mellitus
Reflexes	Reduced ankle reflex	Peripheral neuropathy Medication effect Diabetes mellitus
Gait and posture	Reduced balance	Parkinsonism Arthritis Neuropathies Cervical spondylosis

a chair, to bend over, to reach, and the response to a nudge. The "pull test" is used to test postural instability in parkinsonism. Explain to patients that you will pull them from behind and they are to maintain their balance. Reassure them that you are ready to catch them if they lose their balance. The normal response is to maintain balance in one or two steps. Many of the common findings seen on examination of the elderly and many of the diseases associated with these findings are listed in Table 1–9.

SUGGESTED READING

Applegate, WB, Blass, JP, and Williams, TF: Instruments for the functional assessment of older patients. N Engl J Med 322:1207–1214, 1990.

Brazis, PW, Masdeu, JC, and Biller, J: Localization in Clinical Neurology, ed 2. Little, Brown, Boston, 1990.

DeJong, RN: The Neurologic Examination: Incorporating the Fundamentals of Neuroanatomy and Neurophysiology, ed 4. Harper & Row, Hagerstown, Md., 1979.

Diamond, S, and Dalessio, DJ (eds): The Practicing Physician's Approach to Headache, ed 5. Williams & Wilkins, Baltimore, 1992.

Evans, RW: Diagnostic testing for the evaluation of headaches. Neurol Clin 14:1–26, 1996.

Folstein, MF, Folstein, SE, and McHugh, PR: "Minimental state." A practical method for grading the cognitive state of patients for the clinician. J Psychiatr Res 12:189–198, 1975.

Galetta, SL, Liu, GT, and Volpe, NJ: Diagnostic tests in neuro-ophthalmology. Neurol Clin 14:201–222, 1996.

Kaye, JA, et al: Neurologic evaluation of the optimally healthy oldest old. Arch Neurol 51:1205–1211, 1994.

Knopman, DS, et al: Geriatric neurology. Continuum 2:7–154, 1996.

Mungas, D: In-office mental status testing: A practical guide. Geriatrics 46:54–58, 63, 66, 1991.

Nutt, JG, Marsden, CD, and Thompson, PD: Human walking and higher-level gait disorders, particularly in the elderly. Neurology 43:268–279, 1993.

Odenheimer, G, et al: Comparison of neurologic changes in "successfully aging" persons vs the total aging population. Arch Neurol 51:573–580, 1994.

Samuels, MA, and Feske, S (eds): Office Practice of Neurology. Churchill Livingstone, New York, 1996.

Silberstein, SD, and Lipton, RB: Headache epidemiology. Emphasis on migraine. Neurol Clin 14:421–434, 1996.

Sudarsky, L: Geriatrics: Gait disorders in the elderly. N Engl J Med 322:1441–1446, 1990.

Tangalos, EG, et al: The Mini-Mental State Examination in general medical practice: Clinical utility and acceptance. Mayo Clin Proc 71:829–837, 1996.

Vaughan, VC, III, McKay, J, Jr, and Behrman, RE (eds): Nelson Textbook of Pediatrics , ed 11. WB Saunders, Philadelphia, 1979.

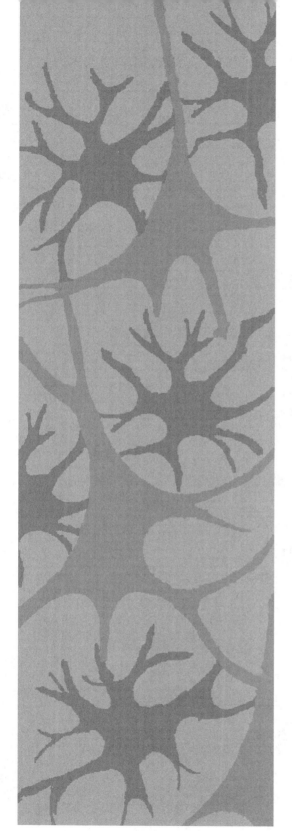

CHAPTER 2

Diagnostic Tests

CHAPTER OUTLINE

**Cerebrospinal Fluid Analysis and
    Lumbar Puncture**
    Indications
    Contraindications
    Procedure
Electroencephalography
Evoked Potentials
**Nerve Conduction Studies and
    Electromyography**
    Nerve Conduction Studies
    Muscle Studies
Neuroimaging
    Computed Tomography
    Magnetic Resonance Imaging
    Angiography
    Myelography

The diagnostic tests used most often to evaluate patients with disease of the nervous system include cerebrospinal fluid (CSF) examination, electroencephalography (EEG), electromyography (EMG), evoked potentials, computed tomography (CT), and magnetic resonance imaging (MRI). These tests should be used to supplement or to extend the clinical examination. Remember that diagnostic tests have technical limitations and the quality of the results depends on the examiner or laboratory performing the test. The results should always be interpreted in view of the patient's clinical presentation.

CEREBROSPINAL FLUID ANALYSIS AND LUMBAR PUNCTURE

CSF usually is obtained by lumbar puncture. Before performing this straightforward but invasive procedure, know its indications and contraindications.

INDICATIONS

Laboratory evaluation of CSF is indicated for the diagnosis and treatment of intracerebral hemorrhage and infectious, neoplastic, and demyelinating diseases of the central nervous system. CSF analysis may become more useful with increasing knowledge about neurodegenerative disorders, prions, and other neurologic disorders.

CONTRAINDICATIONS

Lumbar puncture should not be performed in a patient with known or suspected intracranial or spinal mass, because of the potential for herniation and neurologic compromise with shift in intracranial pressure. In these patients, CT or MRI is recommended before proceeding with lumbar puncture.

However, neuroimaging should not delay the diagnosis or treatment of suspected meningitis. The risk of missing the diagnosis of meningitis is much greater than the risk of herniation. In this life-threatening illness, empiric treatment with antibiotics may need to be started to avoid delay in therapy. Nonfocal findings on neurologic examination and the absence of papilledema are clinical indications that lumbar puncture may be performed safely.

Lumbar puncture is contraindicated in patients taking anticoagulant medication or who have bleeding disorders. Lumbar puncture can cause intraspinal bleeding, with compression of the cauda equina. If CSF analysis is necessary, the patient can be pretreated with fresh frozen plasma, platelets, cryoprecipitate, or the specific factor to correct the hematologic abnormality.

Lumbar puncture should not be performed if there is infection at the puncture site. This is to avoid introducing the infection to the subarachnoid space. In this case, a lateral C1-C2 puncture can be performed by a neurosurgeon to obtain the CSF sample. Despite these contraindications, lumbar puncture is a safe and easy procedure.

PROCEDURE

Explain the procedure to the patient and provide emotional support throughout the procedure to reduce the patient's apprehension. The key to a successful lumbar puncture is proper positioning of the patient. The patient should be in the lateral decubitus position, with the back at the edge of the bed or table to provide back support. The patient's shoulders should be aligned and the spine parallel to the edge of the bed. The patient should assume the fetal position, bringing the knees to the chin. The L3-L4 vertebral interspace is in the midline at the level of the superior iliac crest (Fig. 2–1). In adults, the caudal end of the spinal cord is at vertebral level L1-L2, so vertebral level L3-L4

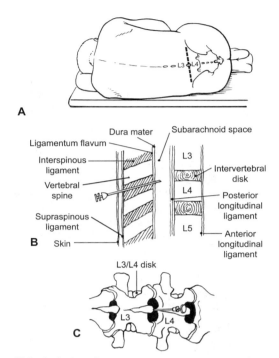

FIG. 2–1. Lumbar puncture. (A) Position of patient and location of L3-L4 interspace. **(B)** Section through vertebral column. **(C)** Lumbar needle in L3-L4 interspace. (Modified from Patten, J: Neurological Differential Diagnosis. Springer-Verlag, New York, 1977, pp 262–264, with permission.)

or the one above or below can be punctured safely. In infants and children, the caudal end of the spinal cord is lower relative to the vertebral column, and it is best to use the L4-L5 or L5-S1 vertebral interspace.

Perform the puncture with strict aseptic technique. Cleanse the skin with an iodine solution three times, starting at the puncture site and washing outward in concentric circles. Often, alcohol is used to remove the iodine, and sterile gloves are changed to avoid introducing iodine into the subarachnoid space. Apply the sterile drape, and prepare all the equipment before inserting the needle. To anesthetize the skin, use a small intradermal needle to inject lidocaine into a small wheal over the puncture site. Warn the patient that this step can cause a stinging sensation. Deeper structures can be anesthetized, but this may be more uncomfortable than the spinal needle.

For adults, use a 20-gauge lumbar puncture needle with stylet because it is rigid enough to penetrate the ligamentum flavum, it provides for an accurate pressure reading, and it is large enough to collect the CSF rapidly. The stylet needs to be in place on insertion to avoid the rare complication of implanting an epidermoid tumor into the subarachnoid space. The needle with stylet should be directed with the bevel parallel to the long axis of the spine to spread or to split the dural fibers that run longitudinally. This minimizes leakage of CSF into the subdural space. Steadily direct the needle toward the umbilicus until there is a "give," or a reduction in resistance, as the needle pierces the dura mater.

Remove the stylet, and check for CSF return. If no fluid is obtained, rotate the needle. If no fluid appears, replace the stylet and advance the needle in small, 1- to 2-millimeter increments, checking for CSF with each advance. Inserting the needle too far injures the venous plexus anterior to the spinal canal; this is the most common cause of a "traumatic tap." If bone is encountered, the needle should be withdrawn to the level of the skin (to avoid following the same path of the first puncture) and redirected. Repeated puncture of the skin should be avoided because of the increased risk of infection and subcutaneous bleeding. If the patient complains of pain down one leg, the needle needs to be directed more medially. If the patient cannot tolerate lying on the side or cannot be positioned properly, the puncture can be done with the patient sitting, leaning forward over a table. This position does not permit an accurate pressure reading, but the patient can be repositioned in the lateral decubitus position for this measurement. If the puncture is unsuccessful, a different interspace can be used or the procedure can be performed with fluoroscopic guidance.

After CSF has been obtained, attach the manometer to the hub of the needle and record the opening pressure. The patient should be encouraged to relax and to breathe normally to avoid a falsely high pressure reading. The meniscus should show minimal fluctuation related to pulse and respiration. Collect the CSF in four separate vials (labeled "1" through "4"), and remove the needle without the stylet to avoid trapping any nerve roots. Traditionally, the patient was instructed to remain flat or prone for some time to reduce the risk of post–lumbar puncture headache. However, according to recent studies, remaining flat is not a significant factor. In a large outpatient study, thin young women had the highest risk for post–lumbar puncture headache. The duration of recumbence and the amount of CSF obtained did not influence the risk for headache.

Post–lumbar puncture headache is the most frequent complication of lumbar puncture, with a reported frequency of 10% to 38%. The headache usually responds to a short period of bed rest. A persistent headache can be treated with an epidural injection of autologous blood at the site of the puncture. Other complications of lumbar puncture are rare and include diplopia, infection, backache, and radicular symptoms.

A "traumatic tap," that is, bleeding into the subarachnoid space from injury to small blood vessels, can compromise the interpretation of CSF results. A CSF sample with traumatic blood often clears as the fluid is collected and fewer erythrocytes are found in vial 4 than in vial 1. The opening pressure in a traumatic tap will be normal, compared with the pressure in subarachnoid hemorrhage or meningitis. The supernatant of centrifuged CSF should be clear if the tap was traumatic and xanthochromic (yellow) if blood has been present for several hours and has undergone hemolysis. Blood from a traumatic tap will increase the number of erythrocytes and leukocytes and the amount of protein. The formula used to estimate the increase is that 700 erythrocytes can account for an increase of 1 leukocyte and 1 milligram of protein.

CSF analysis is essential for diagnosing many disorders of the central nervous system (Table 2–1). Removal of CSF can also be therapeutic, as in pseudotumor cerebri and normal-pressure hydrocephalus. In a patient with normal-pressure hydrocephalus, improved gait after removal of CSF indicates that a shunt may be beneficial. The clinical value of CSF analysis is discussed further in the chapters on neurologic infections and neuro-oncology.

ELECTROENCEPHALOGRAPHY

The most important feature of EEG is that it is a physiologic test that provides information about function instead of structure. An example that emphasizes this point is the case of a child with a head injury and altered behavior and normal findings on neuroimaging. The normal neuroimaging results cannot explain the child's abnormal level of consciousness. However, EEG reveals the problem—namely, nonconvulsive status epilepticus, amenable to anticonvulsant therapy. EEG is noninvasive and relatively inexpensive. It is an extension of the clinical examination, and the information obtained through EEG should be interpreted in view of the patient's clinical presentation. Normal EEG findings do not exclude neurologic disease, and abnormal EEG findings may be of no clinical consequence.

The quality of the test results depends on the skill of the EEG technician and the electroencephalographer. Accreditation of the EEG laboratory and certification of the technician and electroencephalographer indicate that the recording meets acceptable standards. Eighteen to 21 recording channels are recommended. An electrocardiogram line should be used because it provides useful information about cardiac rhythm. This feature is particularly helpful in the evaluation of a patient with spells and other transient disorders. Activation procedures, including hyperventilation, intermittent photic stimulation, and sleep, should be part of the EEG study to increase the frequency of epileptogenic activity. Hyperventilation is an activation procedure that is particularly useful in patients with absence seizures. Hyperventilation should be used with care in patients with cardiopulmonary disease.

EEG is indispensable in the evaluation of patients with seizures. It can be critical in diagnosing seizures, determining the probability of recurrent seizures, and selecting the best treatment for seizures. The sensitivity of a single EEG recording for identifying specific epileptiform activity is reportedly about 50%. This increases to 90% with three EEG recordings. Prolonged EEG recording with video monitoring increases diagnostic sensitivity. Ambulatory EEG monitoring can be useful, but excessive artifact can complicate these studies.

TABLE 2–1. CEREBROSPINAL FLUID FEATURES IN VARIOUS DISEASES

Condition	Clinical Findings	Appearance	Opening Pressure	Protein	Glucose	Cell Count
Normal		Clear, colorless	50–200 mm H$_2$O	15–45 mg/100 mL	45–80 mg/mL (2/3 of serum)	RBCs, 0 WBCs, 0–5/mm^3 (lymphocytes or monocytes)
Subarachnoid hemorrhage	"Worst headache of life," stiff neck, negative CT	Blood tinged, xanthochromic	Increased	Increased	Normal	Same as blood
Bacterial meningitis	Headache, mental status change	Opalescent, purulent	Increased	Increased	Decreased	Increased WBCs (PMNs)
Viral meningitis	Headache, mental status change	Normal or opalescent	Increased or normal	Increased	Decreased	Increased WBCs (lymphocytes)
Carcinomatous meningitis	Headache, cranial nerve signs, seizures	Cloudy	Increased or normal	Increased	Decreased	Increased, malignant cells
Multiple sclerosis	Multiple signs and symptoms	Normal	Normal	Normal, increased IgG	Normal	Normal or increased lymphocytes Oligoclonal bands
Pseudotumor cerebri	Headache, papilledema, normal CT	Normal	Increased	Normal	Normal	Normal
Guillain-Barré	Ascending paralysis	Normal	Normal	Increased	Normal	Normal

CT, computed tomography; PMNs, polymorphonuclear neutrophils; RBCs, erythrocytes; WBCs, leukocytes.

EEG can be clinically useful for many transient disorders or "spells." In disorders of altered consciousness, EEG can determine whether the process is diffuse, focal, or multifocal. Serial EEG recordings can help determine prognosis in coma and encephalopathy. EEG may be indicated for distinguishing dementia from pseudodementia, diagnosing sleep disorders, and determining brain death. When requesting an EEG, the clinical question should be stated clearly and the electroencephalographer should attempt to answer that question within the limitations of the test. Common EEG findings and their anatomical and clinical correlates are summarized in Table 2–2.

EVOKED POTENTIALS

An evoked potential is an electrical response of the nervous system to an external stimulus. Evoked potentials measure conduction in nerve pathways from the periphery through the central nervous system. In clinical practice, this includes the visual, auditory or brainstem, and somatosensory pathways. Evoked potentials are not used frequently in primary care practice. However, they are noninvasive tests that provide valuable physiologic infor-

mation about the nervous system. For example, they are sensitive to demyelination and have been used to detect clinically silent lesions in patients with multiple sclerosis.

Visual evoked potentials extend the physical examination of the visual system and are useful in diagnosing optic nerve disease and determining the prognosis of visual recovery. If an ophthalmologic problem has been excluded, abnormal visual evoked potentials indicate an optic nerve or optic chiasm lesion. Visual evoked potentials reportedly are 100% sensitive in cases of optic neuritis, even with visual recovery, and they can be useful in assessing visual function in infants and uncooperative subjects.

Auditory, or brainstem, evoked potentials are sensitive to anatomical disturbances of brainstem pathways. These potentials are not affected by the level of consciousness, drugs, or metabolic disturbances. Auditory evoked potentials can be used to assess brainstem pathways in infants and in unresponsive and uncooperative patients. They also are helpful in evaluating complaints of vertigo, hearing loss, and tinnitus. Auditory evoked potentials can identify hearing impairment in infants and are used to screen for acoustic neuromas. They also are valuable in intraoperative monitoring during posterior fossa surgery.

TABLE 2–2. COMMON ELECTROENCEPHALOGRAPHIC (EEG) FINDINGS AND LOCALIZATION AND CLINICAL CORRELATES

EEG Finding	Localization	Clinical Correlate
Generalized spike and wave	Diffuse cortex	Absence, generalized tonic-clonic seizure
Focal spike and wave, spikes, sharp waves	Focal cortex	Partial epilepsy
Diffuse slowing	Diffuse cortex	Encephalopathy
Focal slowing	Focal cortex	Focal structural lesion
Periodic lateralized epileptiform discharges (PLEDs)	Localized or hemispheric dysfunction	Acute or subacute process (e.g., herpes encephalitis)
Triphasic waves	Diffuse cortex	Encephalopathy (e.g., hepatic)

Somatosensory evoked potentials are useful in assessing peripheral nerves, the spinal cord, and the cerebral cortex. They can be used to confirm an organic disease process in a patient with sensory complaints. They also are valuable in intraoperative monitoring to protect neural structures.

NERVE CONDUCTION STUDIES AND ELECTROMYOGRAPHY

It cannot be overemphasized that electrophysiologic studies are extensions of the clinical examination and that the quality of the studies is operator dependent. EMG can be indispensable in the evaluation and treatment of patients with muscle, neuromuscular junction, peripheral nerve, or motor neuron disease. It provides functional information and often supplements information from structural tests such as CT and MRI. EMG may provide the most critical information in a patient with low back pain and radicular symptoms in whom MRI reveals multiple-level degenerative changes. Many abnormalities on MRI are not clinically significant. The results of the EMG will indicate which level is symptomatic. Also, EMG is essential in the confirmation of motor neuron disease.

When ordering this test, it is important to understand the kind of information that can be obtained by EMG and the limitations of this test. EMG results will be more meaningful if the clinical question is clear and the electromyographer knows the clinical question to be answered. The timing of the study is critical. Abnormalities of peripheral nerves may not be demonstrable by EMG until 2 to 6 weeks after an acute injury. It is helpful if the patient is prepared for the test and understands what it involves.

NERVE CONDUCTION STUDIES

Nerve conduction can be measured in sensory and motor nerves. Nerve conduction studies can test only medium- to large-diameter myelinated fibers. These include motor fibers and the sensory fibers that convey vibratory sensation and proprioception. Small unmyelinated fibers that conduct pain and temperature sensation cannot be evaluated with EMG. Patients with small fiber neuropathies often have normal EMG findings.

The motor nerves commonly tested are the median, ulnar, peroneal, and posterior tibial nerves. A recording electrode is placed on the muscle, and the nerve is stimulated with a mild electrical shock at distal and

Nerve conduction

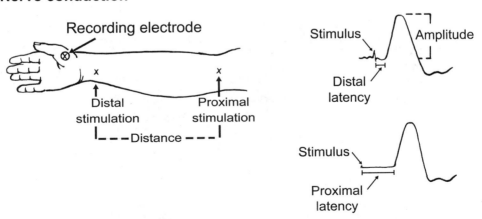

FIG. 2–2. Set-up for recording median nerve conduction. Motor nerve conduction velocity, reported in meters per second, $= \dfrac{\text{Distance}}{\text{Proximal latency} - \text{Distal latency}}$.

proximal sites (Fig. 2–2). Important values include the distal latency, conduction velocity, and conduction amplitude. The time measured from stimulating the nerve at the distal site to contraction of the muscle is called the *distal latency*. The time measured from stimulating the nerve at the proximal site to contraction of the muscle is called the *proximal latency*. For the median nerve, a prolonged distal latency supports the diagnosis of carpal tunnel syndrome. *Conduction time* is the speed of the nerve impulse. It is measured by the length of the nerve segment divided by the difference between the distal and proximal latencies.

Conduction velocity is related to the diameter (myelination) of the nerve. Slow nerve conduction velocities indicate demyelinating peripheral neuropathies. The amplitude of the motor unit potential is related to the number of axons. Reduced amplitudes indicate axonal polyneuropathies (Table 2–3).

MUSCLE STUDIES

The electrical activity in muscles is recorded by inserting a small needle electrode into the muscle. Information is obtained during the insertion of the needle, with the muscle at rest, and with voluntary contraction. The clinical indication for EMG determines which muscles are tested. To facilitate the study, provide the electromyographer with the necessary clinical information. The electromyographer needs to know if the patient is taking an anticoagulant agent or has a bleeding diathesis.

The brief discharge that occurs when the needle is inserted into the muscle is called *insertional activity*. Insertional activity is increased in neurogenic disorders, such as peripheral neuropathies, that cause abnormal excitability of muscle. At rest, a normal muscle has no spontaneous activity (excluding end-plate activity). Abnormal spontaneous activity is seen in neurogenic lesions associated with denervation and inflammatory myopathies. Motor unit action potentials are recorded when the muscle is contracted voluntarily and analyzed for amplitude, duration, phases, and recruitment. With continued muscle contraction, the motor units summate and the response is referred to as the "interference pattern." EMG features of clinical disorders are summarized in Figure 2–3.

NEUROIMAGING

COMPUTED TOMOGRAPHY

CT imaging of the nervous system offers many advantages. It usually is the best test in emergency situations, such as head trauma, stroke, and sudden change in level of consciousness (Fig. 2–4). In a patient with stroke, it is the first test performed to exclude hemorrhage. CT is

TABLE 2–3. COMPONENTS OF NERVE CONDUCTION STUDIES		
Component (Unit of Measure)	**Is a Function of:**	**Is Abnormal in:**
Distal latency (milliseconds)	Conduction rate	Compressive neuropathies (carpal tunnel syndrome)
Amplitude Motor (millivolts) Sensory (microvolts)	Number of axons	Axonal neuropathies (diabetic neuropathy)
Conduction velocity (meters/second)	Axon diameter, myelination	Demyelinating neuropathies (hereditary sensory motor neuropathy, chronic inflammatory demyelinating polyradiculoneuropathy)

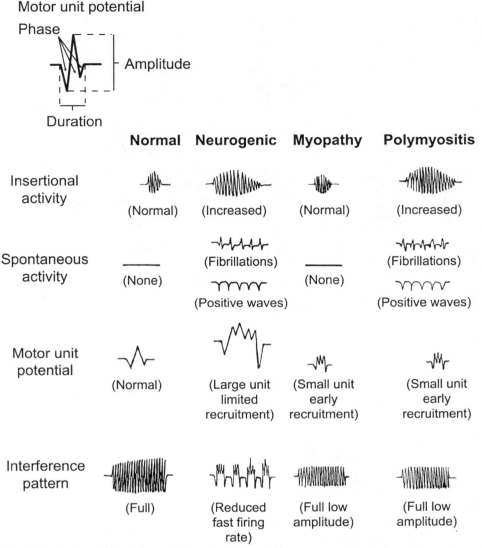

FIG. 2–3. Comparison of normal electromyographic patterns with those in neurogenic disorders, myopathy, and polymyositis. (Modified from Kimura, J: Electrodiagnosis in Diseases of Nerve and Muscle: Principles and Practice, ed 2. FA Davis, Philadelphia, 1989, p 252, with permission of Oxford University Press.)

relatively inexpensive, readily available, and useful in patients who are uncooperative or medically unstable. CT is more sensitive than MRI to calcification, and this can be important in diagnosing craniopharyngiomas, meningiomas, dermoids, aneurysms, and cysticercosis. CT is a very poor choice for visualizing the posterior fossa and is insensitive to demyelination.

MAGNETIC RESONANCE IMAGING

MRI is the preferred imaging test for evaluating the posterior fossa, neoplastic disease, meningeal disease, subacute hemorrhage, seizures, and demyelinating disease. Images can be obtained easily in several planes (Fig. 2–5). The contrast agent gadolinium is safe, and anaphylactic reactions are extremely

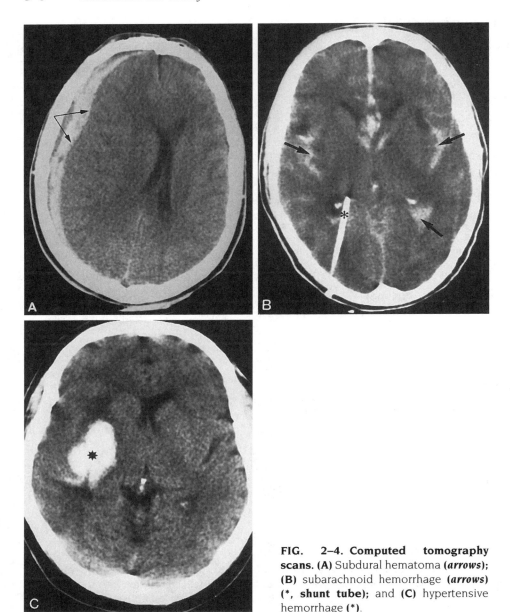

FIG. 2–4. Computed tomography scans. (A) Subdural hematoma **(arrows)**; **(B)** subarachnoid hemorrhage **(arrows)** **(*, shunt tube)**; and **(C)** hypertensive hemorrhage **(*)**.

rare. MRI is more expensive than CT and is insensitive to calcification. An absolute contraindication to MRI is the presence of magnetic intracranial aneurysm clips or cardiac pacemakers. Women in the first trimester of pregnancy and metal workers with metal fragments in the eye are usually excluded from the test. The imaging study preferred for specific clinical indications is shown in Table 2–4.

MRI is also advantageous for imaging flowing blood. Magnetic resonance angiography (MRA) is a noninvasive method for evaluating cerebral vasculature and can detect aneurysms as small as 3 to 4 millimeters (Fig. 2–6). This technique is becoming more sensitive. The use of functional neuroimaging using MRI (functional MRI) is expected to expand to include presurgical mapping and drug studies, monitoring of patients

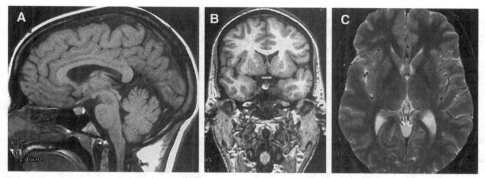

FIG. 2–5. Magnetic resonance imaging of normal brain. (A) Midline sagittal view; **(B)** coronal view; **(C)** axial view.

with stroke and head injuries, and evaluation of cognitive function and seizures.

ANGIOGRAPHY

Angiography is the test preferred for evaluating cerebrovascular disease, including aneurysms, vascular malformations, and vasculitis (Fig. 2–7). Advances have included safer digital imaging, smaller catheters, and better radiographic contrast agents. The risk of serious morbidity has decreased and the rate of stroke resulting from the procedure should be less than 0.5% when it is performed by a skilled practitioner. Therapeutic

uses have expanded to include use in thrombolytic therapy. The most common adverse effect of angiography is a groin hematoma.

MYELOGRAPHY

Myelography is a radiographic test that allows the spine to be visualized after a radiopaque substance has been injected into

TABLE 2–4. INDICATIONS FOR SELECTING CT OR MRI	
Indication	Preferred Method
Acute trauma	CT
Acute stroke (intracranial hemorrhage)	CT
Cost	CT
Bone, calcification	CT
Demyelinating disease	MRI
Mental status changes after trauma	MRI
Seizures	MRI
Tumor	MRI
Metastatic disease	MRI
Meningeal disease	MRI
Dementia	MRI
Uncooperative/medically unstable patient	CT

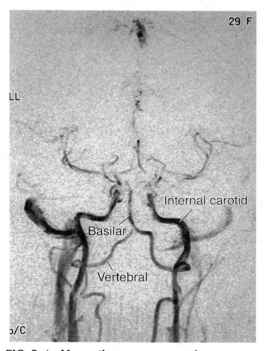

FIG. 2–6. Magnetic resonance angiogram.

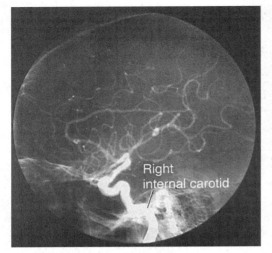

FIG. 2–7. Normal angiogram.

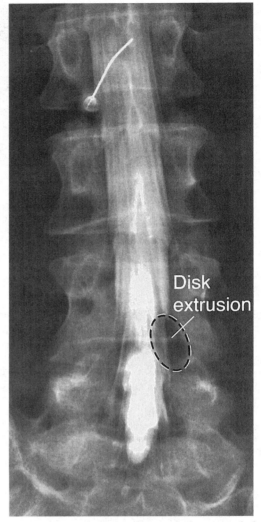

FIG. 2–8. Lumbar myelogram showing disk extrusion.

the spinal arachnoid space. This test is helpful in diagnosing diseases of the spine, such as herniated disk and spinal stenosis (Fig. 2–8). Myelography is invasive and has the same contraindications as lumbar puncture. MRI of the spine has the major advantage of being noninvasive and may be more sensitive for detecting metastatic disease of the spine and cord compression syndromes. With the advent of better contrast agents, myelography has become safer and is associated with fewer adverse reactions. Myelography may be helpful when the results of CT or MRI are ambiguous.

SUGGESTED READING

Evans, RW (Guest Ed): Diagnostic testing in neurology. Neurol Clin 14:1–254, February 1996.

Fishman, RA: Cerebrospinal Fluid in Diseases of the Nervous System. WB Saunders, Philadelphia, 1980.

Gilmore, R (Guest Ed): Evoked potentials. Neurol Clin 6:649–951, November 1988.

Kimura, J: Electrodiagnosis in Diseases of Nerve and Muscle: Principles and Practice, ed 2. FA Davis, Philadelphia, 1989.

Knight, JA: Advances in the analysis of cerebrospinal fluid. Ann Clin Lab Sci 27:93–104, 1997.

Kuntz, KM, et al: Post–lumbar puncture headaches: Experience in 501 consecutive procedures. Neurology 42:1884–1887, 1992.

Members of the Mayo Clinic Department of Neurology, Mayo Clinic and Mayo Foundation, Rochester, Minnesota: Mayo Clinic Examinations in Neurology, ed 7. CV Mosby, St. Louis, 1998.

Samuels, MA (ed): Manual of Neurologic Therapeutics: With Essentials of Diagnosis, ed 5. Little, Brown, Boston, 1995.

Wallach, JB: Interpretation of Diagnostic Tests; A Handbook Synopsis of Laboratory Medicine, ed 3. Little, Brown, Boston, 1978.

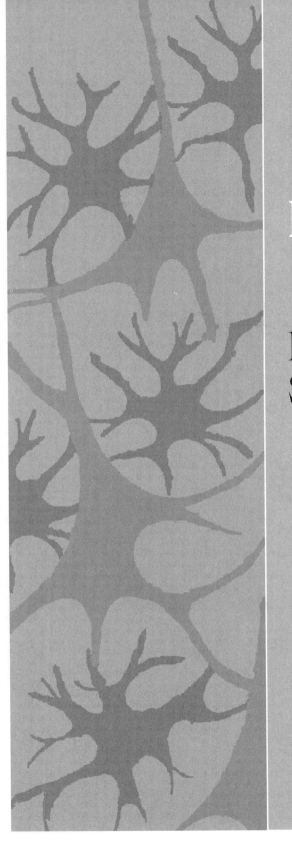

PART II

Neurologic Symptoms

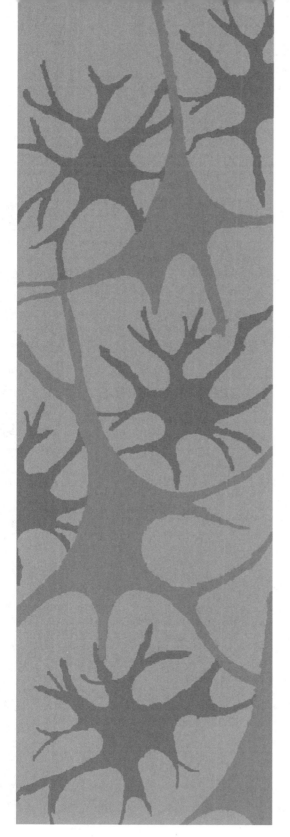

CHAPTER 3

Headache

Chapter Outline

Headache Red Flags
Diagnostic Testing
   Neuroimaging
   Electroencephalography
   Lumbar Puncture
   Other Tests
Classification
Principles of Therapy
Migraine Headache
   Phases of Migraine
   Types of Migraine
   Associations of Migraine
   Medications
Tension-Type Headache
   Tension-Type Headache and Migraine
   Treatment
Chronic Daily Headache
Cluster Headache
   Treatment
Headaches of Short Duration
Post-traumatic Headache
Temporal Arteritis
Facial Pain
   Trigeminal Neuralgia
   Glossopharyngeal Neuralgia
   Occipital Neuralgia

(continued)

Atypical Facial Pain
Herpes Zoster and Postherpetic
    Neuralgia
Temporomandibular Joint
    Dysfunction

A young woman complains of recurrent headache and frustration about her previous medical evaluations. Daily, she has a generalized headache and takes 4 to 6 tablets of aspirin or acetaminophen. Once or twice a month, usually about the time of her menstrual period, the headache is so bad she cannot go to work and she stays home and vomits. She used to go to the local emergency room for an injection, but this made her "feel like a drug addict." She says she has taken all the medicines prescribed for headache and nothing has been effective; in fact, many of them have made her ill. Her previous doctor suggested that she make an appointment with a psychologist, and the only reason she has come to a primary care practitioner is that her chiropractor, who has helped her the most, suggested further evaluation.

Although this case is hypothetical, it is common. The complexities involved in the diagnosis and management of headache are discussed in this chapter, and this hypothetical case is used to illustrate common pitfalls in the treatment of headache.

Headache is a universal problem, with a lifetime prevalence of 99%. It is second to fatigue as the most common presenting complaint to primary care practitioners. Headache may be of little clinical significance or it may represent the onset of a life-threatening illness. To the patient, the symptom is always of major concern, and the relationship you establish with the patient at the initial visit will determine the success of treatment.

The importance of this relationship cannot be overstated. It is essential that you convey to the patient that you believe the patient's symptoms are real and you are concerned about the patient's welfare. You must understand who the patient is, how the headache affects the patient's life, and what the patient's expectations, fears, and concerns are. You must educate the patient about headache, treatment options, and reasonable expectations. The patient must also take responsibility in the treatment plan as both of you work toward the mutual and realistic goal of decreasing the frequency and severity of headache.

HEADACHE RED FLAGS

Most headaches are "primary headaches"—ones without an underlying illness. These include migraine, cluster, and tension-type headaches. "Secondary headaches"—headaches caused by an underlying disease process or condition—are rare but are the initial focus in the diagnostic evaluation of headache. An experienced clinician will seek out the alarming features in the medical history and examination, and this will direct subsequent work-up. These warnings are summarized in Table 3–1.

The temporal profile of the symptom of headache is important. Sudden onset of headache suggests a vascular cause. The most serious diagnostic considerations include subarachnoid hemorrhage, hemorrhage from an arteriovenous malformation, pituitary apoplexy, and bleeding into a mass lesion. The characteristic complaint of a patient with a subarachnoid hemorrhage is that it is "the worst headache of my life." Emergency neuroimaging is advised, and computed tomography (CT) without a contrast agent is usually the most expedient test. Negative CT findings do not exclude the possibility of hemorrhage, and if the findings are not diagnostic, lumbar puncture should

TABLE 3–1. HEADACHE RED FLAGS

Headache Warning	Possible Diagnoses	Evaluation
Sudden onset of headache	Subarachnoid hemorrhage Hemorrhage from mass or arteriovenous malformation Pituitary apoplexy Mass lesion (especially in posterior fossa)	Neuroimaging, lumbar puncture
New onset of headache after age 50	Temporal arteritis Mass lesion	Erythrocyte sedimentation rate, neuroimaging
Papilledema	Mass lesion Pseudotumor cerebri	Neuroimaging, lumbar puncture
Headache with fever, rash, systemic illness, stiff neck	Meningitis Encephalitis Systemic infection Collagen vascular disease Lyme disease	Neuroimaging, lumbar puncture,* blood tests
New onset of headache in patient with cancer or HIV	Metastasis Meningitis Brain abscess	Neuroimaging, lumbar puncture*
Accelerating pattern of headaches	Mass lesions Subdural hematoma Medication overuse	Neuroimaging

HIV, human immunodeficiency virus.

*Lumbar puncture should be performed after neuroimaging. If meningitis is suspected and there are no focal findings and/or papilledema, lumbar puncture should be performed immediately.

be performed to look for blood in the cerebrospinal fluid (CSF). According to estimates, up to 25% of subarachnoid hemorrhages may be missed by CT. Other causes of sudden explosive headache can include vasospasm from migraine and an unruptured aneurysm. If subarachnoid hemorrhage is excluded by CT and CSF analysis, a neurologist should be consulted to direct further evaluation of this type of headache. Angiography or magnetic resonance angiography (MRA) (or both) may be needed to complete the evaluation of these patients.

Another alarming profile is an accelerating pattern of headaches. Most commonly, this pattern is seen in patients who have been overusing an analgesic medication, but the possibility of an enlarging mass lesion such as a tumor or subdural hematoma needs to be considered. CT with a contrast agent or magnetic resonance imaging (MRI) may be warranted. A "new" headache in a patient

with cancer or one who is immunocompromised should always be investigated. Metastasis, carcinomatous or infectious meningitis, and brain abscess are the diagnostic concerns in these patients, and neuroimaging and CSF analysis should be performed.

A patient with headache who has fever, stiff neck, rash, or other signs of systemic illness should be evaluated thoroughly for an infectious disease. Meningitis, encephalitis, Lyme disease, and systemic infections are associated with headache. Collagen vascular disease should also be considered in the setting of systemic illness. The diagnostic evaluation should include neuroimaging, CSF analysis, and blood tests. Focal neurologic symptoms and signs that are not part of a typical migraine aura may indicate a mass lesion and suggest the need to evaluate the patient for a tumor, arteriovenous malformation, stroke, or collagen vascular disease. Papilledema may indicate a mass lesion or pseudotumor cerebri. If imaging study results are negative, lumbar puncture is needed. Pseudotumor cerebri is diagnosed on the basis of negative findings on neuroimaging but increased CSF pressure.

DIAGNOSTIC TESTING

Diagnostic testing in headache can be complicated not only by the medical indications but by the demands of cost containment, medical-legal issues, and patient expectations. Diagnostic testing is indicated to confirm the diagnosis, to exclude serious diagnoses, to establish the presence of comorbid disease that may complicate treatment, and to evaluate the patient's status before initiating treatment. Tests to reassure the patient may be an integral part of the treatment plan. However, diagnostic tests should

never replace the clinical evaluation and education of the patient.

NEUROIMAGING

The diagnostic tests most often used in the evaluation of headache are CT and MRI (Table 3–2). CT is useful in an emergency setting to evaluate for the presence of hemorrhage. With the use of a contrast agent, CT can detect most mass lesions that can cause headache. MRI is more sensitive than CT for detecting tumors and infarcts. MRI is also more sensitive for detecting nonspecific abnormalities. Clinically insignificant white matter changes and atrophy have been reported to occur more frequently in patients with migraine than in age-matched controls. The patient's clinical presentation should dictate how much emphasis to put on the

TABLE 3–2. NEUROIMAGING IN HEADACHE

Indication	Neuroimaging*	Clinical Considerations
First or worst headache	**CT** without contrast or MRI	Hemorrhage
Change in clinical features (frequency or severity)	CT with contrast or MRI	Mass lesion
Abnormal examination	CT with contrast or MRI	Mass lesion
Progressive	CT with contrast or MRI	Mass lesion
Neurologic symptoms atypical for migraine	CT with contrast or MRI	Mass lesion
Persistent neurologic deficits	CT with contrast or MRI	Mass lesion
Focal EEG findings	CT with contrast or **MRI**	Focal lesion
Seizures	CT with contrast or **MRI**	Focal lesion
Orbital bruit	CT with contrast or **MRI/MRA**	Arteriovenous malformation
Same-sided pain with focal deficit	CT with contrast or MRI	Mass lesion
Anxious or doubting patient	CT with contrast or MRI	Reassurance, aid in therapy

CT, computed tomography; EEG, electroencephalography; MRA, magnetic resonance angiography; MRI, magnetic resonance imaging.
*Boldface type indicates preferred method.

imaging studies, but neurologic consultation may be helpful in determining whether the findings are significant.

On the basis of a review of the evidence and expert opinion, the American Academy of Neurology issued a summary statement about the use of neuroimaging in patients with headache who have normal findings on neurologic examination. In adult patients with recurrent headache that has been defined as migraine with no recent change in pattern, no history of seizures, and no other focal neurologic signs or symptoms, the routine use of neuroimaging is not warranted. In patients with atypical headache patterns, a history of seizures, or focal neurologic signs or symptoms, CT or MRI may be indicated.

Headache from an expanding aneurysm, arteriovenous malformation, or vasculitis requires angiography. Noninvasive MRA is useful but can miss aneurysms smaller than 3 millimeters in diameter. MRA is a reasonable test to perform in patients who have a sudden headache but negative findings on CT and CSF analysis.

ELECTROENCEPHALOGRAPHY

Electroencephalography (EEG) generally is not useful in the evaluation of headache. However, many associations have been described between seizures and migraines, including postictal headache and migraine aura–inducing seizures. A patient can have both migraine and epilepsy. The indications for EEG in evaluating headache include alterations in or loss of consciousness, transient neurologic symptoms, suspected encephalopathy, and selection of medications. An anticonvulsant (e.g., valproic acid) may be better for a patient with migraine and seizures than a medication that potentially could induce seizures (e.g., a tricyclic antidepressant).

LUMBAR PUNCTURE

Lumbar puncture, after neuroimaging, is indicated if the patient has the worst headache of his or her life or a severe, recurrent headache with a rapid onset. Lumbar puncture can be useful in evaluating a progressive headache and a chronic headache that is intractable or atypical. The diagnosis of CSF hypotension can be made with lumbar puncture in a patient with a postural headache. Patients with postural headache complain that the headache increases when they stand and decreases when they lie down. Lumbar puncture can be used also to confirm pseudotumor cerebri in a patient with papilledema and negative results on imaging studies. Headache from Lyme disease, chronic fungal meningitides, and carcinomatosis meningitis requires CSF analysis for diagnostic confirmation.

OTHER TESTS

Other laboratory tests may be needed to evaluate headache. Diagnostic tests are needed to make a diagnosis, to establish a baseline status before initiating treatment, and to monitor for compliance and toxic side effects. Some of the diagnostic tests used in the evaluation of headache and their indications are summarized in Table 3–3.

CLASSIFICATION

The International Headache Society has published a detailed classification for headaches. Although this classification has been widely used in clinical research, it is cumbersome in clinical practice. A more practical classification system—one that is useful for diagnosis, for devising a treatment plan, and for educating patients—divides headache into three major categories: vascular, tension-type, and traction/inflammatory. The traction/inflammatory category includes all the secondary types of headache. Many patients have several types of headaches, and a meaningful question to ask is "How many types of headache do you have?"

Frequently, a patient who has head pain is alarmed about the possibility of a brain tumor and is relieved to learn that the brain is not sensitive to pain and that headache is a

TABLE 3–3. DIAGNOSTIC TESTING IN HEADACHE

| Test | Indication for Test | | | Cause of Headache |
	Diagnosis	Baseline	Compliance/Toxicity	
Complete blood count with differential cell count	•	•	•	Anemia, sepsis
Erythrocyte sedimentation rate	•			Temporal arteritis
Chemistry profile	•	•	•	Chronic renal failure, hypoglycemia, hypercalcemia, hypernatremia
Electrocardiogram		•	•	β-Blockers in heart failure, vasoconstrictors in coronary artery disease
Blood gas analysis	•			Hypercapnia, hypoxia
Thyroid function	•		•	Thyrotoxicosis, contraindication of ergotamines
Serology	•			Lyme disease, HIV, syphilis
ANA, lupus anticoagulant, anticardiolipin antibodies	•			Collagen vascular diseases
Drug screen/level	•		•	Drug abuse, drug compliance

ANA, antinuclear antibody; HIV, human immunodeficiency virus.

physiologic process, such as a vasospasm or muscle contraction, and not a structural problem like a tumor. For these patients, the analogy of a "charleyhorse" is helpful—it is a muscle contraction (a physiologic process) that causes severe pain, in the absence of a structural problem. Unnecessary neuroimaging may be avoided.

Vascular structures are pain-sensitive and include all the intracranial and extracranial arteries and veins and dural venous sinuses. Pain-sensitive nonvascular structures of the head, face, and neck are the arachnoid membrane adjacent to the cerebral arteries and veins, the dura mater adjacent to the meningeal arteries and dural venous sinuses, the mucous membranes of the mouth, nasal cavity and paranasal sinuses, the teeth, the extracranial muscles and skin, the temporo-

mandibular and zygapophyseal joints, the intraspinous ligaments, and the intervertebral disks. All these structures can be categorized as musculoskeletal, vascular, and meningeal and described to patients as "muscles," "blood vessels," and "coverings of the brain and spinal cord."

PRINCIPLES OF THERAPY

The relationship established with the patient at the initial visit is important for successful management of headache. The case at the beginning of this chapter illustrates this point. The patient was frustrated with her previous doctors, likely because she thought they were not listening to her or did not seem interested in her problems. She had a better relationship with her chiropractor. Note that although she still had headache, she thought she was being helped by the chiropractor and was following the chiropractor's advice. The patient's fears and expectations must be considered, and the best way to do this is to educate the patient about the diagnosis and treatment plan. If you establish a good relationship at the beginning, the patient is more likely to follow up with you. Continuity of care is essential for effective management of headache.

Psychologic issues may be prominent in headache patients. It may be more effective to approach these issues on follow-up visits, after rapport has been established. Depression and anxiety frequently coexist with headache and need to be discussed because of the implications for treatment. A discussion about the potential side effects of a medication may be helpful in approaching this topic. For example, a migraineur with depression may prefer a tricyclic antidepressant medication to a β-blocker when given a choice of prophylactic agents.

Before a therapeutic regimen is established, it is important to know all the medications the patient is taking, including over-the-counter drugs, and the dosages, the duration of use, and the specific side effects the patient has had. Knowing what over-the-counter drugs the patient is taking is critical because patients take them on the basis of advertising information and not because of medical or pharmaceutical advice. For example, patients may be mistakenly taking "sinus" medicine for migraine. Overuse of over-the-counter analgesic drugs leads to rebound headache and makes prophylactic treatment less effective.

If a patient is not able to provide information about the dose of the drug and how long it has been taken, it generally indicates that the patient was not appropriately educated about the drug. Treatment with the same medication could be attempted again, with education and adequate dosing and duration of treatment. Lack of patient compliance, insufficient dose, inadequate duration of treatment, and side effects frequently are the culprits when therapy fails. The patient in the hypothetical case study may have "taken all the medicines," but if she stopped taking a

tricyclic antidepressant after 1 week of treatment because of drowsiness, the medication did not receive an adequate trial to dismiss its potential benefit. Patients and clinicians both need to know that few patients react in the same way to a treatment and that medication regimens need to be individualized.

The goals of treatment must be clearly defined. It is unrealistic to expect that the headache will be eliminated completely or that the medication will not have side effects. A reasonable goal is to decrease the frequency and severity of the headache so there is minimal disruption of the patient's work and quality of life. The patient must be an active participant in the treatment program and may need to make significant lifestyle changes to accomplish the goal. The patient needs to stop smoking, to exercise regularly, to avoid certain foods and alcohol, to decrease caffeine consumption, and to maintain regular schedules of sleeping and eating. Encourage patients to keep a headache log to monitor their response to a medication and to reveal potential modifiable headache triggers. If biofeedback, relaxation techniques, and cognitive therapies are part of the therapeutic regimen, they need to be practiced and performed regularly. When patients are actively engaged in their health care, they are more compliant, have more realistic expectations, and have better results. Some of the major pitfalls of effective headache treatment are listed in Table 3–4.

Medication regimens, as mentioned above, need to be individualized. Initially, give all medications at a low dose to reduce the chance of side effects. Increase the dosage to the highest dose that is tolerable and effective without causing ill effects. The patient should have an active role in the selection of medications. The cost of a medication is an important factor, but the cost of loss of work time and emergency room visits also should be considered. An emergency room is not the place to treat recurrent headache.

The frequency of a headache is the major factor in determining whether to prescribe an abortive or a prophylactic medication. For infrequent headache, many abortive medications are effective. The patient needs to know that overuse of analgesics can cause

TABLE 3–4. MAJOR PITFALLS OF HEADACHE TREATMENT

Clinician

1. Rapport with patient not established
2. No patient education provided
3. Recurrent headache treated with narcotics, leading to rebound headache
4. Abortive medications prescribed for frequent headache, leading to rebound and chronic daily headache: ergotamines, butalbital-analgesic-caffeine combination products
5. Initial dose of medication too high
6. Dose of medication not changed on basis of patient's response
7. Medication discontinued before an adequate trial is achieved

Patient

1. Overuse of over-the-counter analgesics
2. Overuse of caffeine
3. Smoking
4. Avoidance of exercise
5. Inadequate sleep
6. Improper diet
7. Unrealistic expectations

rebound headache. Overuse (more than 2 days/week) of aspirin, acetaminophen, ergotamines, barbiturates, caffeine, or opioids can cause frequent headache. Rebound headache is less likely with long-acting nonsteroidal anti-inflammatory drugs and dihydroergotamine. Prophylactic medication is recommended when the frequency of the headache is two or more times per month or when the headache results in extended disability (more than 3 days). When prescribing prophylactic medication for women of childbearing age, be aware of the possibility of pregnancy and the potential of the medication for teratogenic effects. Many of the common abortive and prophylactic medications used in headache are listed in Tables 3–5 and 3–6.

MIGRAINE HEADACHE

Migraine is an episodic headache with neurologic, gastrointestinal, and autonomic changes. Genetic factors are important in migraine, but the specific inheritance pattern has not been defined. The International Headache Society classifies migraine into seven subtypes. "Migraine without aura" was previously called "common migraine." The diagnostic criteria include two of the following: unilateral headache, throbbing or pulsating pain, moderate-to-severe pain that may inhibit or restrict ability to function, and pain aggravated by routine physical activity. Associated symptoms include nausea and/or vomiting or photophobia and phonophobia (aversion to light and sound). "Migraine with aura" was previously called "classic migraine." This headache has the same diagnostic criteria as migraine without aura, but it has an associated aura. Auras include visual, sensory, motor, or language symptoms.

Several theories have been proposed for the pathogenesis of migraine. According to the standard vascular theory of migraine, vasoconstriction accounts for the aura and vasodilatation causes the pain of the headache, but this theory has not been supported by recent studies. Currently, it is thought that the pain in migraine and other primary headaches is generated centrally by serotonergic and adrenergic pain-modulating systems. Also, through inhibitory and facilitatory descending pain-modulating systems, the central nervous system controls the information coming from peripheral pain receptors. More is being learned about the pathogenesis of migraine, and this knowledge should help with the development of more effective medications to treat this common disorder.

PHASES OF MIGRAINE

The five phases of migraine are the (1) premonitory phase, (2) aura, (3) headache, (4) headache resolution phase, and (5) postdromal phase. The premonitory phase affects 40% to 60% of patients with migraines and includes behavioral, emotional, autonomic, and constitutional disturbances that occur 1 or 2 days before the headache. These disturbances may include sleep disruption, food cravings, fatigue, yawning, depression, and

TABLE 3–5. ABORTIVE MEDICATIONS FOR VASCULAR AND TENSION-TYPE HEADACHES

Drug	Initial Dose	Rebound Headache*
Acetaminophen	1,000 mg PO	+++
Aspirin	1,000 mg PO	+++
Butalbital combination (Fiorinal)	2 tabs PO	+++
Butorphanol nasal spray (Stadol)	1 mg IN	+++
Caffeine adjuvant	60 mg PO	+++
Codeine	30 mg PO	+++
Dihydroergotamine (DHE 45)	1 mg IM, SC, IV, 2 mg IN	+
Ergotamine (Ergomar)	1 mg PO, 2 mg PR	+++
Ibuprofen (Motrin)	800 mg PO	+++
Indomethacin (Indocin)	50 mg PO	+
Isometheptene combination (Midrin)	65 mg PO	+++
Meperidine (Demerol)	100 mg PO, IM	+++
Naproxen (Naprosyn)	500 mg PO	+
Sumatriptan (Imitrex)	6 mg SC, 50 mg PO, 10 mg IN	++

*+++, high rebound potential; ++, medium rebound potential; +, low rebound potential.

IM, intramuscular; IN, intranasal; IV, intravenous; PO, orally; PR, per rectum; SC, subcutaneous.

euphoria. Common migraine triggers are possible components of the premonitory phase.

The aura usually precedes the headache but can accompany it. Diagnostic criteria for the aura include three of the four following characteristics: (1) one or more reversible symptoms, (2) aura symptoms develop over 4 minutes, (3) the aura lasts no longer than 60 minutes, and (4) headache onset is within 60 minutes after the aura ends.

The headache is usually unilateral but can be bilateral in 40% of patients. Many symptoms can accompany the headache, such as nausea, vomiting, and visual disturbances. Autonomic symptoms include hypertension, hypotension, nasal stuffiness, peripheral vasoconstriction, tachycardia, and bradycardia. Other symptoms include fatigue, emotional changes, mental dullness, sensory abnormalities, and fluid retention. The length of time for the headache phase can vary from 4 to 72 hours. The postdromal phase often includes symptoms of fatigue and mental confusion that last for 1 or 2 days.

TYPES OF MIGRAINE

Basilar migraine is a type of migraine that occurs more frequently in children and young adolescents than in adults. Clinical characteristics involve brainstem symptoms of ataxia, diplopia, vertigo, tinnitus, dysarthria, visual field defects, bilateral motor and sensory disturbances, and depressed level of awareness. *Retinal migraine* is a rare headache condition that is preceded or accompanied by monocular visual disturbance. *Ophthalmoplegic migraine* is a headache accompanied by paresis of the extraocular muscles. The third cranial nerve is usually involved, and the patient has ptosis, mydriasis, and difficulty moving the eyes in any direction except laterally.

TABLE 3–6. PROPHYLACTIC MEDICATIONS FOR HEADACHE

Drug Type (Example)	Example of Initial Dose*	Type of Headache	Clinical Comment
β-Blockers (propranolol)	80 mg PO	Vascular	Not indicated in asthma, some heart diseases
Calcium channel blockers (verapamil)	240 mg PO	Cluster	Care in cardiac conduction defects Adverse effect: constipation
Tricyclic antidepressants (amitriptyline)	10–25 mg PO	Migraine, tension-type, mixed	Adverse effects: drowsiness, dry mouth, weight gain
Anticonvulsants (valproate)	750 mg PO	Migraine	Adverse effects: teratogenic effects, weight gain
Antiserotonin (methysergide)	6 mg PO	Vascular	Adverse effects: fibrotic complications, rebound on withdrawal
Nonsteroidal anti-inflammatory drugs (naproxen sodium)	750 mg PO	Migraine, tension-type	Adverse effect: gastrointestional irritation

PO, orally.
*Doses need to be individualized, and all potential adverse effects and contraindications should be reviewed. Start at the lowest dose and advance according to the patient's response.

"Migraine equivalents" and "acephalic migraines" describe episodes of migraine aura without headache. All types of auras can occur, but visual symptoms are the most common. In patients who present with these symptoms and who have no previous history of migraine, the diagnosis can be very difficult. Transient ischemic attacks are the most important differential diagnosis and should be excluded before attributing these symptoms to migraine.

ASSOCIATIONS OF MIGRAINE

A strong association between migraine and estrogen is suggested by the increased incidence of migraine with menarche, menstruation, use of oral contraceptive agents, pregnancy, and menopause. Menstrual migraine is defined as migraine attacks that occur regularly on or between days −2 to +3 of the menstrual cycle. The proposed mechanism of these headaches is related to decreased levels of estrogen. If patients with menstrual migraine do not have a response to the usual migraine treatment strategies, hormonal treatment may be effective (Table 3–7).

The frequency of migraine generally changes during pregnancy, but 25% of women experience no change. Headaches may increase in frequency during the first trimester and then decrease in the last two trimesters, perhaps related to the sustained high level of estrogen. Despite this decrease in headache frequency, the management of migraine during pregnancy is complicated. Potential adverse effects of drug therapy on the fetus need to be balanced with the frequency of headache and associated complications. Medications should be limited during pregnancy but should be considered if the headache poses a risk to the fetus. Nonpharmacologic treatment should be attempted first, for example, massage, ice packs, intravenous hydration, and inhalation of oxygen. Analgesic medications should be

TABLE 3–7. SUGGESTED TREATMENT OF MENSTRUAL MIGRAINE

Nonsteroidal anti-inflammatory drugs for 5–7 days around vulnerable period

Estrogen therapy
  Percutaneous estradiol 1.5 mg daily from 3 days before menses, for 6 days
  Transdermal estradiol 1 × 100 μg patch on day −3, day −1, and day +2 of menses

Synthetic androgens
  Danazol 200–600 mg daily started before onset of headache and continued through menses

Antiestrogens
  Tamoxifen 5–15 mg daily for days 7 through 14

Dopamine agonists
  Bromocriptine 2.5 mg 3 times daily

cerebral venous thrombosis, eclampsia, and subarachnoid hemorrhage.

The use of oral contraceptive agents can influence migraine, but no consistent pattern has been detected. Women taking oral contraceptive agents have reported an increase, a decrease, and no change in frequency of migraine attacks. This emphasizes the importance of individualized treatment.

The prevalence of migraine decreases with advancing age, but some women experience an increase in migraine frequency during menopause. Hormone replacement therapy can also increase the frequency of migraine attacks. Strategies to treat estrogen-replacement headache include reducing the estrogen dose. A change in the type of estrogen is also recommended, that is, changing from a conjugated estrogen to estradiol, synthetic estrogen, or a pure estrone. Continuous dosing may be preferable to interrupted dosing. Compared with an oral preparation, a parenteral preparation may reduce the headache. Also, adding an androgen to the medication regimen may prevent estrogen-replacement headache.

A daily or almost daily headache can develop in a person with episodic migraine. This

used on a limited basis if the patient does not respond to other measures. Prophylactic medication should be used only as a last resort. The various migraine medications and associated risks during pregnancy are listed in Table 3–8. It is important to remember that several serious causes of headache can occur during pregnancy, for example, stroke,

TABLE 3–8. MIGRAINE MEDICATION AND PREGNANCY RISK

Medication	Pregnancy Risk
Aspirin	Risk to humans has not been ruled out
	Positive risk if used at end of third trimester
Acetaminophen	No evidence of risk but no controlled human studies
Ibuprofen, naproxen	No evidence of risk but no controlled human studies
	Positive risk if used at end of third trimester
Codeine	Risk to humans has not been ruled out
	Positive risk if used at end of third trimester
Meperidine	No evidence of risk but no controlled human studies
	Positive risk if used at end of third trimester
Ergotamine, dihydroergotamine	Contraindicated in pregnancy
Sumatriptan	Risk to humans has not been ruled out
Prochlorperazine	Risk to humans has not been ruled out
Propranolol	Risk to humans has not been ruled out
Amitriptyline	Positive evidence of risk to humans
Verapamil	Risk to humans has not been ruled out
Valproic acid	Positive evidence of risk to humans

is called *transformed migraine*, which often is related to medication overuse or rebound headache. This type of headache is discussed below with chronic daily headache.

The relationship of migraine and stroke is complicated and can be confusing to clinicians. Stroke and migraine can coexist. Furthermore, migraine can also induce stroke, and stroke can occur with clinical features of migraine (symptomatic migraine and migraine mimic, Chapter 11). A large-scale epidemiologic study showed an association between migraine and stroke and concluded that migraine should be considered a risk factor for stroke. The risk of stroke in a young woman with migraine is low, even if she is taking an oral contraceptive. However, if the patient has a prolonged aura, it is best to avoid oral contraceptives or vasoconstrictive agents that make the risk unacceptably high. This emphasizes the importance of avoiding other risk factors for stroke, especially smoking.

The treatment of migraine should follow the recommendations discussed above on principles of therapy. Your relationship with the patient is crucial to successful management of recurrent headache. Patient education about the cause of the pain and about the medications (both prescription and over-the-counter drugs) is essential. The patient needs to have a realistic expectation about the treatment regimen and be an active participant.

Achieving the goal of reducing the frequency and severity of headache begins with an improvement in general health. This includes a regular exercise program, a well-balanced diet with meals at regular intervals, regular sleeping habits, and not smoking. Any potential trigger factors for headache that the patient has noted, such as alcohol or certain foods, should be avoided. If possible, eliminate any medications that could cause or contribute to the headache (Table 3–9).

MEDICATIONS

Many abortive medications are available for treating migraine. It should be emphasized to the patient that frequent use of abortive medications can cause rebound headache

TABLE 3–9. DRUGS THAT CAN CAUSE OR CONTRIBUTE TO HEADACHE

Cardiovascular and Antihypertensive Drugs

Nifedipine
Atenolol, metoprolol, propranolol
Nitroglycerin
Isosorbide
Captopril
Methyldopa

Gastrointestinal Drugs

Cimetidine, ranitidine

Nonsteroidal Anti-inflammatory Drugs

Indomethacin, piroxicam, diclofenac

Antibiotics, Anti-infective Drugs

Trimethoprim-sulfamethoxazole
Metronidazole

Hormones

Estrogens
Danazol
Corticosteroids

(see Table 3–5). Abortive medications that are more likely to cause rebound headaches include aspirin, acetaminophen, butalbital products, ergotamines, ibuprofen, and narcotics. These agents should not be used more often than 2 times per week. The chronic use of any medication should be scrutinized for the possibility of habituation and renal and liver disease. The elimination of chronically used medications may obviate prophylactic therapy.

Nonsteroidal anti-inflammatory drugs (NSAIDs) can be useful in treating symptoms of mild to moderate migraine. Overuse of NSAIDs can lead to rebound headache. This problem is less likely with longer-acting medications. Contraindications to NSAIDs are hypersensitivity to the drug or a history of allergy to aspirin or other anti-inflammatory agents. NSAIDs should be prescribed carefully for patients with a history of gastrointestinal ulceration, bleeding, or perforation or renal or liver dysfunction. Nausea, abdominal pain, diarrhea, and fluid retention are some common side effects. Ketorolac can be given parenterally in the emergency room for migraine. However, it has a high incidence of adverse effects, and it should be used sparingly. Naproxen sodium and ibuprofen have a strong safety profile and are available as over-the-counter drugs.

The combination of isometheptene mucate, dichloralphenazone, and acetaminophen (Midrin) is effective for symptomatic treatment of mild to moderate migraine. It is contraindicated for patients with glaucoma, renal disease, hypertension, organic heart disease, and liver disease and for patients receiving monoamine oxidase inhibitor therapy. The few adverse reactions reported include transient dizziness and skin rash in sensitive patients. Overuse of this product can cause rebound headache.

A new class of medications, the 5-hydroxytryptamine (5-HT$_1$) receptor agonists, has revolutionized acute treatment of migraine. Currently available 5-HT$_1$ receptor agonists include sumatriptan, zolmitriptan, naratriptan, and rizatriptan. The effect of these agents on the 5-HT$_1$ receptors located on intracranial blood vessels and peripheral sensory nerve endings results in cranial vasoconstriction and decreased release of inflammatory neuropeptides. The most common adverse effects are paresthesias, a feeling of chest tightness, nausea, dizziness, and somnolence. Because of the possibility of cardiovascular and cerebrovascular disease, these medications should be avoided in patients with ischemic heart disease and uncontrolled hypertension. The manufacturers recommend that these agents be used with caution in men older than 40 years, postmenopausal women, and persons with other cardiac risk factors such as diabetes mellitus, obesity, cigarette smoking, hypercholesterolemia, or a family history of coronary artery disease. An ergot-containing drug should not be taken within 24 hours before or after taking a 5-HT$_1$ receptor agonist because of the potential for increasing the prolonged vasoconstrictive action of the drug. Similarly, monoamine oxidase A inhibitors should not be taken within 2 weeks of taking a 5-HT$_1$ receptor agonist. Caution should be used for patients taking selective serotonin reuptake inhibitors. Cimetidine and oral contraceptives may in-crease the serum concentration of 5-HT$_1$ receptor agonists (Table 3–10).

Ergotamine tartrate and dihydroergotamine mesylate are 5-HT$_1$ receptor agonists that have been available for more than 50 years to treat acute migraine. Ergotamine tartrate is available in oral, sublingual, inhalation, and rectal suppository dosage forms (with and without caffeine). Because of the poor oral absorption of ergotamine and the frequent association of nausea and vomiting with migraine, the rectal suppository preparation is recommended. These suppositories can be hardened in the refrigerator and sliced along their length into halves or quarters. The dose that does not cause nausea should be used at the onset of headache. Ergotamine tartrate in appropriate doses is safe and effective in the treatment of migraine in adults. Contraindications for the use of ergotamine tartrate include pregnancy, sepsis, coronary artery disease, cerebral or peripheral vascular disease, liver or renal insufficiency, and uncontrolled hypertension. The major adverse reactions are paresthesias, nausea, and cramps. If the patient has a feeling of chest tightness, discontinue treatment with the medication and investigate possible heart disease. Ergotamine should be limited to no more than 10 mg/week. Overuse can lead to rebound headache and ergotism, consisting of vomiting, diarrhea, muscle cramps, peripheral ischemic gangrene, muscle tremors, and headache.

Dihydroergotamine is a potent venoconstrictor that, unlike ergotamine, minimally constricts peripheral arteries. Its advantages over ergotamine include the absence of physical dependence and no problem with rebound headache. The contraindications are similar to those for ergotamine. Dihydroergotamine is an effective abortive therapy for migraine. An antiemetic (25 mg promethazine, 5 mg metoclopramide, 10 mg prochlorperazine) is frequently given in conjunction with dihydroergotamine to avoid nausea. Repetitive intravenous injections of the drug are indicated in the management of status migrainosus and transformed migraine (Table 3–11).

Status migrainosus is a prolonged migraine attack that lasts longer than 72 hours

TABLE 3–10. 5-HT$_1$ RECEPTOR AGONISTS FOR TREATMENT OF ACUTE MIGRAINE

Drug	Dose
Sumatriptan (Imitrex)	
Subcutaneous, 6-mg self-dose kit	6 mg at onset, can repeat in 1 hr; maximum, 2 injections/day
Oral, 25- and 50-mg tablets	50 mg at onset, can repeat (up to 100 mg) in 2 hr; maximum, 300 mg/day
Nasal spray, 5- and 20-mg spray	5 mg in each nostril at onset, may repeat in 2 hr; maximum, 40 mg/day
Zolmitriptan (Zomig): oral, 2.5- and 5-mg tablets	2.5 mg (or less) at onset, can repeat in 2 hr; maximum, 10 mg/day
Naratriptan (Amerge): oral, 2.5-mg tablets	2.5 mg at onset, can repeat in 2 hr; maximum, 10 mg/day
Rizatriptan (Maxalt): oral, 5- or 10-mg tablets or wafers	5 or 10 mg at onset, can repeat in 2 hr; maximum, 30 mg/day
Dihydroergotamine (DHE 45)	
Intramuscular, 1 mg = 1 ampule	1 mg at onset, can repeat in 1 hr; maximum, 3 mg/day
Intravenous, 1 mg = 1 ampule	0.5 to 1 mg at onset, can repeat in 8 hr; maximum, 3 mg/day
Intranasal (Migranal), 0.5 mg/spray	0.5 mg each nostril at onset, repeat in 15 min; maximum, 3 mg/day
Ergotamine tartrate (Ergomar, Ergostat): 2-mg rectal suppositories	¼ to 1 suppository at onset, can repeat in 1 hr; maximum, 4 mg/day, 10 mg/wk

and is associated with nausea and vomiting. Hospitalization is often required. Repetitive intravenous injections of dihydroergotamine are indicated for status migrainosus and provide relief in up to 90% of patients in 2 to 3 days (Table 3–11). Fluids given intravenously and oxygen therapy are useful adjunctive measures. Corticosteroids are prescribed sometimes, but their effectiveness has not been firmly established.

Phenothiazines are useful in treating acute migraine. Intravenous injections of prochlorperazine and chlorpromazine have been given in an emergency room to avoid injections of narcotics. Prochlorperazine, 10 mg, is administered by slow intravenous infusion over 2 minutes. The most frequent side effects are dizziness and drowsiness. Dystonic reactions may occur and are treated with benztropine mesylate, 1 mg given intramuscularly. Pretreatment with 500 mL of isotonic saline is recommended before intravenous injection of chlorpromazine, 12.5 mg. The dose can be repeated every 30 minutes, to a total dose of 37.5 mg. Orthostatic blood pressure should be monitored after every dose and 1 hour after treatment has been completed. Hypotension is the primary adverse reaction, and it is best to keep patients supine for at least 4 hours. Dystonic reactions may occur and are treated with benztropine mesylate or diphenhydramine.

Most migraine attacks can be treated without narcotic analgesics. Narcotics should be avoided because more effective agents are available; also, narcotics produce rebound headache and can cause habituation. However, for patients with headaches unresponsive to 5-HT$_1$ receptor agonists or for whom these agents are contraindicated, narcotics can be

TABLE 3–11. REPETITIVE INTRAVENOUS DIHYDROERGOTAMINE (DHE) FOR STATUS MIGRAINOSUS

Test dose: metoclopramide 10 mg and DHE 0.5 mg

Nausea or headache ceases within 1 hr: repeat 0.5 mg DHE every 8 hr for 2 days

No nausea and headache persists: give additional 0.5 mg DHE and then 1 mg DHE and 10 mg metoclopramide every 8 hr for 2 days (metoclopramide stopped after 24 hr)

Nausea after second dose: 0.3 mg DHE every 8 hr

TABLE 3–12. STEPS IN THE ABORTIVE TREATMENT OF MIGRAINE

1. **Nonsteroidal anti-inflammatory agents**
   Naproxen sodium
   Ibuprofen
   Indomethacin
   Ketorolac
   or
   Combination products
   Isometheptene-dichloralphenazone-acetaminophen
2. **5-HT$_1$ agonists**
   Sumatriptan
   Zolmitriptan
   Naratriptan
   Ergotamine
   Dihydroergotamine
3. **Neuroleptic agents**
   Prochlorperazine
   Chlorpromazine
4. **Parenteral narcotics**
   Meperidine

prescribed. Intravenous meperidine is often given in conjunction with an antiemetic medication. Butorphanol, an opioid agonist-antagonist available in an intranasal dosage form, is sometimes prescribed. Although it has abuse potential, the potential is reportedly low because of its dysphoric effect. Treatment with narcotic analgesics requires that you carefully discuss the possible risks with the patient. Guidelines for the treatment of nonmalignant pain with narcotics are discussed in Chapter 10. Steps in the abortive treatment of migraine are suggested in Table 3–12.

The decision to treat migraine prophylactically should be based on several factors, including the frequency of the headaches, the severity of the attacks, prolonged time of attack, inadequate symptomatic treatment, and the patient's ability to cope with the migraine. If the patient is overusing analgesics, prophylactic treatment may not be needed if the patient stops taking the agents. Prophylactic therapy should not be considered in patients who anticipate becoming pregnant.

The choice of prophylactic medicine should be individualized and made on the basis of the side effects and contraindications. The various medications and potential side effects should be discussed with the patient. If a patient is an active participant in the selection process, he or she is more likely to be compliant with the medication. It is very useful for the patient to maintain a headache log or calendar to follow the frequency and severity of the headache in response to the medication. If the medication

is successful, it is reasonable to withdraw it after 1 year to determine whether it is still necessary. The knowledge that the medication is to be used for a limited time is often reassuring to the patient. The steps in the prophylactic treatment of migraine are listed in Table 3–13.

Certain β-blockers are effective prophylactic medications for the treatment of migraine headache. The ones that are effective lack partial agonist activity. These include propranolol, atenolol, metoprolol, nadolol, and timolol. Failure to respond to one of these does not imply failure to respond to all β-blockers. For example, if the patient does not have a response to propranolol, it is reasonable to try atenolol. Contraindications to β-blockers include cardiogenic shock, sinus bradycardia, greater than first-degree heart block, bronchial asthma, and congestive heart failure. Remember that β-blockers can mask symptoms of hypoglycemia in patients with diabetes mellitus. Potential adverse effects include fatigue, cold extremities, dizziness, and depression. There is no standard dose, and it is reasonable to start low and increase to the highest tolerated dose without side effects. Propranolol should be given twice a day. A long-acting preparation is available and is more convenient for pa-

TABLE 3–13. STEPS IN THE PROPHYLACTIC TREATMENT OF MIGRAINE

1. **β-Blockers**
   Propranolol
   Atenolol
   or
   Tricyclic antidepressants
   Amitriptyline
   Nortriptyline
2. **Anticonvulsant agent**
   Valproate
3. **Calcium channel blocker**
   Verapamil
4. **Combination of the above**
5. **Monoamine oxidase A inhibitor**
   Phenelzine
   or
   Ergot derivative
   Methysergide

tients. If β-blocker treatment needs to be discontinued, gradually withdraw the drug over 1 week.

Tricyclic antidepressants that inhibit the uptake of serotonin and norepinephrine (e.g., amitriptyline and nortriptyline) are effective for prophylactic treatment of migraine. They are most useful for patients with mixed headaches or those who have features of vascular and tension-type headaches. It is extremely important for the patient to understand that it will take at least 6 weeks of continuous therapy before the therapeutic effect can be judged. The time spent educating the patient about the potential side effects is worthwhile and greatly improves compliance. The common side effect of drowsiness can be beneficial for patients with a concomitant sleep difficulty. Dry mouth, constipation, and weight gain are common with these agents. Special attention should be given patients who have urinary retention, seizures, angle-closure glaucoma, or cardiovascular abnormalities, because the medication can potentially aggravate these conditions. Amitriptyline treatment can be started at 10 to 25 mg at bedtime and increased as tolerated. In most adults, 100 mg is the maximal amount. Nortriptyline is as efficacious as amitriptyline and has fewer anticholinergic side effects.

The dose of nortriptyline is the same as that of amitriptyline.

Recently, the anticonvulsant divalproex sodium was approved for the prophylactic treatment of migraine. The benefit of divalproex in epilepsy and some psychiatric disorders may make it the preferred agent in patients with migraine and coexisting seizure disorders, anxiety, or mania. Common side effects include tremor, weight gain, and alopecia. More serious problems are hepatitis and pancreatitis, and the guidelines for monitoring should be followed. Anticonvulsant levels do not correlate with clinical efficacy. Women of child-bearing age should be reminded of the potential teratogenic effects of this medication.

NSAIDs can be given for migraine prophylaxis (e.g., naproxen sodium, 500 mg twice daily, or indomethacin, 25 mg three times daily [75 mg/day, sustained release]). For menstrual migraine, naproxen sodium 1 week before and the week of the menstrual period can be effective. Several headache syndromes, such as the headaches of short duration, are particularly responsive to indomethacin, and, except for these syndromes, NSAIDs are best prescribed for short-term therapy.

The efficacy of calcium channel blockers in the prophylactic treatment of migraine is disappointing. Nifedipine often causes a dull, persistent headache. Nimodipine, approved for the treatment of vasospasm in subarachnoid hemorrhage, is not a practical long-term agent, because it is expensive. Verapamil may be helpful for patients with migraine and coexisting Prinzmetal angina or Raynaud phenomenon. It should be considered for patients who have a prolonged aura or complicated migraine or who have not had a response to other, more efficacious medications. Contraindications include severe left ventricular dysfunction, hypotension, sick sinus syndrome, second- to third-degree atrioventricular block, and atrial flutter or fibrillation. Constipation, hypotension, edema, congestive heart failure, and heart block are potential side effects. The starting dose for verapamil is 40 mg three times daily, with gradual 40-mg increments per week, to a maximum of 480 mg/day. It may take 2 to 3 months to assess its therapeutic effect.

Treatment with multiple medications increases the risk of untoward side effects, but combination therapy may be reasonable for migraine. The combination of a β-blocker and a tricyclic antidepressant may be successful when monotherapy fails. β-Blockers, tricyclic antidepressants, divalproex sodium, and calcium channel blockers can all be given in combination. Product information guidelines should be consulted for possible drug interactions.

Methysergide is an ergot medicine effective in preventing migraine attacks. Its potential serious side effect of fibrotic complications limits its value. To avoid this complication, a 1-month drug holiday is recommended after 6 months of continuous therapy. Contraindications include pregnancy, peripheral vascular disease, arteriosclerosis, hypertension, coronary artery disease, pulmonary disease, collagen disease, and valvular heart disease. In addition to fibrotic complications, patients may experience weight gain, peripheral ischemia, hallucinations, or peptic ulcer disease. The initial dose can be 0.5 mg twice a day, with a gradual increase to a maximum of 2 mg four times a day.

Monoamine oxidase inhibitors can be effective treatment for patients with headaches refractory to more standard treatment. Some headache specialists refer to phenelzine sulfate as "pharmacologic last rites." The list of foods and medications that cannot be taken in conjunction with this medication is extensive, and patients should be made aware of these interactions. Phenelzine can potentiate sympathomimetic substances and cause a hypertensive crisis. Contraindications include liver disease, pheochromocytoma, and congestive heart failure. Constipation, orthostatic hypotension, and weight gain are side effects. The initial dose is 15 mg at bedtime, and this is increased to a maximum of 60 mg/day.

The treatment of migraine headache in children has not been universally established. The problem is that many drugs have not been studied in younger age groups. Treatment with aspirin, acetaminophen, NSAIDs, and other analgesics is reasonable. Cyproheptadine, an antihistaminic and antiserotonergic agent, has some efficacy in childhood migraine. This drug is contraindi-

cated in newborn or premature infants and elderly debilitated patients and in patients with glaucoma, peptic ulcer disease, or prostatic hypertrophy. The common side effects are sedation and weight gain. The dosage is based on weight and can be initiated at 0.25 mg/kg daily and adjusted according to the patient's response. Children have been treated with other agents described for treating adult migraine, but appropriate precautions regarding dosage and effect on growth and development should be considered for the pediatric age group.

TENSION-TYPE HEADACHE

Tension-type headache is the International Headache Society's designation for what was called "tension," "muscle contraction," "stress," or "psychogenic" headache. Abnormal neuronal sensitivity and pain facilitation and not muscle contraction are thought to cause tension-type headache. Myofascial pain receptors may become hypersensitive and lead to pain from noxious and nonnoxious stimuli. Tension-type headache can be episodic or chronic.

Episodic tension-type headache is the most common type of headache, and patients usually self-medicate with over-the-counter analgesics. It generally is a headache of mild to moderate intensity that does not interfere with activity. The headache is described as a nonpulsatile pressure or tightening sensation. The International Headache Society criteria of episodic tension-type headache include at least 10 previous headache episodes, with fewer than 180 per year or 15 per month. The headache duration can vary from 30 minutes to 7 days. Nausea and vomiting are not associated with this type of headache, but anorexia is. Photophobia and phonophobia are usually absent.

TENSION-TYPE HEADACHE AND MIGRAINE

The diagnostic criteria suggest that migraine and tension-type headache are separate entities, and many authors support the contention that the headaches are distinct, with separate causes and comorbid conditions. The distinction has not been defined clearly. However, other authors consider migraine and tension-type headache to be the same, distinguished only by the intensity of the pain. Both headache disorders are episodic, nonthrobbing, unilateral or bilateral, and associated with anorexia, photophobia, or phonophobia. They may respond to the same medications, and many patients have both types of headaches. Whatever the difference is between these two types of headache, the clinical emphasis should always be on the patient.

TREATMENT

The principles of treating episodic tension-type headache are similar to those discussed above. General health measures should be discussed with the patient. Regular exercise is important and should become part of the patient's everyday routine. Most patients respond to exercise, stretching, and simple analgesics. The most important factor to emphasize to patients is the risk of chronic daily headache from the overuse of medication. If the patient does not have a response to these measures, prophylactic treatment should be considered. Tricyclic antidepressants are efficacious for tension-type headache. When depression is present, patients may respond to other antidepressant agents, including selective serotonin reuptake inhibitors. The prophylactic agents described above for migraine are all reasonable alternatives for patients with difficult-to-control episodic tension-type headache (see Table 3–6).

CHRONIC DAILY HEADACHE

Chronic tension-type headache is one type of chronic daily headache. Not all chronic daily headaches are chronic tension-type headache. The most common cause of chronic daily headache is transformed migraine. Patients with transformed migraine have a history of episodic migraines that develop into a daily headache with features of both migraine and tension-type headache. This condition can be caused or aggravated by the overuse of symptomatic medication.

The patient described at the beginning of this chapter exemplifies this problem. Episodic tension-type headache can develop into chronic tension-type headache. Two other types of primary chronic daily headache are hemicrania continua and new daily persistent headache. *Hemicrania continua* is an infrequent headache disorder characterized by mild to moderately severe unilateral pain that is continuous and fluctuating, with occasional jabs or jolts of pain. This type of headache responds to indomethacin. In *new daily persistent headache*, the symptoms begin acutely, and the patient has no previous history of episodic headache. The character of this headache type is like that of transformed migraine.

Chronic daily headache can also be secondary. Causes include trauma, cervical spine disease, vascular conditions such as subdural hematoma, nonvascular disorders such as infection or neoplasm, temporomandibular joint disease, and sinusitis. These potential causes or triggers of chronic daily headache should be looked for and treated accordingly.

Patients with chronic daily headache are the most challenging headache patients to treat. Overused symptomatic medications need to be discontinued. Frequently, this results in a withdrawal syndrome, with an increase in headache. However, if the patient can endure this process, the headache will improve and be more responsive to prophylactic agents. Hospitalization may be necessary if detoxification from symptomatic medication is severe. If so, repetitive intravenous injections of dihydroergotamine can be effective (see Table 3–11).

Patients with chronic daily headache may have an increased frequency of depression, personality disorder, emotional dependency, or low frustration tolerance. The patient's emotional and psychologic needs must be addressed. Psychiatric or psychologic consultation may be necessary.

CLUSTER HEADACHE

Cluster headache is a distinct primary headache characterized by severe, excruciating, unilateral periorbital pain that can last from 15 to 180 minutes. Associated autonomic symptoms include conjunctival injection, lacrimation, nasal congestion, rhinorrhea, forehead and facial sweating, miosis, ptosis, and eyelid edema. The frequency of the attacks can vary from one every other day to eight per day. The attacks occur in "clusters," which can last for weeks to months, separated by headache-free remissions.

Cluster headache is distinct from migraine in many ways. Cluster headache is not associated with an aura, nausea, vomiting, photophobia, or phonophobia. A patient with cluster headache is up and active during an attack, unlike a migraine patient, who prefers to lie down in a quiet dark room. Cluster headaches occur more frequently in men than in women and attacks can continue into late life. In most patients with cluster headache, the pain remains on the same side of the head. The uncommon variant of migraine-cluster headache syndrome confuses these distinctions. Autonomic symptoms readily distinguish cluster headache from tension-type headache and trigeminal neuralgia. The autonomic symptoms and periodicity of the attacks often lead patients with cluster headache to attribute their symptoms to sinus disease or allergies. It is important to think of cluster headache when a patient seeks medical advice because of a severe sinus problem or allergies.

The pathophysiology of cluster headache is not known. The pain is thought to be due to activation of the trigeminal vascular system (i.e., the trigeminal nerve and intracranial blood vessels) and the parasympathetic nervous system. The cause of the periodicity of cluster headache also is not known. Evidence suggests that cyclic hypothalamic dysfunction may impair sympathetic neuronal activity, making the patient susceptible to a cluster attack.

Paroxysmal hemicrania is a variant of cluster headache. The symptoms are comparable to those of cluster headache, but the attacks are more frequent and shorter. The most characteristic feature of paroxysmal hemicrania is that it responds readily to treatment with indomethacin.

TREATMENT

The treatment of cluster headache should include both symptomatic and prophylactic treatments. The observation that high altitude and strenuous exercise precipitated cluster attacks led to the use of oxygen inhalation for abortive therapy. Although oxygen is very effective, it can be inconvenient. The oxygen should be administered by face mask at 7 L/minute until the attack is aborted. The time should not exceed 20 minutes, but if the attack is not aborted during this time, the treatment can be repeated after a 5-minute break. Other medications for aborting cluster headache are listed in Table 3–14.

Prophylactic treatment is essential to decrease the length of the cluster period and to avoid over-treatment with abortive medications. The selection of medication depends on many factors, including the patient's previous experience, the contraindications, the frequency and timing of the attacks, and the expected length of the cluster period. Prophylactic medications most frequently prescribed include verapamil, lithium, indomethacin, ergotamines, methysergide, divalproex sodium, and corticosteroids (Table 3–15). Maintain treatment with the prophylactic medication for at least 2 weeks after cessation of the cluster, followed by gradual taper of the agent. Combination therapy may be needed for patients with chronic cluster, for attacks lasting 1 year without remission, or for a remission of fewer than 14 days. Specialty consultation should be considered for patients with chronic cluster headache or those with headaches that are refractory to treatment.

HEADACHES OF SHORT DURATION

Several headache syndromes are triggered by common external stimuli and characterized by relatively brief attacks of head pain. They are benign and often respond to treatment with indomethacin. Headaches of short duration include benign cough (or exertional), coital, ice pick, and hypnic headaches. Paroxysmal hemicrania, mentioned above, is included in this category.

The transient head pain that occurs with coughing, weight-lifting, bending, stooping, or sneezing is called "benign cough headache" or "benign exertional headache." The head pain begins within seconds after the

TABLE 3–14. ABORTIVE THERAPIES FOR CLUSTER HEADACHE

Therapy	Clinical Comment
Oxygen inhalation, 7 L/min by face mask	Patient should be seated, leaning forward
Sumatriptan 6 mg SC, may repeat in 1 hr; maximum, 12 mg/day	Do not use concomitantly with ergotamines; Contraindicated in hypertension; heart, vascular, liver, or renal disease; and pregnancy
Dihydroergotamine 0.5–1 mg SC, IM, IV, IN; maximum, 3 mg/day	Administer with an antiemetic; Contraindicated in hypertension; heart, vascular, liver, or renal disease; and pregnancy
Ergotamine One inhalation, may repeat in 5 min; maximum, 6/day and maximum, 15/wk	Contraindicated in hypertension; heart, vascular, liver, or renal disease; and pregnancy

IM, intramuscularly; IN, intranasally; IV, intravenously; SC, subcutaneously.

TABLE 3–15. PROPHYLACTIC MEDICATIONS FOR CLUSTER HEADACHE

Drug	Clinical Comment
Verapamil Titrate up to 480 mg/day	Higher doses may be required. Side effects: constipation, hypotension, edema, congestive heart failure, heart block
Lithium carbonate 300–1,200 mg/day	Lithium level below 1.5 mEq/L to avoid toxicity, use divided dosing; Avoid in renal or cardiovascular disease, tremor
Indomethacin 75–150 mg/day	Use lowest effective dose; Side effects: gastrointestinal
Ergotamine tartrate 1–2 mg every night or 1 mg twice daily	Effective in nocturnal cluster; watch for ergotism
Methysergide maleate 2–8 mg/day	Watch for fibrotic complications, peripheral ischemia, hallucinations, peptic ulcer disease
Divalproex sodium 250–2,000 mg/day	Check liver function before treatment; Side effects: tremor, weight gain, alopecia
Corticosteroids Prednisone, 40 mg/day tapered over 3 wk	Helpful short term, observe general precautions with glucocorticoids

stimulus, can involve any part of the head, and subsides in less than 1 minute. After abnormalities of the posterior fossa are excluded by MRI, the patient can be reassured. The mechanism for this headache is thought to be an increase in CSF pressure. Coughing and lifting result in an increase in intrathoracic and intra-abdominal pressure, which reduces venous return to the right atrium. This increases central venous pressure and intracranial pressure. If treatment is necessary, indomethacin is effective (it reduces CSF pressure). Lumbar puncture also can be an effective treatment. Short duration headache syndromes are summarized in Table 3–16.

POST-TRAUMATIC HEADACHE

A 40-year-old woman was in good health and without medical problems until she was in a motor vehicle accident. Her car was struck from behind while she was stopped at a stop sign. Her head went forward and struck the dashboard, but she did not lose consciousness. She went to work that day and noted a mild headache. The following day she had increasing head and neck pain and went to her local physician. During the following months, she complained of headache, dizziness, neck pain, poor concentration, and depression. The results of MRI of her head and cervical spine were normal, and her physician told her nothing was wrong. She continues to experience severe daily headache, takes 6 to 8 aspirin a day, and "knows something is wrong." Her insurance company wants to settle the case, her employer is concerned about loss of time from work, and her family has found her increasingly irritable. She comes to you for further evaluation.

The case of this woman is all too common. The most frequent symptom after mild head injury is post-traumatic headache. The diagnosis is difficult and often complicated by equivocal clinical findings, limited objective information, and medical-legal issues. Post-

TABLE 3–16. HEADACHES OF SHORT DURATION			
Type of Headache	**Clinical Features**	**Evaluation**	**Treatment**
Cough	Transient head pain with cough	MRI to exclude posterior fossa lesion	Indomethacin, lumbar puncture
Coital	Abrupt severe throbbing headache before/at orgasm, associated with migraine	If 1st episode, CT and CSF analysis to exclude SAH, MRA to exclude aneurysm	Indomethacin, propranolol
Ice pick	Sharp jabs in temples or orbits, associated with migraine	ESR to exclude giant cell arteritis	Indomethacin
Hypnic	Diffuse headache that awakens patient from sleep	MRI to exclude mass lesion	Lithium, indomethacin
Chronic paroxysmal hemicrania	Cluster variant, autonomic symptoms	Primary headache evaluation	Indomethacin

CSF, cerebrospinal fluid; CT, computed tomography; ESR, erythrocyte sedimentation rate; MRA, magnetic resonance angiography; MRI, magnetic resonance imaging; SAH, subarachnoid hemorrhage.

traumatic headache is one of the major features of post-traumatic syndrome, which is also characterized by fatigue, dizziness, anxiety, nausea, weakness, insomnia, depression, cognitive disturbance, impaired concentration, and temperature intolerance. These standard symptoms of the syndrome cannot be correlated with the extent of the head injury.

The specific mechanism of post-traumatic headache is not known. Evidence suggests that head trauma causes injury to neurons, disruption of cerebral blood flow, and neurochemical changes with transmission of nociceptive stimuli to the central nervous system. Whiplash injuries, or flexion-extension injury of the cervical spine, can cause neuronal dysfunction from the acceleration and deceleration of the brain, as opposed to direct impact of the head. Damage to cervical roots, facet joints, and temporomandibular joints contributes to the symptoms of post-traumatic syndrome and post-traumatic headache.

The symptoms of post-traumatic headache may not develop or be recognized immediately after the injury. Head symptoms may be delayed up to 48 hours after injury. The pain patterns found in post-traumatic headache include tension-type, migraine, neuralgia-like, cluster, and mixed. The most frequent type is tension-type post-traumatic headache. The pain is dull, bilateral or generalized, and of variable intensity. Next most frequent is the mixed headache type, which has features of tension-type headache and vascular headache.

After a head injury, patients are confronted with several issues that increase emotional distress. The injury affects their health, relationships with family and friends, and employment. It is difficult for the clinician to determine whether the psychologic symptoms that develop are related to the injury, to the patient's reaction to the injury, or to the patient's premorbid personality traits. The interpretation and treatment of post-traumatic headache are complicated further by the role of litigation. Despite these controversial issues, most patients are looking for a health care professional who will believe their symptoms and explain their cause.

The diagnostic evaluation of a patient with post-traumatic headache is performed to exclude structural and physiologic disturbances of the nervous system. Also, many diagnostic tests are performed for medical-legal reasons. However, these tests do not distinguish between patients with legitimate complaints and those feigning injury, although the latter are in the minority. The diagnostic considerations that need to be excluded are subdural and epidural hematomas, CSF hypotension from a dural tear, post-traumatic hydrocephalus, cerebral vein thrombosis, cavernous sinus thrombosis, and cerebral hemorrhage.

Post-traumatic headache is considered chronic if it persists longer than 8 weeks. Post-traumatic headache is seen in 90% of patients with mild head injury at 1 month after injury, in 35% at 1 year, and in 20% at 3 years. The diagnosis of post-traumatic headache should not be made unless analgesic rebound headache has been excluded.

The treatment principles for post-traumatic headache are the same as those for any type of headache. Be vigilant about the problem of analgesic overuse. Patients often need support and reassurance, and they need to know that you believe them. Medications for tension-type headache and migraine are effective for post-traumatic headache. Antidepressant medications, including tricyclic agents and selective serotonin reuptake inhibitors, are useful when depression is part of the post-traumatic syndrome. The anticonvulsant agents carbamazepine and gabapentin are helpful if there is a neuralgic component to the head pain. Psychologic counseling, biofeedback, relaxation therapy, physical therapy, and cognitive retraining exercises may all be useful in the management of post-traumatic headache.

TEMPORAL ARTERITIS

Temporal arteritis, also called "giant cell arteritis" or "cranial arteritis," is an important diagnosis to consider whenever a patient older than 50 years complains of headache. The disease causes inflammation of medium- and large-sized arteries, which can lead to stenosis and occlusion of the arteries. Temporal arteritis can cause several neurologic problems, but the most significant complications are stroke and blindness.

One-third of the patients with temporal arteritis have headache as the presenting symptom, and it is the most common symptom. The headache can be throbbing, bitemporal to generalized, and associated with scalp tenderness. Other symptoms include malaise, fatigue, jaw claudication, fever, cough, neuropathy, dysphagia, vision loss, and limb claudication. Physical findings may include erythema and tenderness to palpation of the temporal arteries and reduced pulses. The erythrocyte sedimentation rate is usually increased at 85 ± 32 mm/hr (Westergren). Anemia and thrombocytosis may occur.

The erythrocyte sedimentation rate can be normal in 3% to 10% of patients; temporal artery biopsy should be performed to confirm the diagnosis. However, the patchy nature of the disease process may result in negative biopsy results. If the diagnosis is suspected, it is recommended that steroid treatment be started immediately to avoid the risk of blindness. Prednisone, 60 mg daily, will eliminate the headache and systemic symptoms. The dose can be gradually tapered over several months. The patient's condition can be monitored clinically and using the erythrocyte sedimentation rate. Temporal arteritis is self-limited, and steroid therapy can be discontinued after 6 months to 2 years.

There is a strong relationship between temporal arteritis and polymyalgia rheumatica. Polymyalgia rheumatica is characterized by diffuse proximal and axial joint pain and proximal myalgias. Whether it is part of the same disease process as temporal arteritis or a related disorder has not been decided. Also, evidence suggests that temporal arteritis and polymyalgia rheumatica may be more benign than originally thought.

FACIAL PAIN

Several conditions distinct from headache are associated with facial pain or head pain. Frequent nonneurologic causes of facial pain are sinusitis and temporomandibular joint syndrome. Common neurologic conditions that cause facial pain are trigeminal neuralgia and herpes zoster. Other neurologic facial pain disorders are glossopharyngeal neuralgia, occipital neuralgia, tumors,

or aneurysms that compress the trigeminal nerve, infiltrative intracranial disease (e.g., lymphoma), trauma, post-endarterectomy syndrome, and carotid artery dissection. A striking aspect of pain in the head and face is the significant psychologic impact it has on the patient. Strong emotional factors need to be considered when treating a patient with facial pain.

The diagnostic approach to a patient with facial pain can be complicated because of referred pain. The location of the pain may be misleading. Cranial and spinal nerve lesions can be referred to any region of the head and neck. For example, right thoracic and abdominal pain can be referred to the right face and ear. Intracranial pain can be represented extracranially. The character of the pain can be helpful in the diagnosis. Paroxysmal pain suggests neuralgic pain. Musculoskeletal pain has a dull quality, and movement or palpation can elicit pain. Physical medicine modalities are helpful in the treatment of somatic or musculoskeletal pain. Medication is often needed for neurogenic pain.

TRIGEMINAL NEURALGIA

The most common facial pain syndrome is trigeminal neuralgia. The pain is brief, lancinating, and located in one or more branches of the trigeminal nerve (see Fig. 1–7). The repetitive jolts of pain can be triggered by tactile stimulation and activities such as brushing the teeth, talking, chewing, kissing, or shaving. Patients often describe a dull ache between the paroxysms of shock-like pain. Pain in the second (maxillary) or third (mandibular) division of the trigeminal nerve often causes the patient to go to a dentist.

Most cases of primary trigeminal neuralgia occur in persons older than 40 years. A secondary cause is suggested if the person is younger than 40 years and if an abnormality is found on neurologic examination. Investigation involves MRI to exclude the secondary causes of trigeminal neuralgia, such as multiple sclerosis, a mass lesion in the posterior fossa, or an abnormal arterial loop.

There are many options for treating trigeminal neuralgia. Effective medications include sodium channel blockers and gamma-aminobutyric acid (GABA) derivatives. These agents are effective in many neuralgic syndromes (Table 3–17). Most of these medications are anticonvulsant agents, of which many of the newer ones (e.g., gabapentin and lamotrigine) are being evaluated for use in neuralgic pain. Carbamazepine has often been the first treatment option. Other useful anticonvulsants are phenytoin, divalproex sodium, and clonazepam. Baclofen, a muscle relaxant, is also helpful. If medical therapy fails or if the patient cannot tolerate the medication, neurosurgical procedures should be considered, for example, an ablative technique with alcohol or glycerol, radiofrequency gangliolysis, or microvascular decompression.

GLOSSOPHARYNGEAL NEURALGIA

Glossopharyngeal neuralgia, less common than trigeminal neuralgia, is characterized by paroxysmal pain in and around the ear, jaw, throat, tongue, and larynx. The pain can be triggered by swallowing cold liquids, chewing, talking, or yawning. Another pain trigger is tactile stimulation around the ear. Although the glossopharyngeal nerve innervates the carotid sinus (which contains receptors important in regulating blood pressure), syncope is rare in glossopharyngeal neuralgia. The evaluation and treatment of this neuralgia are the same as for trigeminal neuralgia.

OCCIPITAL NEURALGIA

Occipital neuralgia is characterized by paroxysms of pain in the distribution of the greater occipital nerve (see Fig. 1–12). The back of the head may be tender, but it also may be painful in migraine, tension-type headache, and disease of the upper cervical

TABLE 3–17. MEDICATIONS FOR NEURALGIC PAIN

Drug and Mechanism	Dose*	Side Effects (Clinical Comment)
Carbamazepine (Tegretol), sodium channel blocker	100 mg twice daily, increase to maximum 1,200 mg/day	Drowsiness, dizziness, diplopia, ataxia (decreasing response)
Gabapentin (Neurontin), GABA-ergic	100–300 mg/day, titrate up to 2,400 mg/day in 3 divided doses	Drowsiness, weight gain, renal metabolism (few drug interactions, high tolerability)
Lamotrigine (Lamictal), sodium channel blocker	25 mg/day, increase 25 mg every 3rd day to maximum 400 mg/day	Dizziness, ataxia, somnolence, headache (few studies in trigeminal neuralgia)
Phenytoin (Dilantin), sodium channel blocker	300 mg/day, titrate as needed	Allergic reaction, dose-related ataxia, slurred speech
Divalproex sodium (Depakote), GABA-ergic	250 mg twice daily, titrate as needed	Tremor, weight gain, alopecia (check liver function before treatment)
Clonazepam (Klonopin), GABA-ergic	0.5 mg twice daily, titrate as needed	Central nervous system depression, tolerance can develop (withdraw gradually)
Baclofen (Lioresal), GABA-ergic	5–10 mg, three times daily; maximum, 20 mg 4 times daily	Sedation, dizziness (withdraw slowly)

*Before prescribing any medicine, check the product information guide.

cord. Occipital neuralgia is much less common than the primary headache disorders and myofascial pain syndromes. The pharmacologic treatment of occipital neuralgia is the same as for trigeminal neuralgia. Occipital nerve blocks are often effective in treating occipital neuralgia.

ATYPICAL FACIAL PAIN

Facial pain that is present daily and persists for most or all of the day is consistent with "atypical facial pain," or "facial pain of unknown cause." The location of the pain can vary from being confined to one area of the face to including both sides of the face and neck. The pain is deep and poorly localized. There are no associated physical, neurologic, laboratory, or radiographic abnormalities. This disorder is difficult to manage, and neurologic and pain specialty consultation may be needed.

HERPES ZOSTER AND POSTHERPETIC NEURALGIA

Reactivation of latent varicella-zoster virus present in cranial nerve ganglia can cause facial pain. When this involves the first (ophthalmic) division of the trigeminal nerve, it is

FIG. 3–1. Summary of the major types of headache.

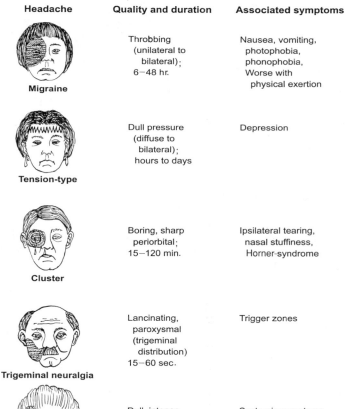

Headache	Quality and duration	Associated symptoms
Migraine	Throbbing (unilateral to bilateral); 6–48 hr.	Nausea, vomiting, photophobia, phonophobia, Worse with physical exertion
Tension-type	Dull pressure (diffuse to bilateral); hours to days	Depression
Cluster	Boring, sharp periorbital; 15–120 min.	Ipsilateral tearing, nasal stuffiness, Horner-syndrome
Trigeminal neuralgia	Lancinating, paroxysmal (trigeminal distribution) 15–60 sec.	Trigger zones
Temporal arteritis	Dull, intense (temporal to diffuse) Increasing in frequency to continuous	Systemic symptoms Elevated sedimentation rate

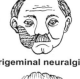

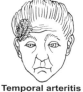

called *herpes zoster ophthalmicus*. If the facial nerve is involved, there may be facial weakness and vesicular eruption in the external ear canal; this is called *Ramsay Hunt syndrome*. Pain that persists longer than 6 months after the herpetic eruption meets the criterion for "chronic postherpetic neuralgia."

Fever, malaise, and gradual onset of paresthesias of the affected dermatome may precede the acute illness. The rash may erupt 2 to 3 days later and consist of erythematous macules, papules, and vesicles. Serious complications of herpes zoster ophthalmicus include eye damage, cranial nerve palsies, meningoencephalitis, and stroke.

Acute treatment of cephalic herpes zoster may include antiviral agents, analgesics, local anesthetic creams, antidepressants, anticonvulsants, and corticosteroids. The suggested regimen is famciclovir, 500 to 750 mg orally three times a day for 1 to 2 weeks, or acyclovir, 800 mg orally five times a day for 10 days. In immunocompromised patients, parenteral antiviral medication may need to be considered. The use of corticosteroids in this condition has not been established. Many clinicians restrict corticosteroid treatment to immunocompetent patients in severe pain or patients with zoster complicated by meningitis or vasculitis. The treatment

of postherpetic neuralgia is discussed in Chapter 10.

TEMPOROMANDIBULAR JOINT DYSFUNCTION

Temporomandibular joint dysfunction can be a source of facial and head pain. The patient may complain of pain of the jaw, face, ear, or surrounding area. The diagnostic criteria for temporomandibular joint disease include two of the following: pain in the jaw precipitated by movement, decreased range of motion, noise during joint movement, and tenderness of the joint capsule.

The temporomandibular joint should be palpated while the patient opens and closes the jaw. Inflammation of the joint will be painful, and any crepitus or noise can be observed. The normal opening range of the jaw is approximately the width of three fingers.

Treatment for temporomandibular joint dysfunction includes bite guards, soft diet, local heat, NSAIDs, and relaxation therapies. Dental and orthodontic consultation may be needed if none of these treatments is effective.

The clinical features of the major types of headache are summarized in Figure 3–1.

SUGGESTED READING

Capobianco, DJ, Cheshire, WP, and Campbell, JK: An overview of the diagnosis and pharmacologic treatment of migraine. Mayo Clin Proc 71:1055–1066, 1996.

Caselli, RJ, Hunder, GG, and Whisnant, JP: Neurologic disease in biopsy-proven giant cell (temporal) arteritis. Neurology 38:352–359, 1988.

Evans, RW: Diagnostic testing for the evaluation of headaches. Neurol Clin 14:1–26, 1996.

Headache Classification Committee of the International Headache Society: Classification and diagnostic criteria for headache disorders, cranial neuralgias and facial pain. Cephalalgia 8(Suppl 7):1–96, 1988.

Herzog, AG: Continuous bromocriptine therapy in menstrual migraine. Neurology 48:101–102, 1997.

Lunardi, G, et al: Clinical effectiveness of lamotrigine and plasma levels in essential and symptomatic trigeminal neuralgia. Neurology 48:1714–1717, 1997.

MacGregor, EA: Menstruation, sex hormones, and migraine. Neurol Clin 15:125–141, 1997.

Marks, DR, and Rapoport, AM: Diagnosis of migraine. Semin Neurol 17:303–306, 1997.

Mathew, NT: Cluster headache. Neurology 42(Suppl 2):22–31, 1992.

Mathew, NT (Guest Ed): Advances in headache. Neurol Clin 15:1–238, February 1997.

Mathew, NT: Serotonin 1D (5-HT$_1$D) agonists and other agents in acute migraine. Neurol Clin 15:61–83, 1997.

Mathew, NT: Transformed migraine, analgesic rebound, and other chronic daily headaches. Neurol Clin 15:167–186, 1997.

Merikangas, KR, et al: Association between migraine and stroke in a large-scale epidemiological study of the United States. Arch Neurol 54:362–368, 1997.

Olesen, J, Tfelt-Hansen, P, and Welch, KMA: The Headaches. Raven Press, New York, 1993.

Packard, RC: Posttraumatic headache. Semin Neurol 14:40–45, 1994.

Pavan-Langston, D: Herpes zoster ophthalmicus. Neurology 45(Suppl 8):S50–S51, 1995.

Raskin, NH: Repetitive intravenous dihydroergotamine as therapy for intractable migraine. Neurology 36:995–997, 1986.

Raskin, NH: Short-lived head pains. Neurol Clin 15:143–152, 1997.

Report of the Quality Standards Subcommittee of the American Academy of Neurology: Practice parameter: The utility of neuroimaging in the evaluation of headache in patients with normal neurologic examinations (summary statement). Neurology 44:1353–1354, 1994.

Sheftell, FD: Role and impact of over-the-counter medications in the management of headache. Neurol Clin 15:187–198, 1997.

Silberstein, SD: Tension-type and chronic daily headache. Neurology 43:1644–1649, 1993.

Silberstein, SD: Migraine and pregnancy. Neurol Clin 15:209–231, 1997.

Silberstein, SD: Drug-induced headache. Neurol Clin 16:107–123, 1998.

Silberstein, SD, and Merriam, GR: Estrogens, progestins, and headache. Neurology 41:786–793, 1991.

Silberstein, SD, et al: Headache and facial pain. Continuum 1(5):8–111, November 1995.

Tfelt-Hansen, P: Prophylactic pharmacotherapy of migraine. Some practical guidelines. Neurol Clin 15:153–165, 1997.

Turnbull, J: Temporal arteritis and polymyalgia rheumatica: Nosographic and nosologic considerations. Neurology 46:901–906, 1996.

Warner, JS, and Fenichel, GM: Chronic post-traumatic headache often a myth? Neurology 46:915–916, 1996.

Ziegler, DK: Opioids in headache treatment. Is there a role? Neurol Clin 15:199–207, 1997.

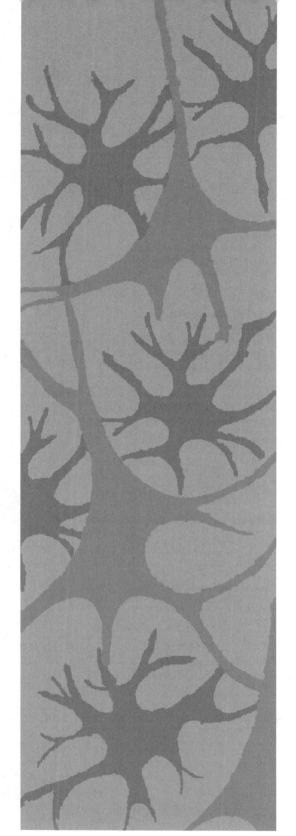

CHAPTER 4

Spine and
Limb Pain

CHAPTER OUTLINE

Spinal Anatomy
Evaluation of Spine Pain
Diagnostic Tests
Radiculopathy
Spinal Stenosis
Cervical Spondylosis
Whiplash
Spinal Surgery
Plexopathy

A 45-year-old laborer injures his lower back lifting a 70-lb object onto a truck. He goes to the doctor's office 1 week after the injury, complaining of low back pain radiating into the left buttock, with occasional tingling into the great toe. The patient prefers to stand in the waiting room. On examining him, you note that he leans slightly to the right when standing. The left lower extremity at the inferior medial buttock and the popliteal fossa is tender when you palpate it. Straight leg raising on the left side causes pain in the buttock at 75 degrees. Strength, sensation, and reflexes are normal. Does the patient have a radiculopathy? Should any tests be performed? Is surgery indicated?

Spine pain is a frequent presenting complaint of patients evaluated by primary care clinicians. Low back pain is estimated to occur in up to 80% of adults and is the greatest cause of lost workdays in the United States. The cause of acute back pain is usually musculoskeletal. The differential diagnosis of back pain is listed in Table 4–1. Most patients with back pain can be cared for by their primary care provider without needing specialist consultation or diagnostic tests.

Chronic back pain is most often caused by degenerative disease of the spine. Neurologists are frequently consulted about back pain and asked about neurologic involvement of the nerve roots, spinal cord, spinal stenosis, and the need for surgery. Neurologic consultation is often requested for patients with intractable back pain.

Pain in the upper and lower extremities is often related to problems of the spine. In addition to limb pain from spinal disease, this chapter reviews limb pain due to plexopathy. Common mononeuropathies are discussed in Chapter 6.

TABLE 4–1. CAUSES OF BACK PAIN

Musculoskeletal/Mechanical

Muscle strain
Degenerative spondylosis
Degenerative disk disease
Osteoarthritis

Tumor

Primary spinal cord tumor
Metastatic tumor
Plasmacytoma or multiple myeloma
Primary bone tumor
Retroperitoneal tumor

Vascular Lesion

Arteriovenous malformation
Spinal dural arteriovenous fistula

Infection

Diskitis
Osteomyelitis
Epidural abscess
Urinary tract infection

Intra-abdominal or Pelvic Disease

Abdominal aortic aneurysm
Posterior perforating duodenal ulcer
Endometriosis

Metabolic Bone Disease

Osteoporosis
Paget disease

Rheumatologic Disease

Ankylosing spondylitis
Rheumatoid arthritis

Congenital

Spina bifida
Tethered cord
Intraspinal lipoma

Trauma

Fracture
Dislocation

SPINAL ANATOMY

The spinal column consists of 7 cervical, 12 thoracic, 5 lumbar, 5 sacral (the sacrum), and 4 coccygeal (the coccyx) vertebrae. The pain-sensitive structures of the spine include the ligaments, facet joint capsules, peripheral fibers of the annulus fibrosus, periosteum of the vertebral bones, spinal nerves, and muscle (Fig. 4–1).

The relationship of the spinal nerves to the vertebrae is important in understanding disk protrusion and its effect on the exiting nerve root. Cervical nerve roots C2 through C7 exit above their respective vertebrae, and the C8 nerve root exits between C7 and T1 (because there are 8 cervical nerve roots but only 7 cervical vertebrae). Note that cervical nerve root C1 usually has no sensory component. The rest of the nerve roots (i.e., T1-Coc 1) exit below their respective vertebrae. Thus, lateral disk protrusion at the C6 level usually affects the C6 nerve root, and lateral disk protrusion at the L4–L5 level usually affects the L5 nerve root. A midline disk protrusion at the L4–L5 level may affect the L5 and sacral nerve roots (Fig. 4–2).

In adults, the spinal cord (conus medullaris) terminates at the level of the L1 vertebra. The conus medullaris consists of the lower lumbar and sacral segments of the spinal cord. This anatomical relationship is important to remember in performing lumbar puncture and in understanding spinal cord syndromes involving the conus medullaris and cauda equina. You need to recognize the clinical syndrome of the cauda equina because it requires emergent surgical treatment (Fig. 4–3).

EVALUATION OF SPINE PAIN

The first step in evaluating a patient with spine pain is to determine whether the problem is complicated or uncomplicated. Most spine pain is uncomplicated; that is, it does not require immediate attention or diagnostic testing. Complicated back pain, which includes fractures, cancer, infection, systemic diseases, and spine pain associated with neurologic deficit, requires further attention. The diagnosis of uncomplicated or complicated back pain can be determined with a careful history and physical examination. The important points, or red flags, associated with complicated back pain are summarized in Table 4–2.

The history of a patient with spine pain should include special reference to the quality of the pain, location, radiation, and factors and activities that exacerbate or relieve the pain. Nerve root pain is usually sharp, "shooting," and brief and is increased by coughing or straining. Pain from the nerve or plexus is described as "burning," "pins and needles," "asleep," or "numb." Other important characteristics of back pain are given in Table 4–3. It is essential to ask questions about weakness and bowel and bladder control. Ask about work activity, trauma, disability, and litigation. Inconsistencies of activity and overreaction may indicate a problem that is more psychologic than physical.

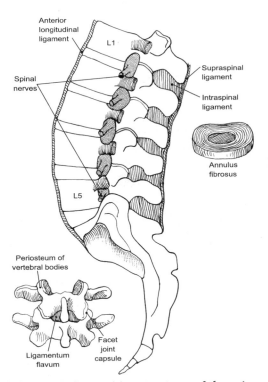

Anterior longitudinal ligament

L1

Spinal nerves

Supraspinal ligament

Intraspinal ligament

Annulus fibrosus

L5

Periosteum of vertebral bodies

Facet joint capsule

Ligamentum flavum

FIG. 4–1. Pain-sensitive structures of the spine.

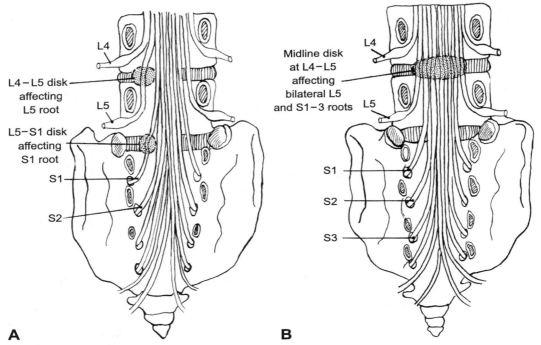

FIG. 4–2. Herniated nucleus of vertebral disk compressing spinal roots. (A) Lateral herniation of a lumbar or sacral disk compresses the nerve root below the disk (e.g., lateral herniation of L4-L5 disk compresses ipsilateral spinal root L5). **(B)** In comparison, midline herniation of a lumbar disk compresses several spinal roots bilaterally (e.g., midline herniation of disk L4-L5 compresses spinal roots L5 and S1-S3 bilaterally. (Modified from Keim, HA, and Kirkaldy-Willis, WH: Low back pain. Copyright 1980. Novartis. Reprinted with permission from Clinical Symposia, Vol 32/6. Illustrated by Frank Netter, M.D. All rights reserved.)

The temporal profile and the presence or absence of red flags will determine whether further diagnostic evaluation is needed. Acute back pain of less than 6 weeks' duration is usually caused by musculoskeletal factors and will resolve without further investigation. Back pain that persists after 6 to 12 weeks warrants further investigation. Subacute back pain raises the possibility of osteomyelitis, neoplasm, or spondylosis. The evaluation at this time may include laboratory testing, spine radiography with oblique views, bone scans, and other spine imaging. If the chronic pain lasts longer than 12 weeks, magnetic resonance imaging and specialist consultation may be needed.

The sudden onset of symptoms in relationship to lifting, bending, or twisting is usually the result of stress on the musculoskeletal structures, as in lumbosacral strain or acute disk herniation. Mechanical pain is suggested when the pain is associated with movement. Radicular pain radiates down the extremity and is aggravated by an increase in intraabdominal pressure. An increase in pain with spinal extension may suggest spinal stenosis. If the pain increases with rest, you need to consider malignancy or infection.

Most spine pain is musculoskeletal; however, back pain can be a feature of serious systemic disease. You should be aware of the signs and symptoms of serious back pain (see Table 4–2). Aggressively evaluate any elderly patient with constitutional symptoms or any immunosuppressed patient. Back pain associated with a neurologic deficit needs to be evaluated. Evaluate for inflammatory spondyloarthropathy when the clinical history suggests that the back pain began before the patient was 30 years old, has

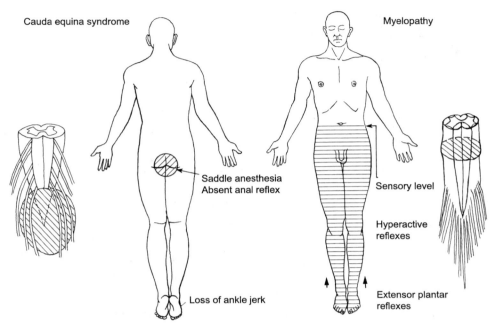

Cauda equina syndrome

Myelopathy

Saddle anesthesia
Absent anal reflex

Sensory level

Hyperactive
reflexes

Loss of ankle jerk

Extensor plantar
reflexes

FIG. 4–3. Comparison of deficits associated with cauda equina syndrome and myelopathy.

lasted several months, increases with rest, and decreases with activity.

It is crucial to ask about any change in bowel or bladder control. Incontinence or retention can occur with any lesion that involves the cauda equina or spinal cord bilaterally. If the patient has bowel or bladder problems and back pain, the sacral dermatomes and anal reflex should be examined. To test the anal reflex, gently scratch the skin around the anus and either observe the contraction of the anal ring or palpate with a gloved fingertip. Spinal cord segments S2–S4 in the conus medullaris and sacral nerve roots of the cauda equina supply the anal sphincter. If a lesion involves the conus medullaris or sacral nerve roots bilaterally, the anal reflex will be absent, the lower extremities will be weak, the lumbosacral area will be anesthetic, and ankle reflexes will be reduced or absent. In comparison, a more proximal lesion of the spinal cord is associated with a spastic bladder and long tract signs, including hyperreflexia, bilateral extensor plantar reflexes, and a sensory level (Fig. 4–3). The flaccid and spastic

types of neurogenic bladder occur in patients with disorders of the spine. The three types of neurogenic bladder are summarized in Table 4–4.

The physical examination of a patient with spine pain should include a general evaluation, with attention to the neurologic, joint, abdominal, and rectal examinations. Observing the patient sitting, standing, and walking before the formal evaluation is often more revealing than it is during the examination. The gait of a patient with back pain frequently is described as painful or antalgic. A patient with an antalgic gait walks slowly, with small steps, while holding the back stiffly in a specific position. A patient with lower extremity pain lists to the asymptomatic side while standing and walking. A patient with L5 weakness may walk with a foot slap because of weakness of the anterior tibialis muscle. With weakness of the gluteus medius muscle, another L5 muscle, the contralateral pelvis drops on stance phase, causing a Trendelenburg gait. When this happens, patients often lean to the symptomatic side. You can detect subtle weakness of muscles innervated by L5 by having pa-

TABLE 4–2. RED FLAGS OF BACK PAIN

Complicated Back Pain	Red Flags
Fracture or dislocation	Trauma: major in young patients, minor in elderly
	Bone disease: osteoporosis, osteomalacia, Paget disease
	Steroid therapy
	Congenital anomalies
Infection	Fever
	Immunosuppressed status
	Intravenous drug use
	Urinary tract infection
	Spinal surgery
	Penetrating wound
Neoplasm	History of cancer
	Pain at rest, causing movement
	Weight loss
	Unexplained blood loss
	Constitutional symptoms
Neurologic deficit	Major strength loss
	Bowel and bladder symptoms
Cauda equina syndrome	Bowel and bladder symptoms
	Saddle anesthesia
Inflammatory spondyloarthropathy	Pain increases with rest, decreases with activity, onset before age 30 years, several months' duration

TABLE 4–3. TYPES OF BACK PAIN AND ASSOCIATED CLINICAL CONDITIONS

Pain Type	Cause
Pain at rest	Neoplasm, infection, primary bone disease
Pain increases with movement	Mechanical (e.g., musculoskeletal problem)
Pain increases with rest, decreases with activity	Inflammatory spondyloarthropathy
Pain with fever	Vertebral osteomyelitis, subacute bacterial endocarditis
Pain that causes movement (e.g., writhing to alleviate pain)	Neoplasm, visceral disease (ulcers, pancreatic disease)
Acute pain in patient with cancer	Metastasis
Pain with urinary incontinence or retention	Cauda equina syndrome, myelopathy
Pain radiating down an extremity, increased with Valsalva maneuver	Radiculopathy
Pain increases with spine extension (standing, walking) and decreases with flexion (sitting)	Spinal stenosis

TABLE 4–4. COMPARISON OF FLACCID, SPASTIC, AND UNINHIBITED BLADDER

	Flaccid	Spastic	Uninhibited
Incontinence	Yes	Yes	Yes
Location of lesion	Cauda equina, sacral segments of conus medullaris	Spinal cord (distal to pontine micturition center)	Medial frontal cortex
Retention	Yes	Yes	No
Anal reflex	Absent	Present	Present
Clinical condition	Cauda equina lesion, disk protrusion, tumor	Myelopathy, spinal cord trauma	Hydrocephalus, dementia

tients walk on their heels. If the muscles innervated by S1 are weak, patients have difficulty walking on their toes. Hysterical or malingering gait tends to be bizarre, with excessive movement of the trunk and arms.

Inspect and palpate the spine for localized tender points and muscle consistency. Hair tufts, dimples, or scoliosis may suggest congenital spine defects. The patient's posture can be revealing. Patients with spinal stenosis often stand with flexed posture. Patients with a radiculopathy may list to one side or keep the knee of the symptomatic leg bent; also, they avoid putting weight on the affected heel. Assess spinal mobility. An increase in the pain with any movement indicates musculoskeletal injury. A "corkscrew" motion with forward flexion suggests radiculopathy. Difficulty bending to one side (side flexion) and bending the symptomatic knee with forward flexion also suggest radiculopathy.

Ask a patient with neck and arm pain to flex, extend, rotate, and bend the neck laterally. These maneuvers often increase musculoskeletal neck pain. An increase in arm pain or paresthesias suggests radiculopathy.

Stretching irritated or inflamed nerve roots causes pain. This is the principle behind several provocative tests, including the straight leg raising, or sciatic stretch, test. The straight leg raising test is useful for determining whether a patient with low back pain has an L5 and S1 radiculopathy. With the patient supine, ask him or her to keep the symptomatic leg straight and raise it to a 90-degree angle. This maneuver stretches the nerve root, and the test is considered positive if the patient feels pain before the leg reaches 90

degrees. The smaller the angle of elevation needed to elicit pain, the greater the likelihood that a herniated disk is compressing the root. The location of the pain is meaningful. Pain in the leg or buttock is more suggestive of radiculopathy than pain in the back. Pain in the leg or buttock when the asymptomatic leg is raised is an excellent indication of radiculopathy (the crossed straight leg raising test). A feeling of tightness in the hamstring is not a positive result. Other methods for stretching the L5-S1 nerve roots is to ask a patient who is seated to dorsiflex the foot or, during a straight leg raising test, ask the patient to dorsiflex the foot of the raised leg when the leg is at an angle that pain would not be felt if the foot were not dorsiflexed. Both of these methods help to assess consistency in patients who exaggerate their symptoms. Similarly, the L2, L3, and L4 nerve roots can be tested with stretching the femoral nerve—for example, by having the patient flex the knee while supine.

While evaluating spine and limb pain, also evaluate the hip joint if the patient has low back pain or the shoulder joint if the patient has neck pain. Referred pain from the hip frequently causes low back pain and leg pain. Pain due to flexion, abduction, and external rotation of the lower extremity may indicate a hip lesion. Shoulder disease frequently causes arm and neck pain. If abduction, flexion, extension, or rotation of the shoulder elicits pain, shoulder disease is likely.

The evaluation of muscle strength can be complicated by pain that inhibits function or the conscious or unconscious attempt of the patient to appear weak. The best way to assess strength is to watch the patient move. Toe flexor and extensor weakness usually precedes foot weakness. Watching the patient walk on the toes and heels is useful in assessing the strength of these muscles. If the patient is not able to walk on the toes and heels, determine whether he or she can stand on the toes or heels while you offer support. A good way to assess proximal lower extremity strength is to ask the patient to squat. By encouraging the patient to "break through the pain," you may be able to determine his or her strength. If root pain prevents testing the quadriceps muscle with the leg extended, the muscle can be tested with the patient prone. Atrophy is rare unless symptoms have been present for more than 3 weeks. If atrophy is severe, consider an extradural spinal tumor. Sudden giving way, jerkiness, or involvement of many muscle groups is characteristic of nonorganic weakness.

On sensory examination, a patient with spine pain may have a sensory loss that has a dermatomal distribution. Because the overlap of root distributions is wide, involvement of a single root may cause minimal sensory loss. Assess the sensory level if there is question of myelopathy. Nonanatomical sensory loss is a functional sign of back pain but should be correlated with more objective signs.

Deep tendon reflexes are useful in evaluating patients with spine pain and are not influenced by subjective factors. The symmetry of deep tendon reflexes is important. If the ankle reflex is difficult to elicit, test this S1 reflex while the patient kneels.

Psychologic dysfunction can be prominent in patients with spine pain. Depression, anxiety, and stress can cause and aggravate pain. Several signs suggest that the pain is nonorganic. Waddell and colleagues described five features that suggest nonorganic pain: palpation tenderness, simulation, distraction, regional distribution, and overreaction. The presence of three of these five features is considered significant. Palpation tenderness is excessive if it is widespread or caused by light touch. Simulation involves mimicking but not performing painful tests. An example is the elicitation of pain while you rotate the patient's shoulders and hips together or while you push down on the patient's head (axial loading). An example of distraction is when a straight leg raising test yields a positive result with the patient supine but a negative result with the patient sitting or being "distracted." Regional distribution involves nonanatomical motor or sensory loss. Disproportionate verbalization, wincing, collapsing, and tremor are examples of overreaction.

DIAGNOSTIC TESTS

Two points deserve emphasis: (1) the history and physical examination are the most important diagnostic tests, and (2) asymptomatic imaging abnormalities of the spine are common. The patient's clinical presentation determines which diagnostic tests are needed and the significance of the findings of imaging studies. Common structural abnormalities are degenerative changes, disk narrowing and bulging, spurs, and spondylolisthesis. The high frequency of spine complaints has the potential of causing expensive and unnecessary testing. Finding asymptomatic structural abnormalities may impede recovery from an episode of uncomplicated back pain. For these reasons, the clinical question must be specific before any diagnostic studies are performed. Diagnostic tests should not be performed for uncomplicated back pain if it has not persisted for 7 weeks.

Plain radiographs of the spine are useful for examining the vertebral bodies for bony abnormalities, including fracture, neoplasm, congenital deformity, and rheumatic disease. Oblique views are useful in assessing spondylolisthesis and spondylolysis. Spondylolisthesis is forward displacement of a vertebral body onto the one below it. Spondylolysis, often associated with spondylolisthesis, is the condition in which the posterior portion of the vertebral unit (pars interarticularis) is split (Fig. 4–4). It can be due to abnormal development, trauma, or degenerative disease. If the borders of the split are sclerotic, the fracture is likely chronic and unlikely to heal. A bone scan can also determine whether the spondylolysis is active or chronic. Plain radiographs with the patient in flexion and extension can help assess the stability of the spine. Flexion

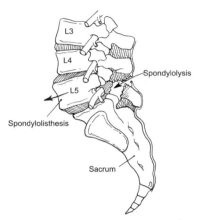

FIG. 4–4. Comparison of spondylolysis and spondylolisthesis in lumbosacral spine. (Modified from Hinton, RC: Backache. In Samuels, MA [ed]: Manual of Neurologic Therapeutics, ed 5. Little, Brown, Boston, 1995, pp 78–88, with permission of Martin A. Samuels and the publisher.)

and extension views are helpful in evaluating stability of the spine in spondylolysis and in patients with previous back surgery. Plain radiography of the spine is the standard for the initial evaluation of trauma.

Disks, nerve roots, and the spinal cord are evaluated best with computed tomography (CT), magnetic resonance imaging (MRI), and myelography with CT. CT is useful for imaging bony detail and can be a reasonable screening test for detecting spinal stenosis and disk herniation. The addition of contrast dye (myelography with CT) provides better visualization of the nerve roots and spinal cord. The disadvantages of myelography are the invasion of the cerebrospinal fluid space and the associated complications.

MRI is superior to CT for evaluating all conditions of the spine. The images can be viewed from several planes, and the variable signal capability provides better images than CT. MRI is noninvasive, uses nonionizing radiation, and is extremely sensitive for detecting tumors and infection. MRI with gadolinium contrast is valuable in distinguishing scar tissue from recurrent disk protrusion in patients with previous back surgery. This highly sensitive test often reveals abnormalities that need to be correlated with clinical findings. MRI can be expensive

and is best used when the anticipated findings will alter management. The diagnostic imaging tests used in imaging the spine are summarized in Table 4–5.

Electromyography (EMG) is a useful extension of the clinical examination and provides physiologic information. It can be helpful when imaging studies show abnormalities at multiple levels. EMG can localize a radiculopathy and determine whether it is active or chronic. This information may be essential if surgery is considered. For a patient with footdrop, EMG can distinguish between a lesion of the L5 root and a peroneal nerve palsy. EMG is discussed in more detail in Chapter 2.

RADICULOPATHY

Radiculopathy is disease of a nerve root. One of the questions neurologists are asked most frequently is whether a patient with spine and limb pain has radiculopathy. The diagnostic approach to the patient depends on the answer to this question (Fig. 4–5).

A spinal nerve consists of a motor component (ventral root), whose axons arise from anterior horn cells, and a sensory component (dorsal root), whose axons rise from cell bodies in the associated dorsal root ganglion. Most diseases of the spinal roots affect both of these components. An exception is herpes zoster, which causes radiculitis of the sensory root. Another, but rare, exception is pure motor polyradiculoneuropathy.

The common causes of radiculopathy are disk herniation and degenerative changes of the spine. Acute radiculopathy can occur in diabetes mellitus, suggesting a vascular cause. Herpes zoster and other infections can affect the nerve roots. A chronic temporal profile suggests degenerative changes or, rarely, a neoplastic cause.

The clinical features of radiculopathy include pain or paresthesia in a sensory dermatome, weakness of the muscles innervated by the nerve root, and reduced or absent deep tendon reflexes mediated by the nerve root. The history and physical examination findings suggest radiculopathy.

TABLE 4–5. DIAGNOSTIC IMAGING TESTS IN SPINE PAIN

Test	Indications	Advantages and Disadvantages
Plain radiographs	Trauma	Inexpensive
Oblique views	Spondylolysis	Disks and nerve roots not well visualized
Flexion and extension	Spinal stability: postsurgical	
Bone scan	Infection	Often adjunctive test
	Neoplasm	
	Bone disease	
	Spondylolysis	
CT	Spinal stenosis	Poor contrast without myelography
	Disk herniation	
		Bone detail is good
Myelography with CT	Disk herniation	Invasive
	Spinal stenosis	Postmyelogram headache
	Cord compression	Entire spinal cord can be evaluated with CSF sample
	Myelopathy	
MRI with gadolinium	Disk herniation	Sensitive, multiplanar, different tissue contrast
	Scar tissue vs. disk	
	Spinal stenosis	Expensive
	Cord compression	Claustrophobia
	Myelopathy	
	Infection/inflammation	
	Neoplasm	

CSF, cerebrospinal fluid; CT, computed tomography; MRI, magnetic resonance imaging.

The important root syndromes are summarized in Figure 4–6. Features suggestive of radiculopathy on clinical examination are listed in Tables 4–6 and 4–7.

More than 95% of herniated disks of the lower back affect either the L5 or S1 nerve roots and cause the clinical syndrome of sciatica. *Sciatica* is the term used to describe pain in the hip and buttock area that radiates down the posterolateral aspect of the leg. This term is not synonymous with *radiculopathy*. Because patients frequently use *sciatica* incorrectly, it is important to have them describe their symptoms without the use of medical terminology.

In the case at the beginning of the chapter, the patient has a radiculopathy. The symptoms described are consistent with L5 radiculopathy due to a herniated disk. In the absence of any neurologic deficit, it is reasonable to follow the patient clinically, pursuing a conservative course, as outlined in Figure 4–5. Most patients with acute back pain, with or without radiculopathy, have improvement after 6 weeks. The recommended period of bed rest is 2 days. Physical medicine may include exercise and the use of modalities (e.g., heat, cold, ultrasound, massage) to reduce pain. Patients, especially those with occupational back pain, may benefit from ergonomic education.

SPINAL STENOSIS

A 66-year-old man with coronary artery disease, hypertension, and tobacco abuse complains of leg pain when he walks. The problem has become progressively worse during the last 6 months and he is not able to walk more than two blocks because of pain in both lower extremities. The clinical question is whether this patient has symptoms due to vascular ischemia (claudication) or spinal stenosis (neurogenic claudication or pseudoclaudication). Features of both disorders can complicate the diagnosis. The differences between vascular and neurogenic claudication are listed in Table 4–8.

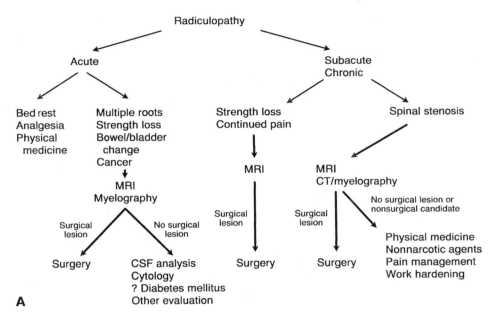

A

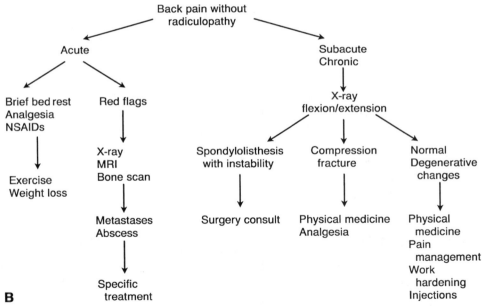

B

FIG. 4–5. Algorithms for evaluation and treatment of (A) radiculopathy and (B) back pain without radiculopathy.

Spinal stenosis is narrowing of the spinal canal. It has several causes, including congenital narrowing of the canal, bulging intervertebral disks, spondylolisthesis, degenerative osteoarthropathies of the spine, or a combination of these. The narrowed spinal canal compresses the nerve roots and, presumably, their vascular supply. The diameter of the spinal canal and the spinal foramina are decreased with standing and walking (extension) and increased with flexion of the spine (Fig. 4–7). Comments that the patient

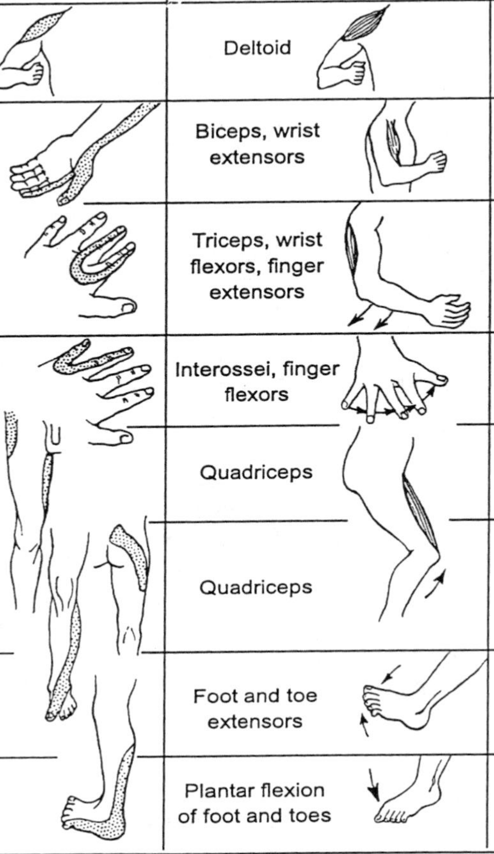

Segment	Sensory loss and pain	Motor weakness	Reflex loss
C3-C4	Shoulder	Diaphragm	
C5	Lateral shoulder	Deltoid	Biceps
C6	Radial side of arm, thumb	Biceps, wrist extensors	Biceps, brachioradialis
C7	2nd & 3rd fingers	Triceps, wrist flexors, finger extensors	Triceps
C8	4th & 5th fingers	Interossei, finger flexors	
L3	Hip, medial thigh	Quadriceps	Knee
L4	Hip, postero-lateral thigh	Quadriceps	Knee
L5	Lateral leg, great toe	Foot and toe extensors	
S1	Back of calf, lateral foot	Plantar flexion of foot and toes	Ankle

FIG. 4–6. Summary of root syndromes.

may make that support spinal stenosis are (1) being able to walk farther when using a shopping cart, (2) leaning on the sink when doing dishes or shaving, and (3) having no difficulty with bicycling. Any activity that flexes the spine reduces the symptoms of neurogenic claudication.

Patients with spinal stenosis often have a flexed posture when standing and walking. The range of motion of the lumbar spine is reduced and can cause leg pain with extension of the back. Other examination findings are normal unless there is impingement of the nerve root.

CT, CT and myelography, and MRI can confirm the diagnosis of lumbar spinal stenosis. If spinal stenosis is diagnosed, surgical consultation may be needed. Nonsurgical management includes physical medicine, nonnarcotic medication, epidural injections, and pain management.

CERVICAL SPONDYLOSIS

Degenerative changes of the cervical spine, including cervical spondylosis, occur with increasing frequency with age. Narrowing of

TABLE 4–6. CLINICAL FEATURES SUGGESTIVE OF LUMBAR RADICULOPATHY

	Radiculopathy			Poor Evidence of Radiculopathy
	Definite	**Probable**	**Possible**	
Location of Pain				
Back			•	
Superior buttock				•
Lateral buttock				•
Medial/inferior buttock		•		
Leg, above knee			•	
Leg, below knee		•		
Associated Paresthesias				
Dorsum of foot, great toe	• (L5)			
Sole of foot, little toe	• (S1)			
Knee, medial calf		• (L4)		
Knee, anterior thigh		• (L3)		
Other				•
Character of pain				
Deep, "toothache"		•		
Electric, "shooting"				•
Postural effect				
Increased with sitting		•		
Onset with extension, relief with flexion	• (spinal stenosis)			
Location of pain with Valsalva effect (strain is more meaningful than cough/sneeze)				
Leg	•			
Buttock		•		
Back			•	
Observations				
List to side	•			
Bent knee, symptomatic leg		•		
Motion				
Unilateral limited side flexion		•		
"Corkscrewing" forward flexion	•			
Bending symptomatic knee with forward flexion		•		
Slow flexion, slow irregular return				•
Palpation tenderness				
Sciatic notch		•		
Popliteal fossa	•			
Spine			•	
Sacrum, gluteal attachments, trochanter				•
Skin				•
Provocation				
Leg pain with SLR		•		

(continued)

TABLE 4–6. CLINICAL FEATURES SUGGESTIVE OF LUMBAR RADICULOPATHY (continued)

	Radiculopathy			Poor Evidence of Radiculopathy
	Definite	**Probable**	**Possible**	
Buttock pain with SLR			•	
Back pain with SLR				•
Opposite leg or buttock pain with SLR	•			
Leg or anterior thigh pain with reverse SLR		• (L3,L4)		
Buttock, back pain with reverse SLR			• (L3,L4)	
Immediate leg pain with back extension			•	
Delayed leg pain with back extension		• (spinal stenosis)		
Buttock, leg pain with back flexion, knees flexed				•

SLR, straight leg raising test.

the spinal canal and the intervertebral foramina can compress the cord and nerve roots. Cervical spondylosis can cause headache, radiculopathy, and myelopathy. Cervical spine disease can cause neck pain or refer pain to the frontal or occipital part of the head, the shoulder, or the interscapular area.

The cervical nerve root most often affected by a herniated disk is C7, and the cervical nerve roots most frequently affected in cervical spondylosis are C5 and C6. Neck and arm pain caused by spondylotic changes occurs more gradually than that due to disk herniation. Patients with cervical spondylosis usually are considerably older than those with a herniated disk.

Cervical spondylotic myelopathy is a difficult clinical problem. The patient may complain of stiff neck, arm pain, leg weakness, and easy fatigability. Numb and clumsy hands are also reported. Neurologic examination may show spastic paraparesis with hyperactive reflexes and bilateral Babinski signs. Amyotrophic lateral sclerosis and vitamin B$_{12}$ deficiency are important disorders in the differential diagnosis of cervical spondylotic myelopathy. Although cervical spondylotic myelopathy has a slow and progressive course, it can develop suddenly in an elderly patient, because of trauma or hyperextension of the neck.

The diagnosis and treatment of cervical spondylotic myelopathy are complicated. Plain radiographs and MRI can readily identify the problem. It is estimated that cervical spondylosis is present by age 59 years in 70% of women and 85% of men and after age 70 in 93% and 97%, respectively. Determining whether the cervical spondylosis is symptomatic may require neurologic consultation and longitudinal follow-up.

The uncertain natural history of cervical spondylotic myelopathy and the 50:50 chance of improvement with surgery complicate treatment. Surgical decompression is performed if there is evidence of progressive myelopathy. Nonsurgical measures include the use of a soft cervical collar, physiotherapy, nonsteroidal anti-inflammatory drugs, and close clinical follow-up.

WHIPLASH

Whiplash is the sudden flexion and extension of the cervical spine that occurs in motor vehicle accidents. Patients with whiplash may experience neck pain, headache, blurring of vision, dizziness, weakness, paresthesias, cognitive difficulty, and psychologic symptoms. Whiplash is often misunderstood because there usually are few radiographic and clinical findings. Litigation issues further

TABLE 4–7. CLINICAL FEATURES SUGGESTIVE OF CERVICAL RADICULOPATHY

	Radiculopathy			Poor Evidence of Radiculopathy
	Definite	**Probable**	**Possible**	
Location of pain				
Neck			•	
Scapula			•	
Shoulder			•	
Proximal arm		•		
Distal arm and hand	•			
Associated paresthesias				
Shoulder	• (C5)			
Thumb and proximal forearm	• (C6) Distinguish from median neuropathy			
3rd finger	• (C7)			
4th & 5th finger	• (C8) Distinguish from ulnar neuropathy			
Character of pain				
Deep "toothache"		•		
Electric, "shooting"				•
Location of pain with Valsalva effect (strain is more meaningful than cough/sneeze)				
Arm	•			
Shoulder		•		
Neck			•	
Provocation (location of pain with neck movement)				
Shoulder		•		
Proximal arm		•		
Individual fingers	•			
Entire upper extremity				•

complicate the problem. Despite negative findings on imaging studies, injury to the zygapophyseal joints, intervertebral disks, muscles, and ligaments has been documented.

The condition of most patients with whiplash improves within the first few months after injury. Patients with chronic symptoms are difficult to treat, and no definitive treatment has been established. Early in the treatment, mobilization is more beneficial than rest. For chronic symptoms, inject corticosteroids into the cervical zygapophyseal joint and prescribe physical therapy. Management of chronic pain is discussed further in Chapter 10.

SPINAL SURGERY

The decision to perform spinal surgery should be made with specific clinical indications and with the consultation of an orthopedic surgeon or neurosurgeon. The indi-

TABLE 4–8. DIFFERENCES BETWEEN NEUROGENIC AND VASCULAR CLAUDICATION

Symptoms and Signs	Neurogenic	Vascular
Pain at rest	Yes, if spine extended	No
Time to relief of symptoms with rest	5–20 min	1–2 min
Distance walked before onset of pain	Variable distance	Same distance
Patient can continue walking after onset of pain	Yes, maybe	No
Vascular history	No	Yes
Leg pain with bicycling	No	Yes
Absent or reduced pedal pulses	No	Yes

cations include compressive radiculopathy, myelopathy, and spinal instability. Acute myelopathy and cauda equina syndrome (see Fig. 4–3) require emergency decompression surgery. Early surgery for radiculopathy with motor deficit optimizes early recovery. Other indications for surgery are increasing neurologic deficit, incapacitating neurogenic claudication, motor weakness, and impaired bladder and bowel function. Surgery for pain only or for a patient with negative findings on imaging studies is ill advised.

Many factors influence surgical outcome. The most important is diagnostic accuracy.

The patient's psychologic and social background are also significant. Patients at risk for a poor surgical outcome have a higher frequency of pending workers' compensation claims, have been on sick leave longer than 3 months, have features of nonorganic pain, or have unsatisfying jobs. Somatization, hysteria, and hypochondriasis are often demonstrated on tests such as the Minnesota Multiphasic Personality Inventory (MMPI).

The possible complications of surgery include diskitis, meningitis, cerebrospinal fluid leak, vascular injury, and neurologic deterioration. Recurrent disk herniation, scarring,

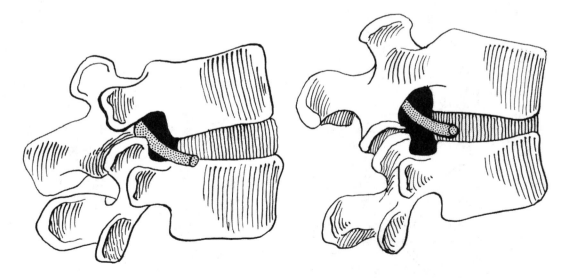

Extension   Flexion

FIG. 4–7. Spine in flexion and extension. The spinal canal and the intervertebral foramen are more open in flexion.

and spinal instability are common postoperative complications. The more accurate the preoperative diagnosis, the better the surgical outcome and the less risk for reoperation.

PLEXOPATHY

Plexopathy is important to consider in patients who have limb pain, weakness, or numbness. Trauma, inflammation, neoplasm, ischemia, and radiation can cause plexopathy, which also can be idiopathic or inherited. The differential diagnosis of plexopathy is limited to involvement of nerve roots or multiple named nerves. The temporal profile of symptoms suggests the cause.

The brachial plexus is derived from cervical roots C5 through T1. C5 and C6 form the upper trunk, C7 the middle trunk, and C8 and T1 the lower trunk (Fig. 4–8). The three trunks divide into anterior and posterior divisions. The posterior divisions come together as the posterior cord and form the axillary and radial nerves. The anterior division of the lower

trunk becomes the medial cord, which gives rise to the ulnar nerve and C8-innervated muscles of the median nerve. The rest of the median nerve and the musculocutaneous nerve come from the lateral cord. Injuries above the clavicle affect the trunks, and those below the clavicle affect the cords. Trauma in the axilla affects the nerve branches.

The upper trunk of the brachial plexus is frequently traumatized in shoulder injuries such as an impact injury (called a "stinger") to the shoulder during a football game or resulting from the recoil of a shotgun. Clinically, an upper trunk brachial plexopathy resembles avulsion of nerve roots C5 and C6. Upper trunk brachial plexopathy is caused by downward traction on the shoulder, such as during a difficult delivery (Erb palsy). Hand strength is strong but the upper arm is weak. The lower trunk of the brachial plexus can be affected by a cervical rib or a tumor of the lung apex (Pancoast tumor). Avulsion of the C8 and T1 nerve roots (Klumpke paralysis) is clinically similar to lesions of the lower trunk. Forceful traction of the arm up-

FIG. 4–8. Brachial plexus. (Modified from Patten, J: Neurological Differential Diagnosis, ed 2. Springer-Verlag, London, 1996, p. 297, with permission.)

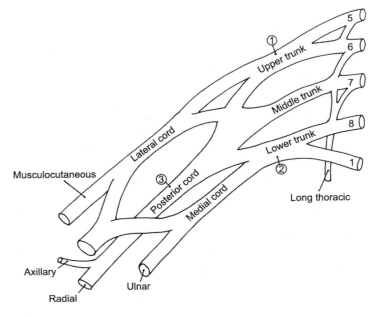

① Upper trunk = weak upper arms, strong hand

② Lower trunk = weak hand

③ Posterior cord = weak elbow, wrist, and finger extension

ward can cause this injury, such as when an adult pulls a child's arm. All intrinsic hand muscles are weak, and Horner syndrome can occur with injury to the sympathetic fibers of T1. Distinguishing between root avulsion and plexus trauma is important. Traumatic injuries to the plexus may be more amenable to surgical repair.

Obstetrical injury to the brachial plexus during delivery has been well described. However, injury can also occur before birth. Performing EMG studies early after delivery may demonstrate that brachial injury occurred before delivery. The medical-legal implications can be significant.

Brachial neuritis, Parsonage-Turner syndrome, and neuralgic amyotrophy are all used to describe a presumed inflammatory condition of the brachial plexus. Evidence suggests that this is an immune-mediated condition. It has been reported following vaccinations and viral illnesses. Males are affected more than females. Shoulder pain is often the first symptom, followed by upper extremity weakness and numbness. The condition can be bilateral, and it usually resolves within 6 months to 1 year. Treatment is primarily supportive.

The brachial plexus is often affected by neoplasm. Also, radiation exposure can cause brachial plexopathy, from days to years after exposure. The distinction between recurrent cancer and radiation-induced plexopathy may require clinical, electrophysiologic, and imaging studies. Plexopathy from recurrent cancer tends to be painful and to affect the lower plexus. In contrast, radiation-induced plexopathy tends to be painless and affect the upper plexus. Myokymic discharges shown on EMG suggest radiation-induced plexopathy. MRI is sensitive for detecting tumor infiltration of the brachial plexus.

Compression of the brachial plexus and the brachial artery and vein at the thoracic outlet describes the thoracic outlet syndrome. Its diagnosis and management are matters of controversy. Compression is caused by an anomalous fibrous band or a cervical rib. Neurogenic thoracic outlet syndrome is extremely rare. The lower trunk of the plexus is affected and the patient should have C8 and T1 weakness and numbness. In patients without neurologic deficit, hand pain may result from compression of the brachial artery. Many believe that this condition is caused by drooping shoulders and that it responds to posture correction and strengthening of cervicoscapular muscles. Surgery is considered when conservative measures fail or when there is a structural anomaly such as a cervical rib.

The lumbosacral plexus is affected by the same types of conditions that affect the brachial plexus, although inflammatory conditions are less likely to affect the lumbosacral plexus. Involvement of the lumbar portion of the plexus mimics a femoral neuropathy, with weak hip flexion and knee extension. However, the two conditions can be distinguished by assessing the function of the obturator nerve (hip adduction). Weakness of hip adduction is not seen in femoral neuropathy. Abdominal surgery can often traumatize the lumbar portion of the plexus. The sacral portion of the plexus can be injured in hip surgery. Symptoms from injury to the sacral portion of the plexus may mimic sciatica.

Ischemic injury to the plexus from diabetes mellitus or other conditions that can cause a mononeuritis multiplex occurs suddenly and is very painful. Radiation-induced plexopathy, as mentioned above, tends to be painless. Lymphoma, leukemia, and tumors of the prostate, rectum, and cervix can affect the lumbosacral plexus, and bleeding into the iliopsoas muscle can cause lumbosacral plexopathy.

The lateral femoral cutaneous nerve, a sensory nerve of the thigh, is a branch of L3 and L2 that innervates the skin of the lateral aspect of the thigh (Fig. 4–9; see also Fig. 1–12). The nerve courses over the iliac crest and can be injured by seat belts, abdominal surgery, and tight clothing. Obesity and pregnancy can predispose patients to lateral cutaneous neuropathy. The syndrome of pain and numbness in the distribution of this nerve is called "meralgia paresthetica." Treatment with tricyclic antidepressants or anticonvulsants can lessen the symptoms. Patient reassurance about this benign neuropathy is usually the most helpful treatment.

Mononeuropathies of the arm and leg can cause limb pain. The sites of common nerve injuries are shown in Figures 4–9 and 4–10. Focal neuropathies are discussed in Chapter 6.

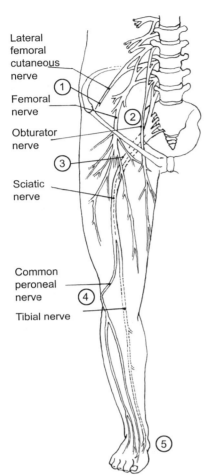

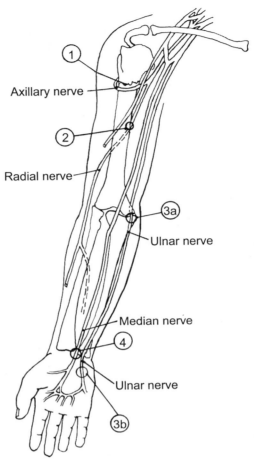

FIG. 4–9. Lower extremity nerves. Common sites of damage (1–5) and associated causes. **1,** Lateral femoral cutaneous: compression at inguinal ligament. **2,** Obturator: complication of pelvic surgery. **3,** Sciatic: complication of hip surgery. **4,** Common peroneal: knee injury: "crossed-leg" palsy. **5,** Tibial: tarsal tunnel syndrome.

FIG. 4–10. Upper extremity nerves. Common sites of damage (1–4) and associated causes. **1,** Axillary: fracture of humeral head, intramuscular injections. **2,** Radial: fracture of humerus, compression: "Saturday night palsy." **3,** Ulnar: **a,** compression; **b,** trauma. **4,** Median: carpal tunnel syndrome. (From Patten, J: Neurological Differential Diagnosis, ed 2. Springer-Verlag, London, 1996, p 283, with permission.)

SUGGESTED READING

Barnsley, L, Lord, S, and Bogduk, N: Whiplash injury. Pain 58:283–307, 1994.

Braddom, RL: Perils and pointers in the evaluation and management of back pain. Semin Neurol 18:197–210, 1998.

Deen, HG, Jr: Diagnosis and management of lumbar disk disease. Mayo Clin Proc 71:283–287, 1996.

Deyo, RA, Diehl, AK, and Rosenthal, M: How many days of bed rest for acute low back pain? A randomized clinical trial. N Engl J Med 315:1064–1070, 1986.

Frymoyer, JW: Back pain and sciatica. N Engl J Med 318:291–300, 1988.

Hadler, NM: Regional back pain (editorial). N Engl J Med 315:1090–1092, 1986.

Haldeman, S: Diagnostic tests for the evaluation of back and neck pain. Neurol Clin 14:103–117, 1996.

Levin, KH, Maggiano, HJ, and Wilbourn, AJ: Cervical radiculopathies: Comparison of surgical and EMG localization of single-root lesions. Neurology 46:1022–1025, 1996.

Paradiso, G, Granana, N, and Maza, E: Prenatal brachial plexus paralysis. Neurology 49:261–262, 1997.

Report of the Quality Standards Subcommittee of the American Academy of Neurology: Practice parameters: Magnetic resonance imaging in the evaluation of low back syndrome (summary statement). Neurology 44:767–770, 1994.

Rowland, LP: Surgical treatment of cervical spondylotic myelopathy: Time for a controlled trial. Neurology 42:5–13, 1992.

Suarez, GA, Giannini, C, and Bosch, EP: Immune brachial plexus neuropathy: Suggestive evidence for an inflammatory-immune pathogenesis. Neurology 46:559–561, 1996.

Thyagarajan, D, Cascino, T, and Harms, G: Magnetic resonance imaging in brachial plexopathy of cancer. Neurology 45:421–427, 1995.

Waddell, G, McCulloch, JA, Kummel, E, et al: Nonorganic physical signs in low-back pain. Spine 5:117–125, 1980.

Wolinsky, AP: The illusion of certainty. N Engl J Med 335:46–48, 1996.

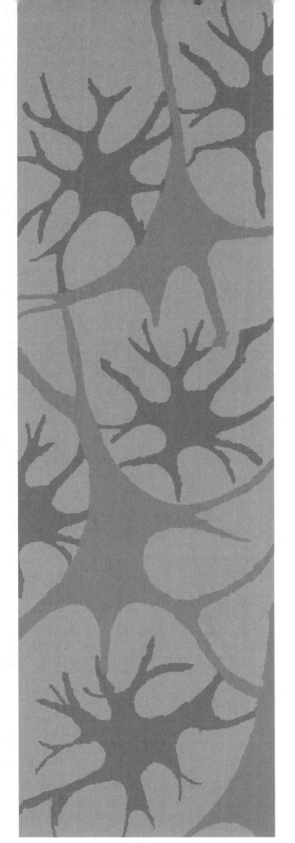

CHAPTER 5

Dizziness

CHAPTER OUTLINE

Diagnostic Approach
Vertigo
    Peripheral Causes
    Central Causes
Presyncope
Disequilibrium
Ill-Defined Dizziness

A 68-year-old man with a history of diabetes mellitus, coronary artery disease, hypertension, and benign prostatic hypertrophy complains of dizziness when he gets up at night to go to the bathroom. He takes the following medications: a diuretic, nitroglycerin patch, finasteride, and a β-blocker. He denies having any auditory or other neurologic symptoms. Pertinent positive physical findings include a 20 mm Hg change in blood pressure from sitting to standing, bilateral cataract changes, bilateral presbycusis, and a mild distal sensory loss in his feet. The patient is given a prescription for meclizine. What type of dizziness does the patient have? Is the therapy appropriate?

Patients frequently complain of "dizziness" and use this term to describe various symptoms. It can be difficult to obtain an accurate history of the symptoms, especially with the time constraints of a busy office practice. The symptom of dizziness requires taking an open-ended history. Direct questions often suggest symptoms to the patient and can lead to a wrong diagnosis. The first 10 questions to ask (or the question that should be asked 10 times) of a patient with a complaint of dizziness should be, "What do you mean by 'dizzy'?"

Dizziness has many mechanisms and causes. The diagnostic approach is simplified by categorizing dizziness into four different types. It is important to remember that the patient may have more than one type of dizziness. The patient described above has several conditions that could explain dizziness: orthostatic blood pressure changes, peripheral sensory loss, and several medications that can cause the symptom.

The first category is "vertigo," that is, a sensation of movement. This type of dizziness implies a problem with the vestibular system and may be peripheral or central. The second category is "presyncope," or the sensation of impending faint. This symptom indicates a disturbance of cardiovascular function. The third category is "disequilibrium," which is a disturbance of postural balance caused by a neurologic disorder. The fourth category is an ill-defined symptom characteristic of psychiatric disorders. The four categories of dizziness, the mechanism associated with each type, and some common clinical examples are listed in Table 5–1.

DIAGNOSTIC APPROACH

The history is the most important aspect of the diagnostic work-up of a patient presenting with dizziness. The situation in which the patient responds, "You know, *dizzy*," is all too frequent and can be trying for both you and the patient. It may help to ask the patient if the sensation compares with anything else he or she has experienced. Inquire about associated symptoms such as auditory, cardiac, neurologic, and psychiatric symptoms. Loss of hearing, tinnitus, and ear fullness may suggest involvement of the vestibulocochlear nerve (CN VIII) in the periphery. Ask about symptoms that indicate brainstem involvement, such as diplopia, dysarthria, visual disturbance, and ataxia. Medications frequently cause dizziness (thousands of drugs are associated with the complaint of dizziness, and hundreds with vertigo). Some of the more common drugs associated with this symptom are listed in Table 5–2. The periodicity and duration of the symptoms, factors that provoke dizziness, and the circumstances associated with it are important historical details. Some of the clinical features associated with common causes of dizziness are listed in Table 5–3.

The physical examination should include measuring orthostatic blood pressure and pulse and examining the ear. Examining the patient's gait is a critical component of the neurologic evaluation. Patients with positional vertigo walk with very limited head

TABLE 5–1. TYPES OF DIZZINESS AND THEIR MECHANISMS AND COMMON CAUSES

Type	Mechanism	Common Causes of Dizziness

Vertigo (sensation of movement)	Disturbance of vestibular function	Peripheral
		  Vestibular neuronitis
		  Labyrinthitis
		  Benign positional vertigo
		  Ménière disease
		Central
		  Vertebrobasilar ischemia
		  Multiple sclerosis
		  Posterior fossa tumors
		  Migraine

Presyncope (sensation of impending faint, lightheadedness)	Diffuse or global cerebral ischemia	Cardiac
		  Arrhythmia
		  Vasovagal
		Orthostatic hypotension
		  Volume depletion
		  Medication effect
		  Autonomic insufficiency

Disequilibrium (disturbance of postural balance)	Loss of vestibulospinal, proprioceptive, or cerebellar function	Ototoxicity Peripheral neuropathy Cerebellar dysfunction Drug intoxication Extrapyramidal syndrome
Ill-defined	Impaired central integration of sensory signals	Anxiety Panic disorders Hyperventilation syndrome Affective disorders

TABLE 5–2. DRUGS ASSOCIATED WITH DIZZINESS

Drug	Mechanism	Type of Dizziness
Aminoglycoside antibiotics	Vestibular hair cell damage	Vertigo, disequilibrium
Antihypertensives, diuretics	Postural hypotension, reduced cerebral blood flow	Presyncope
Anticonvulsants	Cerebellar toxicity	Disequilibrium
Alcohol	CNS depression, cerebellar toxicity	Disequilibrium, vertigo
Tranquilizers	CNS depression	Disequilibrium
Antihistamines	CNS depression	Disequilibrium
Tricyclics	CNS depression	Disequilibrium
Methotrexate	Brainstem and cerebellar toxicity	Disequilibrium
Anticoagulants	Hemorrhage into inner ear or brain	Vertigo
Cisplatin	Vestibular hair cell damage	Vertigo, disequilibrium

CNS, central nervous system.

TABLE 5–3. CLINICAL FEATURES OF COMMON CAUSES OF DIZZINESS

Type of Dizziness	Diagnosis	Clinical Features
Vertigo	Benign positional vertigo	Aggravated by certain head positions, positional nystagmus
	Vestibular neuronitis	Antecedent viral infection, spontaneous nystagmus
	Ménière disease	Fluctuating hearing loss, tinnitus
	Vertebrobasilar insufficiency	Focal neurologic signs and symptoms
Presyncope	Orthostatic hypotension	Occurs with standing, antihypertensive medications, peripheral neuropathy
	Vasovagal	Prolonged standing, heat
	Cardiogenic	Exertion, valvular disease, arrhythmias, angina
	Hyperventilation	Stressful situations, perioral and acral paresthesias
Disequilibrium	Peripheral neuropathy	Trouble walking in dark or on uneven surfaces
	Cerebellar dysfunction	Chronic and continuous
Ill-defined	Panic disorder	Provoked by stress, crowds, panic attacks
Physiologic	Motion sickness	Positive family history, migraine

movement. A wide-based ataxic gait may indicate cerebellar disease, and a slow, flexed, shuffling gait may indicate an extrapyramidal syndrome. Peripheral neuropathy should be suspected if the Romberg sign is present.

Dizziness may be stimulated by several tests. A patient may complain of dizziness if you have him or her hyperventilate for 3 minutes, change position, or perform the Valsalva maneuver. Measuring orthostatic blood pressure and pulse may also cause a complaint of dizziness. Vertigo aggravated by the Valsalva maneuver may suggest a perilymph fistula or a craniovertebral junction anomaly. This maneuver may also aggravate presyncope in patients with cardiovascular disease.

A useful simulation test for positional vertigo is a positioning maneuver called the "Nylen-Bárány" or "Dix-Hallpike" test (Fig. 5–1). It is performed by moving the patient from the sitting to the lying position, with the head extended back by 45 degrees (Fig. 5–1A). This is repeated with the head extended and turned to the right (Fig. 5–1B) and then with the head extended and turned to the left. Examine the patient for positional nystagmus. This maneuver and nystagmus are discussed in the section on vertigo.

The laboratory evaluation of a patient complaining of dizziness may include audiometry, electronystagmography (ENG), posturography, brainstem auditory evoked responses (BAERs), and neuroimaging. Auditory testing is helpful because of the close association between the auditory and vestibular systems from the level of the inner ear to the cerebral cortex. Office evaluation of hearing often includes assessing the patient's response to whisper, conversational speech, and shouting. A tuning fork can be useful in distinguishing between hearing loss due to middle ear disease (conductive) and that due to sensorineural injury. For the Rinne test, place the stem of a vibrating tuning fork on the patient's mastoid process until the vibrations are no longer audible to the

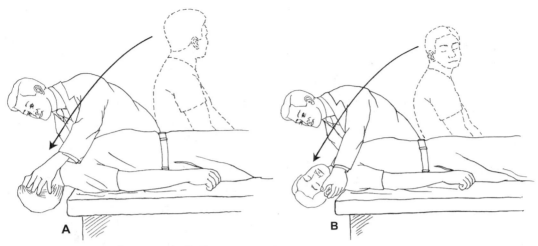

FIG. 5–1. (A and B) Dix-Hallpike maneuver.

patient, then hold the tuning fork next to the ear. Normally, the vibrations are audible when the tuning fork is held next to the ear, because air conduction is better than bone conduction. This is true, too, if the patient has sensorineural hearing loss. However, if the patient has conductive hearing loss, bone conduction is better than air conduction. Thus, the vibrations will not be heard when the tuning fork is moved from the mastoid and held next to the ear. The Rinne test is used in conjunction with the Weber test, in which the stem of the tuning fork is held on the vertex of the head. Normally, the vibrations are heard equally in both ears. This is true also for patients with conductive hearing loss. However, in patients with sensorineural hearing loss, the vibratory sounds are diminished in the affected ear.

Audiometry is a valuable screening test for patients with vertigo, tinnitus, or hearing loss. In conductive hearing loss, all frequencies of sound are affected, but speech discrimination is preserved. If the cochlea or CN VIII is involved, there is hearing loss of high-frequency sounds, and patients have difficulty with speech discrimination, especially if there is background noise. Thus, they may become annoyed at loud speech. The audiograms in Figure 5–2 compare normal findings with those typical of asymmetric sensorineural hearing loss and asymmetric conductive hearing loss.

ENG is used to document a unilateral vestibular lesion and to determine whether it is peripheral or central. A peripheral lesion is suggested by unidirectional spontaneous or positional nystagmus without visual fixation. Direction-changing spontaneous or positional nystagmus with fixation indicates a central lesion. If the patient is not taking any sedating medications, abnormal saccades, abnormal smooth pursuit, and optokinetic nystagmus indicate a central lesion.

For posturography, place the patient on a platform that can be moved, so that the patient moves at the same time as the visual surroundings. This test was designed to assess the vestibular system without involving the visual and somatosensory systems. Instead of being used as a diagnostic tool, this test is better for following a patient's balance function.

BAERs can help distinguish between nerve and cochlear lesions. The absence of all waveforms is not diagnostically useful. However, if all waves are delayed, a conductive or cochlear problem is indicated. Delay of waves I through V indicates a CN VIII or brainstem lesion.

The clinical diagnosis should determine whether neuroimaging is required for a patient who complains of dizziness. Neuroimaging is needed for cases of cerebrovascular disease, intracranial mass, or demyelinating disease, but these conditions rarely occur with vertigo

Normal Audiogram

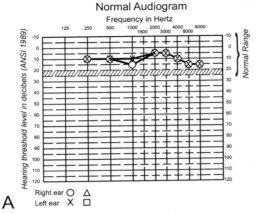

A

Right ear ○ △
Left ear ✕ □

Right Conductive Hearing Loss

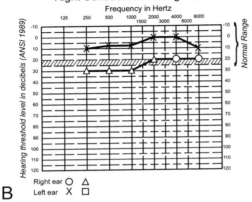

B

Right ear ○ △
Left ear ✕ □

Right Sensorineural Hearing Loss

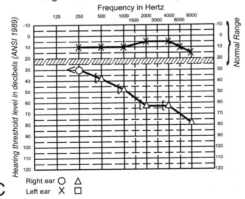

C

Right ear ○ △
Left ear ✕ □

FIG. 5–2. Audiograms. (A) Normal; **(B)** right conductive hearing loss; **(C)** right sensorineural hearing loss.

or disequilibrium in isolation. Neuroimaging results are likely to be negative if other neurologic symptoms or signs are not present.

Magnetic resonance imaging is preferred to computed tomography for evaluating the posterior fossa. However, computed tomography is valuable if an intracranial hemorrhage is suspected.

VERTIGO

Vertigo is the sensation of movement. Its presence implies a problem within the vestibular system (Fig. 5–3). The vestibular receptors are hair cells in the semicircular canals, utricle, and saccule of the inner ear. They are mechanoreceptors that detect changes in the motion and position of the head. This information is conveyed via CN VIII to the vestibular nuclei, which are located at the junction of the medulla and pons. These nuclei also receive input from the visual and somatosensory systems. Vestibular information is distributed widely to the cerebellum, the motor nuclei controlling eye muscles and neck muscles, autonomic centers, and ventral horn cells that innervate skeletal muscles of the extremities and trunk. The cortical representation of the vestibular system is thought to be in the frontal, parietal, and temporal lobes.

If a patient has vertigo, first determine whether the problem is peripheral or central. Peripheral disease involves the cochlea and CN VIII in the internal auditory meatus or cerebellopontine angle. Central disease involves disturbances of vestibular projections in the brainstem, cerebellum, or cerebral hemispheres.

The patient may describe vertigo as "spinning," "falling," or "tilting" and compare the sensation to motion sickness or to being drunk. Head movement and position changes often precipitate the sensation. Symptoms commonly associated with vertigo are nausea, vomiting, and oscillopsia (the subjective sensation of oscillation of viewed objects). Peripheral causes of vertigo are associated with more severe nausea and vomiting than central causes.

A patient with vertigo often has nystagmus. The presence of spontaneous or induced nystagmus is an important physical finding. Nystagmus is the rhythmical oscillation of the

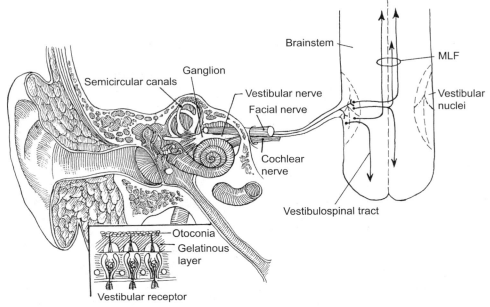

FIG. 5–3. Vestibular pathway. MLF, medial longitudinal fasciculus.

eyes, and it may be horizontal, vertical, or rotatory. The direction of the fast phase designates the direction of the nystagmus. The presence of nystagmus indicates a problem involving the vestibular system, brainstem, cerebellum, or cortical centers for ocular pursuit. The features that distinguish peripheral nystagmus from central nystagmus are listed in Table 5–4.

If a patient has acute vertigo and imbalance, the most serious diagnosis to consider is cerebellar hemorrhage or infarct. Both of these can cause a mass effect that results in brainstem compression and death. Prompt neuroimaging is needed if the patient has profound imbalance, direction-changing nystagmus, or focal neurologic findings. Because cerebellar infarcts may mimic a pe-

TABLE 5–4. COMPARISON OF PERIPHERAL AND CENTRAL NYSTAGMUS

Feature	Peripheral Nystagmus	Central Nystagmus
Location of lesion	Labyrinthine or vestibular nerve	Brainstem or cerebellum
Gaze	Unidirectional	Usually changes direction
Appearance	Horizontal or rotatory	Vertical, horizontal, torsional
Fixation	Nystagmus is inhibited	Little effect
Direction change	Nystagmus increases when looking toward fast phase	Change with convergence
Associated clinical features		
Nausea, vomiting	Severe	Variable
Hearing loss, ear symptoms	Common	Rare
Imbalance	Mild	Severe
Neurologic symptoms	Rare	Common

ripheral vestibular lesion, neuroimaging studies may be needed if the patient has cerebrovascular risk factors and you have difficulty evaluating his or her gait, balance, and eye movements.

The peripheral causes of vertigo include labyrinthitis, vestibular neuronitis, Ménière disease, syphilis, and drug effects (e.g., aminoglycosides). Benign positional vertigo can be due to otolithiasis and perilymph fistula. Acoustic schwannoma and meningioma cause peripheral vertigo. Severe trauma with a basilar skull fracture or vestibular concussion can cause vertigo.

Central diseases that cause vertigo include vascular disease (vertebrobasilar artery disease), migraine, and demyelinating disease (e.g., multiple sclerosis). Anticonvulsant drugs, alcohol, and hypnotic agents can cause vertigo through a depressive effect on the central nervous system. Seizures very rarely cause vertigo. The differences between peripheral and central vertigo are listed in Table 5–5.

PERIPHERAL CAUSES

The differential diagnosis of an acute peripheral vestibulopathy includes viral or bacterial infection, syphilitic labyrinthitis, labyrinthine ischemia, and perilymph fistula. All these disorders can begin abruptly. Viral neuronitis is often associated with a previous flu-like illness. Most patients have a prolonged bout of vertigo that resolves over weeks and does not recur. However, a very small percentage of patients have recurrent episodes. Despite vestibular injury, symptoms resolve because of compensatory mechanisms in the central nervous system. A history of ear infections suggests bacterial labyrinthitis. Bacterial meningitis is a serious complication associated with ear infections. Syphilitic labyrinthitis can lead to recurrent episodes of vertigo, hearing loss, and tinnitus.

Perilymph fistula should be considered if vertigo develops abruptly in association with trauma, heavy lifting or straining, coughing or sneezing, or barotrauma. Perilymph fistula is an abnormal communication between the perilymph of the inner ear and the middle ear. Coughing or sneezing can cause severe vertigo because of the change in pressure that is transmitted directly to the inner ear. Patients with chronic otomastoiditis with cholesteatoma are at risk for this. The fistula test is positive when the Valsalva maneuver produces vertigo. Refer the patient to otolaryngology.

Labyrinthine ischemia has an abrupt onset and is usually associated with other neurologic signs and symptoms. Infarction confined to the inner ear or brainstem is usually the result of intra-arterial thrombosis of the posterior inferior cerebellar, anterior inferior cerebellar, or superior cerebellar artery. Isolated episodes of vertigo may represent transient ischemic attacks and precede infarction of the labyrinth. This diagnosis should be suspected if the patient has cerebrovascular risk factors and suddenly develops hearing loss and vertigo.

TABLE 5–5. COMPARISON OF PERIPHERAL AND CENTRAL VERTIGO

Feature	Peripheral Vertigo	Central Vertigo
Nausea and vomiting	Severe	Variable
Hearing loss, ear symptoms	Common	Rare
Imbalance	Mild	Severe
Nystagmus	Unidirectional, inhibited with fixation	Direction changing, not inhibited with fixation
Neurologic symptoms	Rare	Common
Location of lesion	Labyrinthine or CN VIII	Brainstem, cerebellum

CN, cranial nerve.

CENTRAL CAUSES

Vertigo due to vertebrobasilar insufficiency is usually associated with other neurologic symptoms. However, vertigo can be the only symptom of vertebrobasilar ischemia and should be suspected if a patient has significant cerebrovascular risk factors. Ischemia of the vestibular system in the brainstem should also be suspected if a patient has cerebrovascular risk factors and has unexplained vomiting that seems out of proportion to the symptom of dizziness.

Vertebrobasilar insufficiency can cause recurrent attacks of vertigo. Associated symptoms include visual symptoms, unsteadiness, extremity numbness or weakness, dysarthria, confusion, and drop attacks. The most common cause of vertebrobasilar insufficiency is atherosclerosis of the vertebral, basilar, or subclavian artery. The diagnosis of vertebrobasilar insufficiency is made on the basis of associated clinical signs and symptoms. Vertigo can be an isolated finding but this is very unlikely, especially if the time between episodes is longer than 6 months.

Patients often complain of recurrent episodes of vertigo. The duration of the episode is important. Transient ischemic attacks usually last minutes, as compared with hours for disease of the inner ear. The differential diagnosis of recurrent attacks of vertigo includes vertebrobasilar ischemia, multiple sclerosis, Ménière disease, autoimmune inner ear disease, syphilis, and migraine.

Ménière disease is characterized by recurrent episodes of vertigo, tinnitus, and a fluctuating low-frequency hearing loss. All three of these features may not be present initially. Sudden falling spells, called "otolithic catastrophes," have been reported in this disorder. In Ménière disease, the volume of the endolymph increases, causing distention of the endolymphatic system. Treatment recommendations include a salt-restricted diet, diuretics, and vestibular suppressants. Ablative surgery is performed for intractable cases.

Autoimmune disease of the inner ear can cause recurrent episodes of vertigo. The patient may present with a fluctuating hearing loss, tinnitus, and vertigo suggestive of Ménière disease. Unlike Ménière disease,

autoimmune disease of the inner ear progresses rapidly over weeks to months and involves both ears. This disorder may involve only the inner ear or may be part of a systemic autoimmune disease such as polyarteritis nodosa or rheumatoid arthritis. Inner ear disease in conjunction with interstitial keratitis is called *Cogan syndrome*. These disorders have been treated with corticosteroids, cytotoxic drugs, and plasmapheresis.

Syphilis, acquired or congenital, can cause recurrent episodes of vertigo and hearing loss. Syphilis can cause meningitis involving CN VIII or it can cause temporal bone osteitis with labyrinthitis. The diagnosis is based on positive findings on a fluorescent treponemal antibody absorption test (FTA-ABS). The Venereal Disease Research Laboratory (VDRL) test is positive in only 75% of cases. Treat syphilitic ear infections with penicillin.

- The association between vertigo and migraine is strong, and patients with migraine frequently have vertigo as part of their headache syndrome. Motion sensitivity is reported by more than 50% of patients with migraine. Vertigo without headache can be a symptom of migraine. This diagnosis should be suspected in a patient with recurrent attacks of vertigo who has a history of migraine or a positive family history of migraine.

Positional vertigo is a common problem that is often due to a benign condition, such as viral infection or head trauma. Usually, however, the cause is idiopathic. The mechanism of positional vertigo is attributed to lesions of the otoliths and connections of the vestibular nuclei. Under the influence of gravity, otoliths move from one position to another in the semicircular canals and cause positional vertigo.

In benign positional vertigo, patients experience vertigo with a change in head position. The onset of symptoms often occurs when patients get into or out of bed or when they extend their neck, "the top-shelf syndrome." The diagnosis can be confirmed by eliciting fatigable nystagmus during the positioning maneuver described in Figure 5–1.

Benign positional vertigo is usually caused by otolithiasis of the posterior semicircular canal. A variant involves the horizontal semicircular canal. Patients with this variant often complain that they have vertigo when they turn over in bed or turn their head from side to side while walking.

Benign positional vertigo can be treated effectively by procedures designed to rotate the freely moving otoliths around the semicircular canal. One of these methods is the canalith repositioning procedure (see Fig. 5–4). After the procedure has been performed, have the patient keep the head upright for 48 hours. The maneuver is repeated as needed. The variant of benign positional vertigo also responds to a positioning maneuver—one that rotates the head in the plane of the horizontal semicircular canal.

Central causes of positional vertigo include multiple sclerosis, brainstem tumor, cerebellar tumor or atrophy, and Arnold-Chiari malformation. These conditions are usually associated with other neurologic findings. Nystagmus due to a central cause is nonfatigable.

Use antiemetic and vestibular suppressant medications to treat the symptoms of vertigo: antihistamines, benzodiazepines, and anticholinergic agents. Antihistamines have moderate vestibular suppression capabilities and a minimal antiemetic effect. In comparison, benzodiazepines are more effective vestibular suppressants. The most effective antiemetic agents, such as prochlorperazine (Compazine) and chlorpromazine

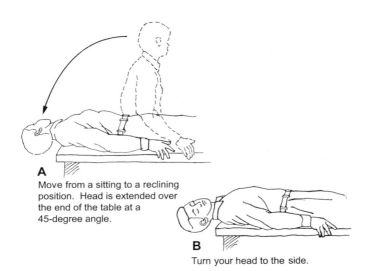

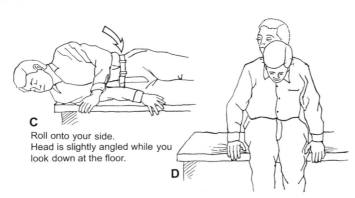

A
Move from a sitting to a reclining position. Head is extended over the end of the table at a 45-degree angle.

B
Turn your head to the side.

C
Roll onto your side. Head is slightly angled while you look down at the floor.

D
Return carefully to a sitting position tilting your chin down.

FIG. 5–4. Canalith repositioning procedure. (Modified from *Mayo Clinic Health Letter*, 12(12): December 1994, with permission of Mayo Foundation for Medical Education and Research.).

(Thorazine), have little vestibular suppressant effect. Droperidol (Inapsine) is an effective antiemetic and vestibular suppressant. Medications for treating the symptoms of vertigo are listed in Table 5–6.

PRESYNCOPE

The sensation of impending faint is often described as "dizziness." This sensation implies a disturbance of cardiovascular function. The mechanism for this type of dizziness is pancerebral ischemia. Cardiac causes of presyncope or syncope include arrhythmias, valvular disease, vasovagal (reflex syncope), and carotid sinus hypersensitivity. Orthostatic hypotension, defined as a decrease in systolic blood pressure of 20 mm Hg or more, can be caused by cardiac dysfunction, decreased intravascular volume, venous pooling, and medications. Common medications that can cause orthostatic hypotension include diuretics, antihypertensive agents, antianginal agents, and tricyclic antidepressants.

Neurologic causes of orthostatic hypotension or autonomic dysfunction include disorders of the central nervous system or peripheral nervous system. Although central nervous system disorders such as pure autonomic failure, dysautonomias, or multiple system atrophy can cause orthostatic hypotension, they are relatively rare. A more common cause of autonomic dysfunction is parkinsonism or cerebrovascular disease.

Most cases of autonomic dysfunction treated by primary care providers involve disease of the peripheral nervous system. Diabetes mellitus, amyloidosis, connective tissue disorders, neoplasia, human immunodeficiency virus infections, and pernicious anemia can cause autonomic neuropathy. In developed countries, diabetes is the most common cause. The symptoms of orthostatic hypotension include dizziness, blurred or tunnel vision, and head and neck discomfort. The clinical features of autonomic neuropathies are protean (Table 5–7).

The management of symptomatic hypotension entails both pharmacologic and nonpharmacologic measures. Patients need to exercise care when changing position, and they need to know that hypotension can be caused by certain stimuli, for example, food, hot ambient temperature, infection, hyperventilation, and lifting. Any unnecessary medications

TABLE 5–6. MEDICATIONS FOR THE SYMPTOMATIC TREATMENT OF VERTIGO

Drug Class	Medication	Dosage	Relative Contraindications
Antihistamines	Meclizine (Antivert)	25–50 mg orally 1–4 times daily	Prostate enlargement, asthma, glaucoma
	Dimenhydrinate (Dramamine)	50 mg orally every 4–6 hr	Prostate enlargement, asthma, glaucoma
	Promethazine (Phenergan)	25 mg orally every 6 hr	History of seizures
Benzodiazepines	Diazepam (Valium)	2–10 mg 2–4 times daily	History of drug addiction
	Lorazepam (Ativan)	1–2 mg orally 3 times daily	History of drug addiction
	Clonazepam (Klonopin)	0.5 mg orally 3 times daily	History of drug addiction
Anticholinergic agents	Scopolamine (Transderm-Scop)	1 patch every 3 days	Prostate enlargement, asthma, glaucoma, liver or kidney disease

TABLE 5–7. CLINICAL FEATURES OF AUTONOMIC DYSFUNCTION

System	Features
Gastrointestinal	Nausea, vomiting, early satiety, postprandial bloating, epigastric pain, constipation, diarrhea (nighttime)
Genitourinary	Urinary retention, inadequate bladder emptying, overflow incontinence Erectile dysfunction
Sudomotor	Anhidrosis (stocking-glove distribution), compensatory hyperhidrosis, gustatory sweating
Cardiovascular	Increased heart rate, fixed heart rate

should be eliminated. Increased sodium intake, the use of elastic or compression stockings, and raising the head of the bed can help prevent hypotension.

Medications used to treat orthostatic hypotension—mineralocorticoids, sympathomimetic amines, prostaglandin synthetase inhibitors, and others—are listed in Table 5–8. The most serious problem with these agents is supine hypertension.

DISEQUILIBRIUM

Many patients who complain of dizziness describe "unsteadiness" or a concern that they might fall. Disequilibrium is a disturbance in postural balance. Postural balance depends on visual, somatosensory, and vestibular sensory input. Disequilibrium may result from a disorder of sensory input or the central processing of this input and the motor response. Causes of disequilibrium are listed in Table 5–9.

Disturbance of two of these three sensory inputs is called *multisensory disequilibrium*. An example is a patient with diabetes who has both a peripheral neuropathy and retinopathy. Disequilibrium is a significant problem, especially among the elderly population, because of the risk of falling. Medications like meclizine that can cause drowsiness and blurred vision are ill-advised for these patients.

Bilateral vestibular dysfunction also causes disequilibrium. The diagnosis should be suspected if the patient complains of unsteadiness and oscillopsia. A history of vertigo or exposure to ototoxic drugs supports the diag-

nosis. Classes of ototoxic drugs include antibiotics (especially aminoglycosides), anti-inflammatory, antimalarial, diuretic, and antineoplastic drugs. The more common ototoxic medications are listed in Table 5–10. On examination, patients with bilateral vestibular

TABLE 5–8. PHARMACOLOGIC AGENTS FOR TREATING ORTHOSTATIC HYPOTENSION

Mineralocorticoids

Fludrocortisone

Sympathomimetic Agents

Clonidine
Dextroamphetamine
Ephedrine
Methylphenidate
Midodrine
Phenylpropanolamine
Pseudoephedrine

Prostaglandin Synthetase Inhibitors

Ibuprofen
Indomethacin
Naproxen

Nonspecific Pressor Agents

Caffeine
Ergot derivatives

β-Adrenergic Blocking Agents

Propranolol

Dopamine Blocking Agents

Metoclopramide

TABLE 5–9. CAUSES OF DISEQUILIBRIUM

Disorders of Sensory Input

Peripheral neuropathy: diabetes mellitus, vitamin B_{12} deficiency, hypothyroidism, syphilis
Myelopathy: cervical spondylosis, subacute combined degeneration (vitamin B_{12} deficiency), tabes dorsalis
Bilateral vestibular loss: ototoxic drugs, meningitis, autoimmune disorders, hydrocarbon solvents, bilateral Ménière disease, bilateral vestibular neuritis

Disorders of Central Processing and Motor Response

Cerebellar dysfunction: chronic alcohol use, cerebellar degeneration, paraneoplastic syndrome
Apractic syndromes: multi-infarct state, hydrocephalus, frontal lobe lesions
Extrapyramidal syndromes: Parkinson disease, progressive supranuclear palsy, striatonigral degeneration

loss are unsteady but do not show any signs of cerebellar dysfunction. In addition to the causes listed in Table 5–9, idiopathic, congenital, familial, and infectious conditions can cause bilateral vestibular loss.

Patients with sensory ataxia often complain of dizziness. Peripheral neuropathies are the most common cause of sensory ataxia. Patients may report that they have increasing difficulty walking in the dark or maintaining their balance in the shower when they close their eyes. Uneven surfaces are frequently more difficult to walk on, and there is a greater tendency to fall. Neurologic examination shows reduced peripheral proprioception, Romberg sign, and reduced ankle reflexes. Peripheral neuropathies are discussed further in Chapter 6. Myelopathies also can cause sensory ataxia.

Many neurologic disorders are associated with disequilibrium. Cerebellar dysfunction can be the source of dizziness. The findings on physical examination of a patient with cerebellar dysfunction are those seen in acute alcohol intoxication. Familiar signs of cerebellar dysfunction are nystagmus, dysarthria, wide-based ataxic gait, intention tremor, and dysdiadochokinesia. Chronic alcohol consumption can lead to similar findings. Cerebellar symptoms in a patient with ovarian cancer or small cell carcinoma of the lung should raise the suspicion of a paraneoplastic syndrome. Many familial degenerative disorders of the cerebellum can present as dizziness. These genetic degenerative disorders progress much more slowly than paraneoplastic syndromes.

Disequilibrium is common in patients with Parkinson disease, parkinsonism, or gait apraxia. Apractic gait is wide-based, with slow and short steps. Patients have difficulty with starting and turning and often appear as though their feet are glued to the ground.

TABLE 5–10. OTOTOXIC DRUGS		
	Effect	
Drug	**Vestibulotoxic**	**Cochleotoxic**
Cisplatin	High	High
Gentamicin	High	Low
Tobramycin	Moderate	Moderate
Amikacin	Low	High
Aspirin	—	Low
Furosemide	—	Low

This type of gait is called a "frontal gait" or "lower body parkinsonism." It is the characteristic gait of patients with normal pressure hydrocephalus, multiple strokes, or a frontal lobe syndrome. Neurologic consultation may be helpful for patients with disequilibrium.

ILL-DEFINED DIZZINESS

Dizziness that cannot be categorized as vertigo, presyncope, or disequilibrium may fall into the "ill-defined" group. This category of dizziness has been called "functional," "psychogenic," "hyperventilation syndrome," "phobic postural vertigo," and "psychiatric dizziness." It has been estimated that 20% to 50% of all patients who complain of dizziness have this type of dizziness. Features that characterize psychiatric dizziness have traditionally included the absence of true vertigo, replication of symptoms by hyperventilation, psychiatric symptoms preceding the onset of dizziness, and the presence of dizziness in anxious or phobic patients.

This concept of psychiatric dizziness has several problems: (1) vertigo does not distinguish psychiatric from otologic disorders, (2) hyperventilation can cause symptoms in many disorders, and (3) patients with psychiatric illness are not immune to otologic disorders. Furthermore, fear and anxiety are common symptoms in patients with vestibular disease. A more restricted definition of psychiatric dizziness is dizziness that occurs in combination with other symptoms as part of a recognized psychiatric symptom cluster that is not itself related to vestibular function.

Panic disorder is the psychiatric diagnosis that includes dizziness, vertigo, or unsteady feelings as a diagnostic criterion. Patients with depressive symptoms may describe the difficulty they have with concentrating as a "dizzy" or "swimming" feeling. Dizziness as part of a conversion disorder or malingering is rare. Dizziness and imbalance are not features of personality disorders.

It is important not to confuse psychogenic overlay, or the amplification of somatic concerns, with psychiatric dizziness. Many patients have a tendency to exaggerate their symptoms and complicate the diagnosis. Patients with hypochondriacal concerns are prone to exaggeration. Psychogenic overlay is seen frequently in patients with depressive, panic, or somatoform disorders. It is important to remember that many patients experience more than one kind of dizziness.

SUGGESTED READING

Baloh, RW, and Jacobson, KM: Neurotology. Neurol Clin 14:85–101, 1996.

Baloh, RW, et al: Neurotology. Continuum 2:9–132, 1996.

Fisher, CM: Vomiting out of proportion to dizziness in ischemic brainstem strokes. Neurology 46:267, 1996.

Furman, JM, and Jacob, RG: Psychiatric dizziness. Neurology 48:1161–1166, 1997.

Gizzi, M, Riley, E, and Molinari, S: The diagnostic value of imaging the patient with dizziness. A Bayesian approach. Arch Neurol 53:1299–1304, 1996.

Gomez, CR, et al: Isolated vertigo as a manifestation of vertebrobasilar ischemia. Neurology 47:94–97, 1996.

Guldin, WO, and Grusser, OJ: Is there a vestibular cortex? Trends Neurosci 21:254–259, 1998.

Lanska, DJ, and Remler, B: Benign paroxysmal positioning vertigo: Classic descriptions, origins of the provocative positioning technique, and conceptual developments. Neurology 48:1167–1177, 1997.

Low, PA: Diabetic autonomic neuropathy. Semin Neurol 16:143–151, 1996.

Robertson, D, and Davis, TL: Recent advances in the treatment of orthostatic hypotension. Neurology 45 (Suppl 5):S26-S32, 1995.

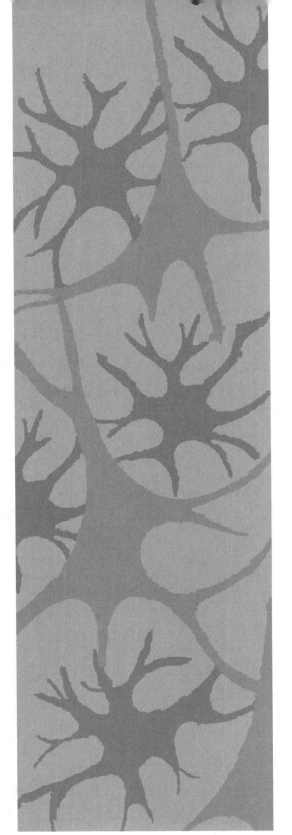

CHAPTER 6

Sensory Loss and Paresthesias

CHAPTER OUTLINE

Diagnostic Approach
Diabetic Neuropathy
    Generalized Sensorimotor
        Polyneuropathy
    Diabetic Autonomic Neuropathy
    Diabetic Polyradiculoneuropathy
    Truncal Neuropathy
    Mononeuropathy
Neuropathy of Other Endocrine
    Disorders
Metabolic Neuropathies
    Nutritional Disorders
    Chronic Renal Failure
    Porphyria
    Critical Illness
Toxic Neuropathies
Connective Tissue Disease
Dysproteinemic Polyneuropathy
Infectious Neuropathy
Inflammatory Neuropathies
    Acute Inflammatory Demyelinating
        Polyneuropathy
    Chronic Inflammatory Demyelinating
        Polyradiculoneuropathy

(continued)

Focal Neuropathies
Carpal Tunnel Syndrome
Other Compression Neuropathies

A 57-year-old woman complains that she has had increasing numbness and tingling in her feet for the last 9 to 12 months. She wants to know what is going on, if her symptoms can be treated, and what she can expect. Examination shows mild orthostatic changes on blood pressure recording, decreased pin and vibratory sensation in the distal lower extremities, absence of ankle reflexes, difficulty with tandem gait, and excessive sway on the Romberg test. Do you perform additional diagnostic testing? What laboratory tests do you order? How do you respond to her questions?

This patient has a clinical history and examination findings consistent with neuropathy, or disease of the peripheral nervous system. The diagnostic possibilities are many and include endocrinopathies, malignancies, infections, and metabolic, toxic, inflammatory, and genetic disorders. Addressing all the potential causes of a polyneuropathy is impractical. Despite a thorough evaluation, it is estimated that a cause will not be identified in almost one-half of patients with neuropathy (13% to 22% at specialty centers). Diagnosis is essential, to avoid missing a correctable neuropathy and to provide accurate prognostic information. This chapter considers the common polyneuropathies and focal neuropathies that underlie patients' complaints of sensory loss and paresthesias (spontaneous abnormal sensations).

DIAGNOSTIC APPROACH

The anatomy of a peripheral nerve is shown in Figure 6–1. Disease of peripheral nerves may involve motor, sensory, and autonomic nerve fibers (axons). Motor fibers and sensory fibers that convey vibration and joint position sensation are large myelinated axons. Autonomic fibers are small myelinated axons, and sensory fibers that convey temperature and pain sensation are small myelinated and unmyelinated axons. The symptoms that a patient with disease of the peripheral nervous system reports and the signs that you may find on examining the patient are summarized in Table 6–1.

In evaluating a patient who has sensory loss or paresthesias, first determine whether there is disease of the peripheral nervous system. Some of the many disorders that may mimic peripheral nerve disease are listed in Table 6–2. After you establish that the patient has disease of the peripheral nervous system, determine whether the pattern of involvement is focal, multifocal, or diffuse. Localization of the neuropathy should answer many questions. Does the process involve an individual nerve, nerve root, plexus, or several nerves? If the neuropathy is diffuse, is it symmetric? Does the process affect distal or proximal aspects of the extremities? Localization is based on the clinical examination and can be supplemented by electrodiagnostic tests. Knowledge of the distribution of individual nerves and patterns of sensory involvement helps you localize the problem (see Figs. 1–11 and 1–12).

Most neuropathies are symmetric, and the patient has distal symptoms and findings. This reflects axonal degeneration, the most common type of pathologic process, with injury to the distal ends of the longest nerves. Thus, patients report sensory loss and paresthesias in their feet. Large-fiber paresthesias are often described as "pins and needles" or an "electric sensation." These neuropathies have the common stocking-glove pattern. The fingers usually are not affected until the "stocking" pattern is at the level of the upper calf. In rare neuropathies like porphyria and some inflammatory demyelinating neuropathies, proximal areas can be involved before distal areas. The common physical

104

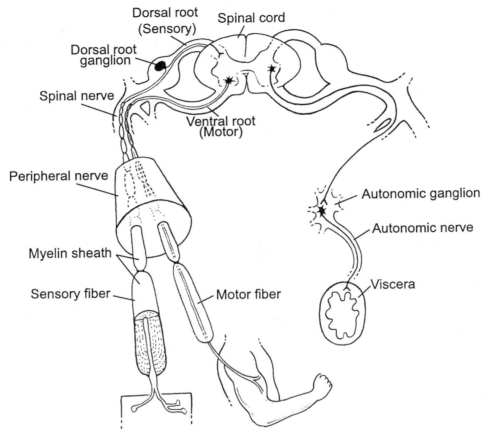

FIG. 6–1. Structure of a peripheral nerve. (Redrawn from Leeson, TS, and Leeson, CR: Histology, ed 4. WB Saunders, Philadelphia, 1981, p 218, with permission.)

TABLE 6–1. GENERAL CLINICAL FEATURES OF PERIPHERAL NERVOUS SYSTEM DISEASE

Nerve	Historical Symptoms	Physical Signs
Sensory	Numbness Tingling, burning, "pins and needles" sensation Clumsiness	Sensory loss, areflexia, hypotonia, ataxia
Motor	Weakness, clumsiness, cramps, muscle twitches	Weakness, atrophy, fasciculations, areflexia, hypotonia, deformities (pes cavus, kyphoscoliosis)
Autonomic	Lightheadedness, fainting, excessive sweating, heat intolerance, impotence, bowel and bladder disturbance	Orthostatic blood pressure changes, hyperhidrosis, anhidrosis, pupil abnormalities

TABLE 6-2. DISORDERS THAT MIMIC PERIPHERAL NERVE DISEASE

Symptom/Sign	Disorder	Distinguishing Clinical Feature
Generalized weakness	Myopathy, myasthenia gravis, motor neuron disease	Normal sensation
Sensory symptoms	Myelopathies	Sensory level
	Multiple sclerosis	Upper motor neuron signs
	Syringomyelia, dorsal column disease (tabes dorsalis)	Sensory dissociation
Multiple symptoms	Conversion disorder, somatoform disorder	Nonanatomical features
	Malingering	Secondary gain, disability issues

findings in a length-dependent axonal neuropathy are reduced sensation distally in the lower extremities, reduced or absent ankle reflexes, Romberg sign, and difficulty performing tandem gait. The woman in the above case study likely has a length-dependent axonal polyneuropathy. If the patient has difficulty walking on the toes and heels, suspect motor involvement. Significant weakness may result in footdrop. Muscle bulk may be reduced in the interossei muscles of the hands or in the extensor digitorum muscles of the feet (Fig. 6–2). Anhidrotic skin, pupil abnormalities, and orthostatic changes in blood pressure and pulse recordings indicate involvement of autonomic nerves.

Patients with small-fiber neuropathies may have few abnormal findings on neurologic examination except for reduced pain and touch sensation in the distal lower extremities. They often complain of painful burning dysesthesias. Other adjectives used to describe their paresthesias include "stinging," "coldness," and "heat." Nonpainful stim-

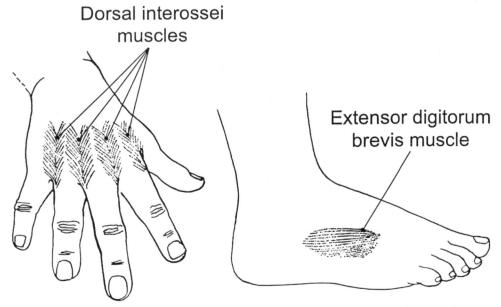

FIG. 6–2. Topography of the interosseous muscles of the hand and the extensor digitorum brevis muscle of the foot.

uli such as a sheet or blanket covering the feet can be painful (allodynia). The findings on electrodiagnostic tests are often normal. Important causes of small-fiber neuropathies are diabetes mellitus, amyloidosis, human immunodeficiency virus (HIV), acquired immunodeficiency syndrome (AIDS), and alcoholic neuropathy. Small-fiber neuropathies involve the autonomic nervous system. Diabetes mellitus is the most common cause of an autonomic neuropathy. If a patient has an autonomic neuropathy but does not have diabetes, consider amyloidosis.

Asymmetry is an important finding and suggests a mononeuropathy multiplex pattern, a superimposed radiculopathy, an entrapment mononeuropathy, or an acquired demyelinating neuropathy. The pattern of mononeuropathy multiplex is distinct from that of a length-dependent "dying back" axonal neuropathy. Individual cranial nerves and peripheral nerves are involved in an asymmetric stepwise progression. Over time, the pattern may become confluent and difficult to distinguish from a generalized polyneuropathy. The temporal profile of symptoms is helpful in this regard. Mononeuropathy multiplex is important to recognize because many of its causes can be treated. Disorders associated with mononeuropathy multiplex include vasculitis, leprosy, sarcoidosis, chronic inflammatory polyradiculoneuropathy, some malignancies, diabetes mellitus, and HIV infection or AIDS.

The patient's history provides the temporal course, or how the neuropathy has evolved over time. Most neuropathies are chronic and slowly progressive; thus, whether the onset is acute or subacute limits the extensive differential diagnosis. Acute inflammatory demyelinating polyradiculoneuropathy, or Guillain-Barré syndrome, has an onset of days to weeks. A mononeuropathy multiplex pattern is suggested if the neuropathy progresses in a stepwise fashion. A history of relapsing and remitting sensory symptoms suggests either autoimmune inflammatory neuropathy or an exposure or intoxication. Neuropathies that can be differentiated by their clinical course are listed in Table 6–3.

The next major distinction to make is whether the neuropathy is acquired or hereditary. This distinction may be difficult because patients with inherited polyneuropathy are asymptomatic for a long time. Inherited neuropathies begin gradually and progress very slowly. The family history may be negative or a family history of "polio" or "arthritis" may in fact represent an inherited neuropathy. The important clues to an inherited neuropathy include skeletal abnormalities of the foot (pes cavus) (Fig. 6–3)

TABLE 6–3. NEUROPATHY DIFFERENTIAL DIAGNOSIS BY TEMPORAL PROFILE

Acute (Days)	Subacute (Weeks to Months)	Relapsing-Remitting Course
AIDP	CIDP	AIDP
Porphyria	Paraneoplastic	CIDP
Infarction (vasculitis)	syndrome	Porphyria
Diabetes mellitus	Continued toxic	HIV/AIDS
(amyotrophy)	exposure	Toxic
Diphtheria	Abnormal metabolic	
Toxins (thallium,	state	
arsenic)	Persisting nutritional	
Tick paralysis	deficiency	
Trauma		
Critical illness		
neuropathy		

AIDP, acute inflammatory demyelinating polyneuropathy; AIDS, acquired immunodeficiency syndrome; CIDP, chronic inflammatory demyelinating polyneuropathy; HIV, human immunodeficiency virus.

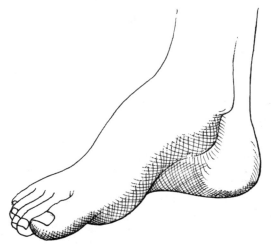

FIG. 6–3. Pes cavus.

and spine (kyphoscoliosis), the absence of positive sensory phenomena, and positive findings in asymptomatic family members. Hereditary motor sensory neuropathies include most of the inherited neuropathies and account for many of the cases in which diagnosis is difficult. The genetic understanding of these disorders is rapidly increasing, and many genetic tests are available. The diagnosis of an inherited neuropathy is important for prognosis and genetic counseling.

Clues to systemic and other medical illnesses associated with peripheral neuropathies are provided by the general history and physical examination findings. It is important to look for historical and physical

evidence of diabetes mellitus and other endocrinopathies, cancer, connective tissue disorders, infections, and deficiency states. The patient's occupational and exposure history is significant in narrowing the differential diagnosis of neuropathy. Alcohol is a frequent cause of a toxic neuropathy. In addition, any prescription and over-the-counter medications can cause neuropathy (Table 6–4). Most of these drugs damage peripheral nerve axons. Amiodarone, chloroquine, and gold cause a demyelinating neuropathy, and cisplatin, pyridoxine, and thalidomide injure neurons.

Electrodiagnostic tests are invaluable in evaluating patients who have sensory loss and paresthesias due to disease of peripheral nerves. Electromyography and nerve conduction studies confirm the presence of a neuropathy, help localize the neuropathy (focal, multifocal, diffuse), determine the fiber type (motor, sensory), and predict the pathologic process (e.g., demyelinating or axonal neuropathy). Electrodiagnostic tests can also provide information about symmetry, chronicity, and severity. The important diagnostic distinction between demyelinating and axonal neuropathies cannot be made without electrodiagnostic tests. Because most neuropathies are axonal, the presence of a demyelinating neuropathy restricts the differential diagnosis. In axonal neuropathy, the amplitude of the nerve action potentials is reduced and, on needle examination, denervation potentials are found in the affected muscles. The findings consis-

TABLE 6–4. COMMON DRUGS ASSOCIATED WITH NEUROPATHY	
Amiodarone (Cordarone)	Gold (Myochrysine)
Amitriptyline (Elavil, Endep)	Hydralazine (Apresoline)
Chloroquine (Aralen)	Immunizations
Cimetidine (Tagamet)	Isoniazid, INH (Nydrazid)
Cisplatin (Platinol)	Lithium (Eskalith, Lithobid)
Clioquinol (nonprescription antidiarrheal medicines) (Vioform)	Metronidazole (Flagyl)
	Nitrofurantoin (Furadantin, Macrodantin)
Colchicine and probenecid (ColBENEMID)	Nitrous oxide
Dapsone (Avlosulfon)	Paclitaxel (Taxol)
Didanosine (Videx)	Phenytoin (Dilantin)
Disulfiram (Antabuse)	Pyridoxine (Beesix)
Ethambutol (Myambutol)	Thalidomide (Synovir)
	Vincristine (Oncovin, Vincasar PFS)

tent with a demyelinating neuropathy include slow nerve conduction velocities, prolonged distal latencies, temporal dispersion, and prolonged F-wave latencies. Hereditary demyelinating neuropathies are characterized by uniform slowing of nerve conduction. Acquired demyelinating neuropathies show nonuniform slowing and can be distinguished further by their temporal profile. Demyelinating neuropathies are listed in Table 6–5.

It is important to remember the limitations of electrodiagnostic tests. Electromyography and nerve conduction studies examine large myelinated nerve fibers. Thus, the findings of these tests can be normal in a patient with a small-fiber neuropathy. Proximal sensory nerves cannot be tested, and in normal elderly subjects, lower extremity sensory responses can be reduced or absent. Remember, electrodiagnostic tests are an extension of the clinical examination and are operator-dependent.

A large number of laboratory tests are available to evaluate polyneuropathy. A reasonable screening evaluation for the common distal symmetric neuropathies includes determining the following values: fasting serum glucose, glycosylated hemoglobin, blood urea nitrogen, creatinine, complete blood count, erythrocyte sedimentation rate, urinalysis, vitamin B_{12}, and thyroid-stimulating hormone. Many neurologists include serum protein electrophoresis in the initial screening evaluation. Other important laboratory tests may be indicated on the basis of the patient's clinical presentation or the results of the screening evaluation. If there is no evidence of connective tissue disease on clinical examination, the diagnostic yield from connective tissue laboratory tests is extremely low. Similarly, paraneoplastic antibodies are less helpful than chest radiography, breast examination, and stool guaiac testing for an underlying neoplasm. The exception to this is testing for anti-Hu or antineuronal nuclear antibody in a patient with a sensory neuronopathy and the possibility of small cell carcinoma of the lung. Many tests are available that detect antibodies to the glycolipids associated with peripheral nerves. Clinically useful tests include myelin-associated glycoprotein antibody (associated with chronic inflammatory demyelinating polyneuropathy) and anti-ganglioside antibody (associated with multifocal motor neuropathy with conduction block). Antibody panels are expensive and can lead to inappropriate treatment. Neurologic consultation may be useful to determine the appropriate clinical setting for these tests. Laboratory tests used in the evaluation of neuropathy are summarized in Table 6–6.

Nerve biopsy is valuable for a limited number of diagnostic possibilities. The rare conditions that demonstrate characteristic findings include vasculitis, amyloidosis, sarcoidosis, leprosy, and leukodystrophies. Progressive demyelinating neuropathies may require biopsy if the diagnosis remains in question after electrodiagnostic testing. The nerve usually selected for biopsy is the sural nerve. Painful dysesthesias and poor healing complicate this procedure.

TABLE 6–5. DEMYELINATING NEUROPATHIES

Hereditary—uniform demyelination

HMSN-I, -III, -IV
Hereditary predisposition to pressure palsy

Acquired—nonuniform demyelination

Acute

AIDP
Acute arsenic intoxication
Diphtheria

Subacute/chronic

CIDP
Multifocal conduction block
Osteosclerotic myeloma
MGUS

AIDP, acute inflammatory demyelinating polyneuropathy; CIDP, chronic inflammatory demyelinating polyneuropathy; HMSN, hereditary motor and sensory neuropathy; MGUS, monoclonal gammopathy of undetermined significance.

DIABETIC NEUROPATHY

"Diabetic neuropathy" describes the many disorders of the peripheral nervous system that are related to diabetes mellitus. Diabetic neuropathy is the most common neuropathy

TABLE 6–6. LABORATORY TESTS USED IN EVALUATION OF NEUROPATHY

Test	Clinical Condition Detected
Glucose	Diabetes mellitus
Glycosylated hemoglobin	Diabetes mellitus
Blood urea nitrogen	Renal, metabolic
Creatinine	Renal, metabolic
Complete blood count	Hematologic, vasculitis
Erythrocyte sedimentation rate, antinuclear antibody, rheumatoid factor, complement, immunoelectrophoresis, hepatitis B antigen and antibody, eosinophil count, antineutrophil cytoplasmic antibody, anti-extractable nuclear antigen, cryoglobulins	Inflammation, vasculitis, other connective tissue disorders
Urinalysis	Renal, metabolic, vasculitis
Vitamin B_{12} methylmalonic acid, homocysteine	Vitamin B_{12} deficiency
Thyroid-stimulating hormone	Endocrine
Serum protein electrophoresis, serum and urine immunoelectrophoresis, skeletal survey, bone marrow aspiration	Hematologic, malignancy, amyloidosis, multiple myeloma, osteosclerotic myeloma, Waldenström macroglobulinemia, cryoglobulinemia, lymphoma, leukemia
Human immunodeficiency virus	Acquired immunodeficiency syndrome
Lyme serology	Lyme disease
Syphilis serology	Syphilis
Anti-neuronal nuclear antibody or anti-Hu antibody	Malignancy
Cerebrospinal fluid	Demyelinating neuropathies, vasculitis
Angiotensin-converting enzyme	Sarcoidosis
Heavy metal screen	Lead, mercury, arsenic
Fat aspirate	Amyloid
Porphyrin, porphobilinogen deaminase, uroporphyrin synthetase	Porphyria
Myelin-associated glycoprotein antibody	Chronic inflammatory demyelinating polyneuropathy
Anti-ganglioside antibody	Multifocal motor neuropathy with conduction block
Phytanic acid	Refsum disease
Molecular genetic analysis	Hereditary motor sensory neuropathy-IA, hereditary neuropathy for pressure palsy, familial amyloid polyneuropathies

in the Western world and, because of its high incidence and significant morbidity and mortality, deserves special attention (Table 6–7).

GENERALIZED SENSORIMOTOR POLYNEUROPATHY

The most frequent type of diabetic neuropathy is generalized sensorimotor polyneuropathy. Although this is common and frequently the cause of neurologic complications, it is prudent to use diabetic neuropathy as a diagnosis of exclusion to avoid missing other serious causes of neuropathy. Generalized sensorimotor neuropathy is length-dependent and has the stocking-glove type of sensory pattern. Patients may be asymptomatic or complain of paresthesias of the feet. Although this neuropathy is related to the severity and duration of diabetes, it can be the presenting symptom of diabetes.

Generalized sensorimotor polyneuropathy usually has a slow and insidious course, with minimal motor involvement. Infrequently, it can be more rapid, painful, and associated

TABLE 6–7. TYPES OF DIABETIC NEUROPATHY AND THEIR CLINICAL FEATURES

Type	Clinical Features
Generalized sensorimotor polyneuropathy	Stocking-glove sensory distribution, paresthesias in feet
	Minimal motor findings
Autonomic neuropathy	Orthostatic hypotension
	Pupil abnormalities
	Gastrointestinal, genitourinary, cardiovascular signs and symptoms
Diabetic polyneuropathy, diabetic amyotrophy, trunk neuropathy (thoracic radiculoneuropathy)	Acute to subacute painful asymmetric proximal nerve involvement
Mononeuropathy	Carpal tunnel syndrome
Mononeuropathy multiplex	Multiple nerve involvement in a stepwise progression
Cranial neuropathy	Pupil-sparing CN III palsy

CN, cranial nerve.

with weight loss. The polyneuropathy affects both small and large fibers, but some patients have predominantly either small- or large-fiber involvement. Sensory symptoms usually develop slowly and begin in the feet and move proximally. Patients complain of burning feet or "pins and needles." The symptoms tend to be more pronounced at night and can interfere with sleep. Although motor involvement is usually minimal, foot-drop can occur. A severe form of osteoarthritis of the feet (Charcot, or neuropathic, joint) may occur because of the loss of pain and proprioception. Diabetic neuropathy is also a major risk factor for the development of foot ulcers.

Treatment of diabetic neuropathy begins with good control of the patient's blood glucose level. Glycemic control affects the development and progression of diabetic neuropathy. Proper care of the feet is extremely important to avoid foot ulcers. Treatment has been directed mainly at symptomatic control of the pain and paresthesias (Table 6–8). The use of aldose reductase inhibitors, essential fatty acids, and antioxidants to treat neuropathy is being investigated.

DIABETIC AUTONOMIC NEUROPATHY

Diabetic autonomic neuropathy is also a length-dependent neuropathy, and the level of the neuropathy is correlated with the severity of somatic nerve findings. Numerous organs are affected by autonomic neuropathy. Because the pupillary light response is abnormal, patients may complain that they have trouble seeing in dim light. Decreased vagal tone causes an increase in resting heart rate. As the neuropathy becomes more severe, orthostatic hypotension may occur. Gastroparesis may cause postprandial nausea, bloating, and early satiety. Other gastrointestinal symptoms are constipation and nocturnal diarrhea. Genitourinary effects of autonomic neuropathy include decreased sensation of bladder filling, incomplete emptying, impotence, and reduced vaginal secretions and lubrication. Sweating is usually decreased in a stocking-glove pattern, and severe compensatory hyperhidrosis may occur on the face and torso.

It can be difficult to treat autonomic neuropathy. The standard initial treatment of orthostatic hypotension includes a high-salt diet (10 to 20 g/day), increased fluid intake (>20 oz/day), elevation of the head of the bed by 4 inches, and use of compressive stockings. Drug treatment is discussed in Chapter 5 (see Table 5–8). Gastroparesis may be helped by having patients eat small meals low in carbohydrates. Metoclopramide and cisapride may be helpful. Diarrhea can be treated with tetracycline, erythromycin, cholestyramine, or clonidine. Constipation may respond to adequate hydration and psyllium. Laxatives may

TABLE 6–8. DRUGS FOR TREATING DIABETIC NEUROPATHIC PAIN	
Drug	**Comment**
Tricyclic Antidepressant Agents Amitriptyline (Elavil) 10–100 mg at bedtime Nortriptyline (Pamelor) 10–100 mg at bedtime	Anticholinergic side effects can aggravate autonomic neuropathy, helpful for sleep
Anticonvulsant Agents Gabapentin (Neurontin) 1,800–3,600 mg/day in 3 divided doses Carbamazepine (Tegretol) 200 mg 3 times daily Phenytoin (Dilantin) 300 mg daily	Best for paroxysmal pain
Topical Agent Capsaicin (Zostrix) 3–4 times daily	Limitations of applying on large surface area
Antiarrhythmic Agents Mexiletine (Mexitil) 150 mg/day, increase 10 mg/kg daily in divided doses	Cardiac arrhythmias, gastrointestinal disturbance, dizziness, tremor
Analgesic Tramadol (Ultram) 50–100 mg every 6 hr	Seizure risk

be necessary. Scheduled voiding and self-catheterization may be needed for trouble with voiding. Seek urologic consultation for treating impotence.

DIABETIC POLYRADICULONEUROPATHY

Diabetic polyradiculoneuropathy includes several clinical syndromes that affect the proximal nerves in an asymmetric fashion. Diabetic amyotrophy (sometimes referred to as "lumbosacral polyradiculoneuropathy" or "Bruns-Garland syndrome") and limb and trunk neuropathies are included in this category. Diabetic amyotrophy usually involves the L2-L4 roots and tends to occur in patients with non-insulin-dependent diabetes who are older than 60 years. It is not related to the duration of the patient's glucose intolerance. Severe pain in the back, hip, buttock, or anterior thigh may be the presenting symptom. Clinical findings include proximal and distal muscle weakness, reduced or absent quadriceps reflex, and atrophy. The temporal course may be acute to subacute, stepwise, or progressive. Typically, improvement occurs in weeks to months. Pain is a promi-

nent feature and often requires treatment with narcotic analgesics. Other diagnoses to consider are intraspinal lesion, lumbar plexopathy, and femoral neuropathy. Electrodiagnostic tests and magnetic resonance imaging of the spine may be needed to exclude other serious diagnostic possibilities.

TRUNCAL NEUROPATHY

Sudden stabbing pain in the chest, abdomen, or thoracic spine may represent a diabetic truncal neuropathy. Patients often attribute the pain to an intra-abdominal process or a heart attack. The absence of any relationship to eating, position, activity, or coughing distinguishes this pain from gastrointestinal, cardiovascular, or pulmonary disease. In most patients, thoracic polyradiculoneuropathy improves within several months to a year.

MONONEUROPATHY

Patients with diabetes have a high incidence of mononeuropathy. Compression, or entrapment, of the median nerve (carpal tunnel) and compression of the ulnar nerve (cubital tunnel) are frequent upper extremity mononeuropathies. Decompression surgery may be necessary to maintain function, even for patients who have both a compression neuropathy and a generalized polyneuropathy. The peroneal nerve at the head of the fibula and the lateral femoral cutaneous nerve are frequently affected in the lower extremity. Diabetes can cause a mononeuritis multiplex.

Cranial nerves affected by diabetes include CN III, IV, and VI. Although CN VII is often included in this list, it is uncertain that it should be because of the high frequency of involvement of CN VII in nondiabetic patients in the general population. The most common cranial neuropathy is the pupil-sparing CN III palsy. A patient with this nerve palsy may complain of periorbital pain, droopy eyelid, and double vision. The affected eye has ptosis and a pupil that is responsive to light; the eye is positioned down and out. Because the pupilloconstrictor fibers are located in the periphery of CN III nerve, pupil sparing is thought to exclude a compressive lesion. Despite this clinical finding, neuroimaging is recommended to exclude other causes. Recovery usually occurs in 2 to 5 months.

NEUROPATHY OF OTHER ENDOCRINE DISORDERS

Peripheral neuropathies are not commonly associated with other endocrine disorders. Hypothyroidism and hyperthyroidism may be associated with carpal tunnel syndrome and, rarely, a distal neuropathy. Acromegaly is also associated with carpal tunnel syndrome and a distal polyneuropathy. Hyperparathyroidism can mimic motor neuron disease, with weakness, sparse sensory abnormalities, and hyperreflexia.

METABOLIC NEUROPATHIES

A large number of metabolic disorders are associated with neuropathy. Most metabolic neuropathies are axonal in type, associated with systemic disease, and demonstrate a length-dependent pattern. In addition to the neuropathies from endocrine disease, metabolic neuropathies are caused by nutritional disorders, chronic renal failure, porphyria, and critical illness polyneuropathy.

NUTRITIONAL DISORDERS

Nutritional disorders in developed countries are due to chronic alcoholism, malabsorption, abnormal diet, or drug toxicity. Malabsorption of vitamin B_{12} (cyanocobalamin) is a common deficiency disorder associated with peripheral neuropathy, myelopathy, and dementia. Defective production of intrinsic factor, the vitamin B_{12} binding protein secreted by gastric parietal cells, is the most common cause. This can result from various gastrointestinal disorders or from a genetic predisposition (pernicious anemia). Pernicious anemia is frequent in African-Americans and northern Europeans.

Patients may have gradual onset of paresthesias in the hands and feet. Large-fiber sensory function is affected preferentially. The neurologic examination may show reduced vibratory and joint position sense in the feet and a Romberg sign. Reflexes may be increased or decreased, depending on involvement of the spinal cord. Distal sensory loss associated with brisk reflexes indicates a peripheral sensory loss and spinal cord involvement. If a patient has reduced distal sensation and extensor plantar reflexes, consider vitamin B_{12} deficiency. This common correctable disorder should be sought in any patient with suspected peripheral neuropathy. A low serum level of vitamin B_{12} confirms the diagnosis. Other supportive laboratory results include increased levels of homocysteine and methylmalonic acid. The Schilling test can evaluate intrinsic factor function. Treatment is 1,000 μg of cyanocobalamin intramuscularly daily for 1 week and then monthly thereafter.

Neuropathies associated with a deficiency of vitamin B_1 (beriberi), vitamin B_2, niacin (pellagra), or vitamin E are rare. Vitamin B_1, or thiamine, deficiency is associated most often with alcoholism. Pyridoxine, or vitamin

B$_6$, deficiency is usually caused by a medication, for example, isoniazid, penicillamine, hydralazine, or cycloserine. Riboflavin, or vitamin B$_2$, deficiency is associated with "burning feet syndrome." Hypophosphatemia from hyperalimentation can cause a subacute neuropathy resembling Guillain-Barré syndrome.

CHRONIC RENAL FAILURE

Peripheral nerve involvement in chronic renal failure includes uremic polyneuropathy, carpal tunnel syndrome, and ischemic mononeuropathy. Ischemic mononeuropathy can occur in relation to the arteriovenous fistula used in hemodialysis.

PORPHYRIA

Porphyrias, rare hereditary disorders of heme biosynthesis, are associated with polyneuropathy and primarily affect motor nerves. Involvement of the facial, bulbar, and proximal arm muscles is common. Porphyria should be considered in a patient with neuropathy who has gastrointestinal and/or neuropsychiatric symptoms.

CRITICAL ILLNESS

Critically ill patients in an intensive care unit often have diffuse neuromuscular weakness. Many of these patients are thought to have a neuropathy of critical illness, although this diagnosis is controversial. Prolonged ventilator dependence, sepsis, and multiple organ failure are associated with this condition.

TOXIC NEUROPATHIES

Many toxins can cause peripheral neuropathy. The most common toxins are pharmaceutical and iatrogenic. Occupational neuropathy is uncommon in North America. Most often, toxic neuropathies are distal axonal neuropathies that demonstrate a length-dependent symmetric sensory and/or motor loss. Most toxic agents show a strong dose-response relationship and a consistent pattern of disease related to the dose and duration of exposure. Neuropathic symptoms coincide or soon follow toxic exposure. After exposure has been eliminated, neuropathic signs and symptoms should improve. Persons with preexistent neuropathies are more susceptible to neurotoxins. Some of the industrial and environmental toxins that cause peripheral neuropathy are listed in Table 6–9.

Chemotherapeutic agents that cause peripheral neuropathies include paclitaxel alkaloids (Taxol), platinum agents (cisplatin), and vinca alkaloids (vincristine and vinblastine). Paclitaxel is used to treat ovarian and breast cancers. The associated neuropathy is primarily sensory. Platinum agents are also associated with a sensory neuropathy, with significant loss of proprioception that results in gait ataxia. Vinca alkaloids affect sensory, motor, and autonomic nerves. The adverse effects of these anticancer drugs can be exaggerated by the presence of coexisting diseases such as diabetes mellitus, renal failure, and nutritional deficits. Other pharmaceutical agents that cause neuropathy are listed in Table 6–4.

CONNECTIVE TISSUE DISEASE

Connective tissue diseases, or collagen-vascular disorders, are systemic illnesses frequently associated with neuropathy. Neuropathy may be the initial manifestation of an undiagnosed connective tissue disease. As with diabetes mellitus, numerous neuropathies are associated with connective tissue disease, including mononeuropathy multiplex, asymmetric polyneuropathy, distal symmetric polyneuropathy, compression neuropathy, trigeminal sensory neuropathy, and sensory neuronopathy. Patients with connective tissue disease may have more than one type of neuropathy, as well.

Connective tissue diseases can be associated with vasculitic neuropathies. These require immediate diagnosis and treatment to improve patient outcome. Vasculitic neuropathy is caused by inflammatory occlusion

TABLE 6–9. OCCUPATIONAL AND ENVIRONMENTAL TOXINS

Toxin	Environmental/Occupational Use or Setting
Acrylamide	Flocculators and grouting agents
Allyl chloride	Pesticides
Arsenic	Suicides and homicides
Carbon disulfide	Production of rayon, cellophane film
Cyanide	Cassava consumption
Ethylene oxide	Sterilization of medical equipment
Hexacarbons	Glue sniffing
Lead	Paint, battery manufacturing, moonshine whiskey
Mercury	Battery manufacturing, electronics
Methyl bromide	Fumigant, fire extinguisher, refrigerant, insecticide
Organophosphates	Insecticides, petroleum additives, flame retardants
Polychlorinated biphenyls	Industrial insulation
Thallium	Rodenticides, insecticides
Trichloroethylene	Industrial solvent
Vacor	Rodenticides

of blood vessels, which leads to ischemic infarction of nerves. It can occur with any of the connective tissue disorders, but it is usually associated with polyarteritis nodosa and rheumatoid arthritis. A vasculitic neuropathy usually has a mononeuropathy multiplex pattern. However, an asymmetric polyneuropathy, multifocal mononeuropathies with partial confluence, or distal sensory polyneuropathies can occur. The peroneal nerve in the lower extremity and the ulnar nerve in the upper extremity are particularly vulnerable to infarction. The first symptom may be aching in the extremity, followed by burning pain, tingling, and sensory and motor loss in the distribution of the affected nerve. The diagnosis is confirmed by finding arteritis in nerve biopsy specimens. In persons with known connective tissue disease who present with mononeuritis multiplex and multifocal axon loss, the diagnosis can be made with electrodiagnostic tests. Treat with immunosuppressive agents.

A sensory neuronopathy is unique to Sjögren syndrome. This neuropathy results from inflammation of dorsal root ganglia. The typical presentation is that of a middle-aged woman with sensory symptoms, clumsiness,

and ataxic gait. Large-fiber sensory loss is predominant, with loss of vibration and joint position sense. Treat with immunosuppressive agents.

Many connective tissue diseases, especially systemic sclerosis and mixed connective tissue disease, are associated with trigeminal sensory neuropathy. The patient may complain of slowly progressive unilateral or bilateral facial numbness. If a patient has facial numbness and negative findings on imaging studies, consider the possibility of connective tissue disease. The various connective tissue disorders and their associated neuropathies are summarized in Table 6–10.

DYSPROTEINEMIC POLYNEUROPATHY

Dysproteinemias, or plasma cell dyscrasias, are frequently associated with peripheral nerve disease. These disorders, also called "monoclonal gammopathies," produce excessive amounts of monoclonal proteins, also called "M proteins" (M spike seen on serum electrophoresis), or immunoglobu-

TABLE 6–10. CONNECTIVE TISSUE DISEASES AND ASSOCIATED NEUROPATHIES

Connective Tissue Disease	Vasculitic Neuropathy	Distal Symmetric Neuropathy	Compression Neuropathy	Sensory Neuronopathy	Trigeminal Sensory Neuropathy
Polyarteritis nodosa	+++	++			+
Rheumatoid arthritis	++	+++	+++		+
Systemic lupus erythematosus	+	++	+		+
Sjögren syndrome	+	++	+	+++	++
Systemic sclerosis	+	+	+		+++
Mixed connective tissue	++	+			+++

+, common; ++, more common; +++, most common.

lins, that may injure a nerve directly by reacting with antigens in the myelin sheaths and axonal membranes. Nerves may also be injured by the deposition of amyloid, a byproduct of M proteins, or paraproteins.

Common plasma cell dyscrasias include monoclonal gammopathy of undetermined significance (MGUS), osteosclerotic myeloma, multiple myeloma, Waldenström macroglobulinemia, cryoglobulinemia, and primary systemic amyloidosis. The clinical presentation of these disorders varies, but most patients have distal neuropathic signs and symptoms. Amyloidosis is unique because of the presence of autonomic symptoms. Serum protein electrophoresis is a reasonable screen for these disorders. However, if the patient has an idiopathic polyneuropathy, perform the more sensitive immunoelectrophoresis or immunofixation on serum and urine. Additional studies include bone marrow evaluation, metastatic skeletal bone survey, and biopsy of other appropriate tissues.

Dysproteinemic neuropathies are important to recognize because they may precede several systemic and lymphoproliferative disorders. For example, a malignant plasma cell dyscrasia develops in 20% to 25% of patients with MGUS. Neuropathies associated with paraproteinemia often respond to treatment (Table 6–11).

INFECTIOUS NEUROPATHY

Several infectious diseases are associated with polyneuropathy. These include leprosy, HIV, Lyme disease, syphilis, and herpes zoster radiculitis or cranial neuritis (shingles). These are discussed further in the chapter covering infectious disease (Chapter 13).

INFLAMMATORY NEUROPATHIES

ACUTE INFLAMMATORY DEMYELINATING POLYNEUROPATHY

A 50-year-old woman complains that she has had numbness and tingling in her extremities for the last week. She also reports having some mild back pain. She had been well except for an episode of gastroenteritis 3 weeks earlier. Examination reveals some mild proximal and distal weakness in her lower extremities, mild facial weakness, and diffuse hyporeflexia. What do you do next?

This patient has the signs and symptoms typical of an acute inflammatory demyelinating polyneuropathy (AIDP) or Guillain-Barré syndrome. She should be hospitalized. AIDP is the most common cause of acute generalized weakness and can occur at any age. Most patients describe an antecedent viral infection. *Campylobacter jejuni* enteritis may be the most common infection, but other precipitants include Epstein-Barr virus, cytomegalovirus, and HIV. Sensory symptoms may be the first sign of the illness, followed by as-

TABLE 6–11. DYSPROTEINEMIC NEUROPATHIES

Disorder	Diagnostic Criteria	Treatment Options for Neuropathy
MGUS	Monoclonal protein, no malignancy or amyloid	Intravenous immunoglobulin, plasma exchange, corticosteroids
Osteosclerotic myeloma	Plasmacytoma(s) with osteosclerotic features	Resection of solitary bone lesion, focused radiation, prednisone, melphalan, cyclophosphamide
Multiple myeloma	Abnormal plasma cells in bone marrow, osteolytic lesions, monoclonal protein	None
Waldenström macroglobulinemia	IgM monoclonal protein, abnormal bone marrow	Plasma exchange, prednisone, melphalan, chlorambucil
Cryoglobulinemia	IgM or IgG	Plasma exchange, prednisone, cyclophosphamide, interferon alfa
Amyloidosis	Light chain amyloid by histology	Melphalan plus prednisone, autologous stem-cell transplantation

MGUS, monoclonal gammopathy of undetermined significance.

cending muscle weakness. The diagnosis requires progressive weakness in more than one limb, with areflexia or hyporeflexia. CN VII and the autonomic nervous system are frequently involved, with the more serious consequences being cardiac arrhythmias, hypotension, hypertension, and hyperpyrexia.

Findings on cerebrospinal fluid (CSF) analysis and electrophysiologic features of demyelination support the diagnosis of AIDP. The CSF has an increased protein concentration and few cells (albuminocytologic dissociation). The diagnosis should be questioned if there are more than 50 cells/mm^3. The results of both CSF and electrophysiologic tests may be normal up to the first week of the illness. Other laboratory tests are not needed unless the patient has questionable features, for example, marked asymmetry of weakness, bowel and bladder dysfunction, a sensory level, or cellular CSF. HIV serologic testing may be reasonable if the patient has the appropriate risk factors. The differential diagnosis for a patient with an acute neuropathy is limited (see Table 6–3), and the presence of other features may dictate further evaluation.

In most patients, progressive weakness develops over 2 to 4 weeks. Patients should be hospitalized because of the potential for respiratory compromise and autonomic dysfunction. Forced vital capacity should be monitored, and the patient should receive ventilatory assistance if there is any sign of fatigue or if the forced vital capacity becomes less than 15 mL/kg. Progressive neck weakness may signal impending respiratory failure. Other supportive measures include compressive stockings and heparin given subcutaneously for protection against deep venous thrombosis, physical therapy to prevent contractures, and a means of communication if the patient is on a ventilator.

Plasma exchange and intravenous immunoglobulin are used to treat AIDP. Both treatments have been shown to be effective, and both are expensive. Intravenous immunoglobulin may be preferred in patients who are hemodynamically unstable or in hospitals where plasma exchange is unavailable. Currently, treatment with corticosteroids is not recommended.

CHRONIC INFLAMMATORY DEMYELINATING POLYRADICULONEUROPATHY

Chronic inflammatory demyelinating polyradiculoneuropathy (CIDP) differs from the acute disease by the temporal profile. The muscle weakness is progressive for at least 2 months, and antecedent infections and autonomic and respiratory involvement are less common than with AIDP.

Several diseases are associated with a syndrome similar to CIDP, including HIV infection, monoclonal gammopathy, chronic active hepatitis, inflammatory bowel disease, connective tissue disease, bone marrow and organ transplantation, lymphoma, hereditary neuropathy, diabetes mellitus, thyrotoxicosis, nephrotic syndrome, and central nervous system demyelination. The diagnostic workup of a patient with CIDP entails looking for these systemic diseases. Treatment options include corticosteroids, intravenous immunoglobulin, plasma exchange, and other immunosuppressive agents.

FOCAL NEUROPATHIES

 A 52-year-old industrial worker is evaluated because of intermittent numbness and pain in his right hand. His symptoms occur during his job, which requires repetitive wrist movement. He also has noticed the symptoms at night and when reading the newspaper or driving. Findings on neurologic examination are normal, but percussion at the wrist causes paresthesias to spread to the thumb and first two digits of the right hand. Is this carpal tunnel syndrome? Are there other diagnostic considerations? What is the relationship of symptoms to work? What treatment do you recommend?

CARPAL TUNNEL SYNDROME

Carpal tunnel syndrome is the result of compression of the median nerve at the wrist by the volar ligament (Fig. 6–4). It is the most common entrapment neuropathy and is associated with several conditions, including pregnancy, diabetes mellitus, hypothyroidism, acromegaly, rheumatoid arthritis, and amyloidosis. The incidence of carpal tunnel syndrome is high among assembly line workers, keyboard operators, and workers whose occupations require forceful repetitive movement of the hand. The relationship of carpal tunnel syndrome to work is not clear, and some evidence suggests that nonoccupational factors such as age are important in its development.

The case described here is consistent with carpal tunnel syndrome. Activity-related and nighttime paresthesias are common in this disorder. Although the median nerve supplies only the palmar surface of the thumb and first two digits, patients often complain of pain and numbness of the entire hand. Radiation of pain into the forearm (and, rarely, the shoulder) can occur. If pain is the most prominent symptom, it is important to consider other diagnoses. Musculoskeletal

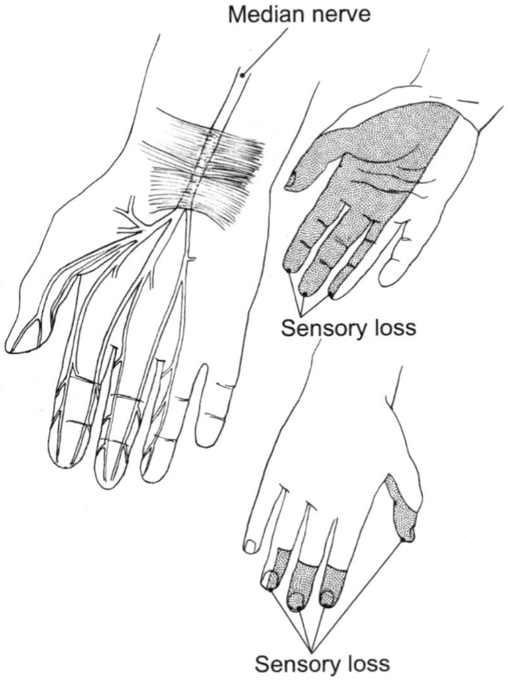

Median nerve

Sensory loss

Sensory loss

FIG. 6–4. Median nerve at the wrist and distribution of sensory loss in the hand.

causes that may mimic carpal tunnel syndrome include tenosynovitis, arthritis, muscle strain, and overuse. Neurologic causes to consider include C6 radiculopathy, thoracic outlet syndrome, and brachial plexopathy.

Examination findings in a patient with mild or moderate carpal tunnel syndrome may be normal. Percussion of a nerve that causes paresthesias in the distribution of the nerve (Tinel sign) indicates a partial lesion of the nerve or early regeneration. Reproduction of the symptoms with wrist flexion (Phalen maneuver) is consistent with a median neuropathy at the wrist. Reduced sensation to pinprick in the thumb and first two digits, weakness, and atrophy of the thenar muscles are seen in moderate-to-severe carpal tunnel syndrome.

Other neurologic findings distinguish carpal tunnel syndrome from other neurologic diseases. Patients with C6 radiculopathy complain of neck pain and may have C6 muscle weakness and reflex loss. Patients with thoracic outlet syndrome develop symptoms and C8 and T1 neurologic deficits (interosseous, hypothenar muscles) when they elevate and abduct the arm. Pronation of the wrist (pronator teres) and flexion of the distal thumb joint (flexor pollicis longus) test median nerve function proximal to the wrist.

Electrophysiologic tests can provide an accurate diagnosis of carpal tunnel syndrome and detect other conditions such as peripheral neuropathy, cervical radiculopathy, or ulnar neuropathy. Electromyography is useful in determining the severity of the condition and the response to treatment. Conservative treatment includes wrist splinting, avoidance of aggravating activities, nonsteroidal anti-inflammatory drugs, and injection of corticosteroid under the volar ligament. If the patient does not respond to conservative treatment and has progressive symptoms, recommend surgery.

OTHER COMPRESSION NEUROPATHIES

Compression or entrapment of nerves often causes paresthesias in the arms and legs. In the upper extremity, the ulnar nerve can be affected at the elbow, as it courses by the medial epicondyle and enters the cubital tunnel under the edge of the aponeurosis of the flexor carpi ulnaris (Fig. 6–5). Numbness and paresthesias occur in the 4th and 5th digits of the hand. If the motor fibers of the ulnar nerve are affected, interosseous muscles become weak and the patient has difficulty spreading the fingers. Atrophy of the 1st dorsal interosseous muscle (the "web" between the thumb and index finger) is frequently seen. Repetitive elbow flexion, leaning on the elbow, prolonged bed rest, and the position of the arm during certain surgical procedures may compress the ulnar nerve at the elbow. The nerve can also be injured at the wrist (see Fig. 4–10). Mechanics who use the heel of their hands as tools may traumatize the nerve in this location.

Radial nerve compression can cause numbness and paresthesias on the dorsum of the hand. The nerve can be injured in the axilla, for example, by the incorrect use of a crutch. Prolonged compression of the upper arm on the edge of a chair may injure the radial

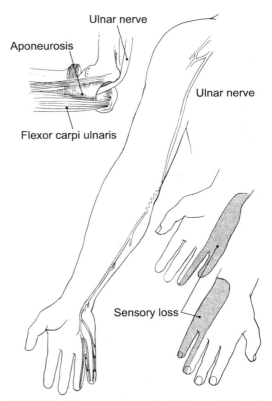

FIG. 6–5. Ulnar nerve at the elbow and distribution of sensory loss in the hand.

nerve along its course in the posterior aspect of the upper arm (spiral groove). This focal neuropathy is often called "Saturday night palsy," for persons who wake up with hand numbness and wristdrop after a night of drinking.

Common focal neuropathies of the lower extremity include those of the lateral femoral cutaneous nerve and the peroneal nerve. It is important to distinguish these from lumbosacral radiculopathies and plexopathies. Compression of the lateral femoral cutaneous nerve, called *meralgia paresthetica*, occurs at the inguinal ligament, for example, with pregnancy, obesity, abdominal surgery, and constrictive clothing. This neuropathy is

characterized by paresthesias of the upper thigh, well-demarcated sensory loss, and no motor involvement. Symptomatic treatment and reassurance are usually effective therapy for this focal neuropathy.

The peroneal nerve can be compressed at the head of the fibula, for example, by crossing the legs, prolonged squatting, and knee injury (Fig. 6–6). Numbness occurs in the dorsum of the foot. Footdrop results from peroneal motor weakness. Both the peroneal nerve and the posterior tibial nerve are derived from the L5 nerve root. Thus, weakness of ankle inversion (posterior tibial nerve) can help distinguish a peroneal neuropathy from an L5 radiculopathy.

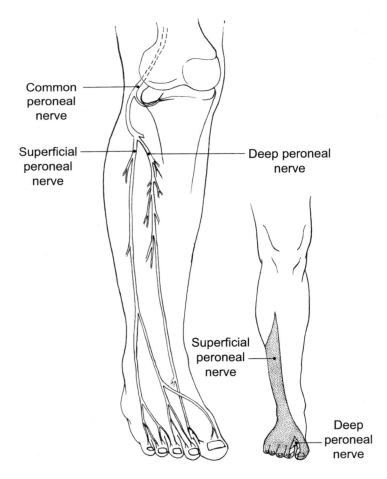

FIG. 6–6. Peroneal nerve and distribution of sensory loss in the foot and lower leg.

Common peroneal nerve

Superficial peroneal nerve

Deep peroneal nerve

Superficial peroneal nerve

Deep peroneal nerve

SUGGESTED READING

Amato, AA, and Collins, MP: Neuropathies associated with malignancy. Semin Neurol 18:125–144, 1998.

Barohn, RJ: Approach to peripheral neuropathy and neuronopathy. Semin Neurol 18:7–18, 1998.

Barohn, RJ, and Saperstein, DS: Guillain-Barré syndrome and chronic inflammatory demyelinating polyneuropathy. Semin Neurol 18:49–61, 1998.

Berger, AR: Toxic Peripheral Neuropathies. In Samuels, MA, and Feske, S (eds): Office Practice of Neurology. Churchill Livingstone, New York, 1996, pp 534–540.

The Diabetes Control and Complications Trial Research Group: The effect of intensive treatment of diabetes on the development and progression of long-term complications in insulin-dependent diabetes mellitus. N Engl J Med 329:977–986, 1993.

Kelly, JJ, Jr: Dysproteinemic polyneuropathy. In Samuels, MA, and Feske, S (eds): Office Practice of Neurology. Churchill Livingstone, New York, 1996, pp 522–528.

Kissel, JT: Autoantibody testing in the evaluation of peripheral neuropathy. Semin Neurol 18:83–94, 1998.

Logigian, EL: Approach to and classification of peripheral neuropathy. In Samuels, MA, and Feske, S (eds): Office Practice of Neurology. Churchill Livingstone, New York, 1996, pp 492–497.

Low, PA, et al: Autonomic function and dysfunction. Continuum 4:59–119, April 1998.

Mendell, JR, et al: Peripheral neuropathy. Continuum 1:7–103, December 1994.

Nathan, PA, et al: Natural history of median nerve sensory conduction in industry: Relationship to symptoms and carpal tunnel syndrome in 558 hands over 11 years. Muscle Nerve 21:711–721, 1998.

Olney, RK: Neuropathies associated with connective tissue disease. Semin Neurol 18:63–72, 1998.

Partanen, J, et al: Natural history of peripheral neuropathy in patients with non-insulin-dependent diabetes mellitus. N Engl J Med 333:89–94, 1995.

Poncelet, AN: An algorithm for the evaluation of peripheral neuropathy. Am Fam Physician 57:755–764, 1998.

Ropper, AH, and Gorson, KC: Neuropathies associated with paraproteinemia. N Engl J Med 338:1601–1607, 1998.

Weinberg, DH: Metabolic neuropathy. In Samuels, MA, and Feske, S (eds): Office Practice of Neurology. Churchill Livingstone, New York, 1996, pp 510–516.

Wilbourn, A, and Shields, RW, Jr: Diabetic neuropathy. In Samuels, MA, and Feske, S (eds): Office Practice of Neurology. Churchill Livingstone, New York, 1996, pp 506–510.

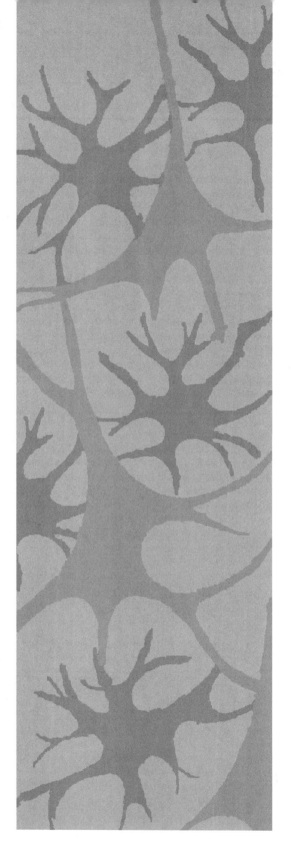

CHAPTER 7

Weakness

CHAPTER OUTLINE

Diagnostic Approach
Family History
Motor Examination
EMG
Muscle Biopsy
Inherited Myopathies
Muscular Dystrophies
Myotonic Dystrophy
Inflammatory Myopathies
Dermatomyositis
Polymyositis
Inclusion Body Myositis
Associated Conditions and Findings
Treatment
**Myopathies Associated With Drugs
and Toxins**
Endocrine Myopathies
**Disorders of the Neuromuscular
Junction**
Myasthenia Gravis
Diagnostic Tests
Treatment
Factors That Exacerbate Myasthenia
Gravis
Lambert-Eaton Syndrome
Botulism
Motor Neuron Disease
Poliomyelitis
Cramps and Fasciculations

123

A 56-year-old woman is evaluated for weakness. During the last several weeks, she has noted soreness in her muscles and trouble with climbing stairs and holding her arms up to fix her hair. She has trouble getting on the examining table. Physical examination findings are notable for mild weakness of the neck flexor, deltoid, and iliopsoas muscles. No rash or skin changes are evident. Muscle stretch reflexes are mildly decreased, and sensory examination findings are entirely normal. What are the diagnostic considerations? Are there associated conditions about which you should be concerned? How do you proceed?

Weakness is a very common complaint. Most patients use the term "weakness" to imply fatigue, general illness, or myalgias. Determining whether a patient has actual neuromuscular weakness can be a diagnostic challenge. Disease of the motor system can occur at all levels of the nervous system. This chapter considers disorders of the lower motor neuron seen in primary care practice, including disorders of muscle, the neuromuscular junction, and motor nerves.

DIAGNOSTIC APPROACH

The history of a patient who complains of weakness is crucial. The first question should be how the weakness has affected the person's activities. This information will help distinguish between neuromuscular weakness and a generalized fatigue or malaise. The pattern of weakness provides diagnostic information (see Table 1–5). The woman in the case study just described reported that she had trouble climbing stairs and elevating her arms. These symptoms as well as trouble getting up from a chair or getting out of a car indicate proximal muscle weakness. Proximal

weakness is the pattern of weakness seen in myopathy. Distal weakness is indicated when a patient reports difficulty with buttoning clothing or opening jars or complains of tripping because of footdrop. Distal weakness is the pattern of weakness seen most often in neuropathy. The absence of sensory symptoms limits the differential diagnosis of distal weakness. Disorders such as motor neuropathy, myotonic dystrophy, and inclusion body myositis can cause distal weakness.

The hallmark of disorders of the neuromuscular junction is fatigable weakness. Patients with myasthenia gravis report increasing weakness and fatigue as the day goes on. Because extraocular muscles are frequently involved, patients complain of double vision and ptosis. Trouble swallowing, chewing (bulbar muscles), and breathing is the most serious problem of neuromuscular junction disorders.

Amyotrophic lateral sclerosis (ALS, Lou Gehrig disease) is the prototypic disorder of motor neurons. Patients with a disorder of motor neurons report the gradual onset of painless weakness. The pattern can be proximal or distal. Many patients may report "jumping muscles," that is, fasciculations. Sensory symptoms are absent, but muscle cramps are frequently reported.

FAMILY HISTORY

It is important to obtain a family history from a patient presenting with neuromuscular disease. After you have determined that the patient has a neuromuscular problem, next determine whether it is acquired or inherited. A thorough family history may avoid an extensive neuromuscular evaluation if there is evidence of a compatible inherited neuromuscular disorder. It may not be sufficient to ask the patient if family members had weakness or difficulty walking. For example, if myotonic dystrophy is suspected, it may be necessary to ask if any

124

member of the family had frontal balding or early cataracts.

MOTOR EXAMINATION

The motor examination is described in Chapter 1. Test proximal muscle strength by asking the patient to squat, to get up from a chair, or to sit up from the supine position without using the hands. Assess neck flexion strength if you suspect the patient has proximal muscle weakness. Normally, neck flexion should not be overcome by the examiner. Assess distal strength by the strength of the grip and by having the patient stand on the toes and heels. To eliminate any problem with balance, support the patient. Perform repetitive muscle testing if there is a history of fatigable weakness. Asking the patient to maintain upward gaze for several minutes may provoke extraocular muscle weakness. Another way to elicit muscle fatigue is to have the patient perform repeated squats or sit-ups. The patient's gait may reveal weakness. Bilateral pelvic abductor weakness produces a characteristic waddling gait, and footdrop causes a high steppage gait.

In lower motor neuron disorders, muscle tone is normal or decreased. Muscle bulk is also normal to reduced (see Table 1–4). Pseudohypertrophy occurs in some muscular dystrophies such as Duchenne muscular dystrophy. Children with this disease may have prominent calves, deltoid muscles, and forearm muscles ("Popeye" arms). The patient needs to be undressed to adequately assess muscle bulk and to check for fasciculations. Fasciculations may be elicited by gently tapping the area over the muscle. In the absence of weakness, fasciculations are normal.

Sensory examination findings are normal in disorders of muscle, the neuromuscular junction, or motor nerves. However, a patient may have both a lower motor neuron disease and a sensory neuropathy. This is possible, considering the high frequency of diabetes mellitus in the general population. In these patients, the weakness will seem out of proportion to the sensory loss. Muscle stretch reflexes in lower motor neuron disease are reduced or absent. In ALS, reflexes

may be increased because of the involvement of upper motor neurons.

Many systemic diseases are associated with neuromuscular weakness. Thus, patients should be evaluated for signs and symptoms of connective tissue disease, toxicity, nutritional disorders, and malignancies.

The diagnostic evaluation of a patient with neuromuscular weakness depends on the clinical presentation. Electromyography (EMG), muscle biopsy, and determination of creatine kinase levels are indispensable in evaluating neuromuscular weakness. Muscle degeneration causes release of creatine kinase into the blood, increasing the level of this enzyme in the plasma. The creatine kinase level should be determined before EMG is performed, to avoid the artifactual increase caused by needle injury to the muscle.

EMG

Myopathies demonstrate short-duration, low-amplitude, and polyphasic motor unit potentials on EMG (see Fig. 2-3). In addition to these EMG features, inflammatory myopathies have increased spontaneous activity. Defects in neuromuscular transmission can be demonstrated by repetitive stimulation. EMG findings in motor neuron disease include large, polyphasic, varying motor unit potentials with fibrillation potentials. Finding these EMG features in two muscles of each limb innervated by a different nerve and root confirms the diagnosis of motor neuron disease.

MUSCLE BIOPSY

Muscle biopsy is a safe diagnostic procedure that can provide a definitive diagnosis in many neuromuscular disorders. Indications for biopsy include suspected inflammatory muscle disease, suspected vasculitis or collagen vascular disease, congenital or metabolic myopathies, and progressive muscular atrophy. The muscle selected for biopsy should have mild to moderate weakness. Biopsy should not be performed on a muscle that has been injured by previous trauma, injections, or EMG needles (within 4 to 6 weeks after EMG). The deltoid muscle is usually avoided because it is frequently used for intramuscular injections. Common muscles used for biopsy include the biceps, triceps, and quadriceps. The extensor carpi radialis and anterior tibialis are selected for biopsy of distal muscles. The pathologist needs to know which muscle is used because of the variation in fiber type in different muscles. The specimen should be prepared for light and electron microscopy and histochemical stains.

INHERITED MYOPATHIES

Disorders of muscle include both acquired and inherited disorders.

MUSCULAR DYSTROPHIES

Inherited disorders include the muscular dystrophies. These disorders are characterized by progressive muscular weakness and loss of muscle bulk. The many forms of dystrophy are distinguished by mode of inheritance, distribution of muscles involved, and speed of progression. Duchenne muscular dystrophy is one of the most severe dystrophies and has a high rate of mortality before adulthood. Some forms of dystrophy are mild and do not significantly impair longevity, for example, facioscapulohumeral dystrophy. Muscular dystrophies are relevant to primary care practice because they frequently are associated with cardiac abnormalities and other general medical concerns. The characteristic features of Duchenne, facioscapulohumeral, and limb-girdle dystrophies are summarized in Table 7–1.

MYOTONIC DYSTROPHY

Myotonic dystrophy is an autosomally dominant inherited neuromuscular disorder associated with various systemic complications. Patients with myotonic dystrophy often seek medical attention because of these systemic symptoms instead of the neuromuscular complications. The pattern of muscle weakness in myotonic dystrophy is different from that in other dystrophies. Patients have ptosis and facial and distal limb weakness. They often interpret the myotonia (the slow relaxation of muscle contraction) as "muscle stiffness" and frequently do not complain about it. Myotonia can be demonstrated by asking patients to clench their hands tightly and then release. Patients with myotonia have a delayed release. The patients also have characteristic facial features, with facial weakness, ptosis, and, in men, frontal balding.

The more serious systemic problems that occur in myotonic dystrophy include cardiac conduction defects and arrhythmias and aspiration pneumonia from involvement of the esophagus and diaphragm. These problems increase the risk of perioperative morbidity in

TABLE 7–1. COMPARISON OF COMMON TYPES OF MUSCULAR DYSTROPHY

Characteristic	Duchenne Dystrophy	Facioscapulohumeral Dystrophy	Limb-Girdle Dystrophy
Inheritance	X-linked	Autosomal dominant	Autosomal recessive
Weakness	Pelvic girdle	Shoulder girdle, face	Pelvic and shoulder girdles
Age at onset	Before 5 years	Adolescence	Adolescence
Progression	Rapid	Slow	Slow
Other features	Pseudohypertrophy	Facial involvement	Heterogeneous disorder
Creatine kinase level	Markedly increased	Normal	Normal or increased
Abnormal ECG findings	Common	Rare	Occasional

ECG, electrocardiographic.

patients with myotonic dystrophy. Cataracts, atrophic testicles, diabetes mellitus, hypersomnia, and mild mental deterioration are also seen in this disorder.

The diagnosis is made on the basis of clinical findings and a positive family history. EMG findings include myopathic changes and myotonic discharges. The pattern of abnormalities seen on muscle biopsy can distinguish this disorder from other myopathies and neuropathies. The gene for myotonic dystrophy has been identified and the diagnosis can now be made on a molecular basis.

INFLAMMATORY MYOPATHIES

Acquired myopathies are seen more frequently than dystrophies in a primary care practice. This category includes endocrine myopathies, inflammatory myopathies, and myopathies due to drugs, toxins, or nutritional deficiencies. Inflammatory myopathies include polymyositis, dermatomyositis, and inclusion body myositis. They are characterized by muscle weakness and inflammatory infiltrates within the skeletal muscle. Medications, viruses, and parasites can also cause muscle inflammation.

DERMATOMYOSITIS

The absence of skin changes in the woman described in the case above is significant. Dermatomyositis has been described as polymyositis with a rash, but it is a separate clinical entity. It occurs in children or adults, with a female predominance. The skin changes consist of a blue-to-violet discoloration of the upper eyelids (heliotrope rash), with edema, erythema, and scaly eruption on the knuckles and a flat red rash on the face and upper trunk. The rash may precede the proximal muscle weakness. Dermatomyositis may occur alone or in association with scleroderma or mixed connective tissue disease. An overlap syndrome has also been described, in which patients have features of dermatomyositis and scleroderma or mixed connective tissue disease.

Compared with other inflammatory muscle disorders, there is an increased association between dermatomyositis and malignant conditions. It is not clear how aggressive the search for an underlying malignancy should be. The work-up should be directed by the patient's clinical presentation. An annual physical examination, with pelvic and rectal examinations, complete blood count, chemistry profile, urinalysis, and chest radiography, is recommended.

POLYMYOSITIS

The diagnosis of polymyositis is based on the exclusion of other neuromuscular conditions. Exclusion criteria include the presence of a rash, positive family history of neuromuscular disease, eye and facial involvement, exposure to myotoxic drugs, and endocrinopathies. Muscle biopsy findings can exclude inclusion body myositis and other neuromuscular disorders.

Polymyositis tends to occur in adults and, as in the woman described in the case above, can progress over weeks to months. Polymyositis is often associated with several systemic autoimmune diseases such as Crohn disease, vasculitis, primary biliary cirrhosis, discoid lupus, and adult celiac disease. A definitive association between polymyositis and malignant conditions has not been demonstrated.

INCLUSION BODY MYOSITIS

Inclusion body myositis is unique among the inflammatory myopathies. It can have early distal muscle involvement, and it is refractory to immunosuppressant therapy. A familial association has been shown in some cases. Connective tissue diseases have been associated with inclusion body myositis, but an association with malignant conditions has not been proved.

ASSOCIATED CONDITIONS AND FINDINGS

Cardiac abnormalities, including conduction defects, arrhythmias, dilated cardiomyopathy, and congestive heart failure, are the more serious conditions associated with the inflammatory myopathies. Pulmonary involvement can include interstitial lung disease. When inflammatory myopathies are associated with connective tissue disease, fever, malaise, weight loss, arthralgia, and Raynaud phenomenon may be present.

Muscle enzyme levels are increased in inflammatory myopathies. The creatine kinase level can be 50 times normal in dermatomyositis and polymyositis, but it may be normal or only slightly increased in inclusion body myositis. Muscle biopsy findings are diagnostic for all three of these conditions.

TREATMENT

Corticosteroids are effective treatment for polymyositis and dermatomyositis. The dose may vary depending on the severity of the symptoms. The recommended dose of prednisone is 1 mg/kg daily. This high dose is continued until the serum level of creatine kinase normalizes and muscle strength improves. Depending on the patient's clinical response and creatine kinase level, the dose can be tapered. If the creatine kinase level remains normal, the dose can be tapered by 25% every 3 to 4 weeks. An increase in the creatine kinase level before an increase in muscle weakness is evidence of relapse. By 6 to 12 months, the majority of patients can be taking a maintenance dose (10 mg/day or 10 to 20 mg every other day).

Prolonged use of corticosteroids can complicate therapy by causing a myopathy. Increasing weakness may indicate increasing disease activity or a steroid-induced myopathy. The creatine kinase level does not increase in steroid-induced myopathy. The creatine kinase level, EMG findings, and the patient's response to a change in dose help determine whether the weakness is due to disease or to treatment.

Other immunosuppressant therapy, for example, methotrexate, azathioprine, or cyclophosphamide, is used for disease that is resistant to corticosteroids or for patients who experience intolerable side effects. Physical therapy is important to prevent disuse atrophy and joint contractures.

MYOPATHIES ASSOCIATED WITH DRUGS AND TOXINS

Many drugs can cause muscle injury. Myotoxic injury is important to recognize to reduce further damage to the muscle. If a patient has muscle weakness, review all the medications that the patient is taking to discover possible myotoxic effects. The mechanism of muscle injury varies with the toxin. D-Penicillamine and procainamide can cause inflammatory myopathy. Diuretics, laxatives, and alcohol can cause hypokalemia, which in turn results in muscle weakness and muscle injury. The majority of toxic substances cause a necrotizing myopathy, for example lipid-lowering agents. Patients may present acutely or subacutely with muscle pain and proximal weakness. The serum level of creatine kinase is increased. If muscle necrosis is severe, myoglobinuria can occur. Many of the drugs and toxins that can cause myopathy are listed in Table 7–2.

Muscle injury is also associated with illicit drug use. Heroin, with impairment of consciousness, can lead to pressure-induced damage of skeletal muscle. Cocaine, amphetamines, and phencyclidine can cause myoglobinuria as a result of agitation, convulsions, and catatonic muscular rigidity. Chronic glue sniffers develop weakness due to metabolic derangements associated with exposure to toluene.

Nutritional deficiencies can cause muscle weakness. There may be a nutritional component to the myopathy seen in alcoholics. Vitamin E deficiency, which can cause peripheral neuropathy, can also cause muscle weakness. This deficiency occurs in patients with lipid malabsorption syndromes such as cystic fibrosis or cholestatic liver disease. Excessive consumption of vitamin E causes muscle injury. Vitamin D deficiency is associated with muscle weakness. Osteomalacia responds to vitamin D treatment.

ENDOCRINE MYOPATHIES

Muscle dysfunction frequently accompanies endocrine disorders, because muscle function depends on hormonal balance. Both hor-

TABLE 7–2. MYOTOXIC AGENTS

Toxin (Brand Name)	Use or Setting
Alcohol	Abuse
Aminocaproic acid (Amicar)	Antihemorrhagic agent
Amiodarone (Cordarone)	Antiarrhythmic agent
Amphotericin B (Abelcet)	Antifungal agent
Chloroquine (Aralen)	Antimalarial agent
Cimetidine (Tagamet)	Histamine antagonist (ulcer/reflux)
Clofibrate (Atromid-S)	Hyperlipidemia
Colchicine and probenecid (ColBENEMID)	Uricosuric agent (gout)
Contaminated tryptophan	Dietary supplement
Prednisone (Deltasone)	Immunosuppressant
Cyclosporine (Neoral)	Immunosuppressant
Gemfibrozil (Lopid)	Hypertriglyceridemia
Vitamin E	Excessive self-medication
Ipecac syrup	Emetic agent
Labetalol (Normodyne)	Antihypertensive agent
Lovastatin (Mevacor)	Hypercholesterolemia
Organophosphates	Insecticide exposure
Penicillamine (Cuprimine)	Heavy metal antagonist (rheumatoid arthritis)
Pravastatin (Pravachol)	Hypercholesterolemia
Procainamide (Pronestyl)	Antiarrhythmic agent
Simvastatin (Zocor)	Hypercholesterolemia
Toluene	Solvent exposure (glue sniffing)
Vincristine (Oncovin)	Antineoplastic agent
Zidovudine (Retrovir)	Antiviral agent

monal excess and deficiency are associated with muscle weakness. Patients with hyperthyroidism frequently have proximal muscle weakness in the course of the illness, and a small percentage have muscle weakness as the initial complaint. The serum level of creatine kinase is not usually increased in hyperthyroidism, but it is in hypothyroidism. Patients with hypothyroidism frequently report muscle weakness, cramps, pain, and stiffness. Myopathic changes on EMG and nonspecific histologic changes in muscle are seen in both hypothyroidism and hyperthyroidism. The muscle weakness resolves with treatment of the thyroid condition.

Hyperparathyroidism can cause proximal muscle weakness and, infrequently, bulbar weakness. Muscle stretch reflexes may be brisk, unlike in other myopathies. The underlying cause of the myopathy may be related to the vitamin D deficiency, hypercalcemia, phosphate deficiency, or neurogenic influ-

ences. Hypoparathyroidism and the associated hypocalcemia can cause tetany (a condition marked by intermittent tonic muscle contractions).

Myopathy associated with corticosteroid excess is described above. The same type of pattern is seen in Cushing syndrome. Adrenocortical deficiency (Addison disease) is also associated with muscle weakness, fatigue, and cramping. Attacks of periodic paralysis can occur in this disorder because of hyperkalemia. Hyperaldosteronism and associated hypokalemia also can cause attacks of periodic paralysis. Muscle weakness is frequently a feature of hyperaldosteronism.

Acromegaly, due to excess growth hormone, is associated with proximal muscle weakness, wasting, and hypotonia. The myopathy resolves with normalization of growth hormone levels. The absence of growth hormone also affects muscle. Muscle fails to develop properly without growth hormone, as in children with pituitary failure. Thyroid deficiency and adrenocortical hormone deficiency in pituitary failure also impair muscle function.

DISORDERS OF THE NEUROMUSCULAR JUNCTION

A 59-year-old man goes to the emergency room because of slurred speech and trouble swallowing. His symptoms began while he was dining with friends at a restaurant. By the time he reached the emergency room, his symptoms had resolved and the examination and electrocardiographic results and computed tomographic scanning of the head were normal. The tentative diagnosis was transient ischemic attack, and 1 aspirin per day was recommended.

The following week, the patient also had slurred speech while giving a presentation at work. He went to his physician, and the results of a neurologic examination were normal. Because both episodes of slurred speech occurred after prolonged talking, the patient was asked to read aloud for 10 minutes. After 5 minutes, progressive dysarthria was apparent. Repetitive muscle testing revealed fatigable weakness. Myasthenia gravis was diagnosed. What further evaluation should be performed? What treatment should this patient receive?

MYASTHENIA GRAVIS

The cardinal feature of neuromuscular junction dysfunction is fatigable weakness. Myasthenia gravis is the most common disorder of the neuromuscular junction. It is an autoimmune disease in which sensitized T-helper cells mediate an IgG-directed attack on nicotinic acetylcholine receptors on muscle cells. Lambert-Eaton myasthenic syndrome and botulism are other neuromuscular junction disorders. Many drugs and toxins can also impair neuromuscular transmission. Although disorders of neuromuscular transmission are rare, they can mimic other disorders, and this is important in primary care. The preceding case emphasizes this point. Although the patient had symptoms compatible with brainstem ischemia, the absence of sensory symptoms or dizziness makes transient ischemic attack a less likely diagnosis.

Myasthenia gravis is characterized by fatigable weakness. The muscles most often affected are the bulbar muscles for speaking, chewing, and swallowing; extraocular muscles; and proximal limb muscles. Thus, patients complain of ptosis, diplopia, dysarthria, dysphagia, and fatigable weakness. The symptoms are least noticeable first thing in the morning after the patient has rested and are worse at the end of the day. In contrast, patients with depression complain of fatigue that is worse at the beginning of the day.

Ophthalmoplegia, with ptosis and diplopia, is a very common sign in myasthenia gravis. However, the pupil is not affected in this disease (although it is affected in most disorders of CN III). Having the patient look upward for several minutes can provoke extraocular muscle weakness. The muscles of mastication may be affected and cause difficulty with chewing. This should not be confused with jaw claudication seen in temporal arteritis.

Diagnostic Tests

If myasthenia gravis is suspected, further testing is needed to confirm the diagnosis. Antibodies to acetylcholine receptors are found in the blood of more than 75% of patients with generalized myasthenia. If these antibodies are detected, the diagnosis is confirmed. If antibodies to acetylcholine receptors are not detected, perform electrophysiologic tests. Repetitive nerve stimulation fatigues the neuromuscular junction by depleting the nerve ending of acetylcholine. A decremental response in the compound muscle action potential of 10% or more is seen in patients with myasthenia gravis. Because other neurologic disorders can also cause a decremental response with repetitive nerve stimulation, neurologic consultation may be helpful.

Intravenous injection of edrophonium (Tensilon test) is a useful test in the diagnosis of myasthenia gravis. Edrophonium, a short-acting cholinesterase inhibitor, must be used with care because of potential serious reactions, including bradycardia and bronchospasm. The test should be conducted only if definite muscle weakness is observed, for example, ptosis. The decision to perform this test should be made only on the basis of physical signs, not subjective symptoms.

Other diagnostic tests that are frequently performed if myasthenia gravis is suspected are thyroid function tests, antinuclear antibody test, anti-striated muscle antibody test, and chest computed tomography or magnetic resonance imaging. Thyroid function tests are useful because autoimmune thyroid disease occurs in approximately 10% of patients with myasthenia. The antinuclear antibody test may indicate other autoimmune disorders; lupus erythematosus is the only disorder in which the acetylcholine receptor antibody test gives false-positive results. Chest imaging is important because of the high incidence of thymic hyperplasia and thymoma in myasthenia gravis. A positive antistriated muscle antibody test suggests thymoma.

Treatment

The treatment of myasthenia gravis includes cholinesterase inhibitors, immunosuppressant drugs, and thymectomy. Pyridostigmine (Mestinon), a cholinesterase inhibitor, is frequently the initial therapy for symptomatic relief. Most patients with myasthenia require additional medication. The side effects of pyridostigmine are symptoms of acetylcholine excess and include muscle cramps, diarrhea, and an increase in oral secretions. The increase in oral secretions may be a very difficult problem for patients with pharyngeal and respiratory weakness.

Because excessive anticholinesterase therapy can cause increasing weakness, instruct patients not to increase the dose of medication without medical direction. Acute weakness is a medical emergency, and the patient should be hospitalized in an intensive care unit and respiratory function monitored. With the patient in the hospital, stop all treatment with anticholinesterase agents to determine whether increased weakness is due to cholinergic excess or to exacerbation

of the disease. Any concurrent infections and electrolyte abnormalities need to be corrected. The patient should be intubated if the respiratory status declines (vital capacity, 15 mL/kg or less) or there is a risk of aspiration. Plasmapheresis or intravenous administration of a high dose of immunoglobulin will provide rapid improvement in the patient's condition.

Immunosuppressant therapy includes the use of corticosteroids, azathioprine, plasmapheresis, and an intravenously administered high dose of immunoglobulin. Remember that corticosteroids may exacerbate myasthenia, and hospitalization is often recommended before corticosteroid therapy is instituted. The side effects of chronic corticosteroid treatment are often the reason to try other immunosuppressant therapy. Azathioprine is effective, but the onset to improvement is slow. Both plasmapheresis and intravenous administration of a high dose of immunoglobulin can cause rapid improvement, but the improvement is of short duration. Intravenous administration of a high dose of immunoglobulin and plasmapheresis are useful for myasthenia crises or preoperative preparation.

Thymectomy improves the condition in the majority of patients, and surgery is often recommended even if there is no thymoma or thymic hyperplasia. Thymectomy is indicated for all patients with thymoma and those younger than 60 years who have generalized myasthenia, and it should be considered for older patients on an individual basis. Young adults with early myasthenia tend to have the best results, with a high rate of remission after the operation.

Factors That Exacerbate Myasthenia Gravis

It is important to be aware of factors that exacerbate myasthenic weakness. These include major physical stress, fever, pregnancy, and heat. Many antibiotics exacerbate myasthenia, for example, aminoglycosides, fluoroquinolone antibiotics, erythromycin, clindamycin, polymyxin B, and tetracycline. Other medications that can also exacerbate myasthenia are phenytoin, lithium, β-blockers, calcium channel blockers, quinine, antiarrhythmic agents, sedatives, and muscle relaxants. Except for penicillamine, which is contraindicated, these medications can be used if necessary. However, be aware of the potential effect, and be prepared to manage an exacerbation of weakness.

LAMBERT-EATON SYNDROME

Lambert-Eaton myasthenic syndrome is a rare autoimmune disorder characterized by fluctuating muscle weakness, autonomic dysfunction, and hyporeflexia. It is often associated with small cell carcinoma of the lung and has been reported in other malignancies. A primary autoimmune nonparaneoplastic form of Lambert-Eaton myasthenic syndrome has been reported. Patients may have trouble walking or have other symptoms of proximal muscle weakness. Unlike myasthenia gravis, some improvement may be noted with exercise. Autonomic symptoms include a dry mouth and, in men, erectile dysfunction. Vague numbness in the thighs is often reported.

Lambert-Eaton myasthenic syndrome is caused by antibodies to voltage-gated calcium channels in motor and autonomic nerve terminals that disrupt calcium influx and decrease acetylcholine release. EMG is used to confirm the diagnosis of this syndrome. A decremental response occurs with repetitive nerve stimulation, similar to that in myasthenia gravis. After a brief period of exercise, facilitation of the compound muscle action potential is seen. An underlying malignancy should be sought and treated. Pyridostigmine, 3,4-diaminopyridine, and various immunosuppressant regimens have been used to treat this syndrome.

BOTULISM

Botulism is caused by the exotoxin of *Clostridium botulinum*. The four types of botulism that have been described are infant, foodborne, wound, and from an undetermined source. The toxin binds to autonomic and motor nerve terminals and blocks the presynaptic release of acetylcholine. Symptoms include progressive muscle weakness that begins in the extraocular or pharyngeal muscles and then affects other muscles. Gastrointestinal symptoms are prominent. Dilated unreactive pupils and dry mucous membranes indicate autonomic involvement. An antitoxin is available, and treatment with it should be initiated as soon as the diagnosis is made.

Neuromuscular junction problems can be caused or unmasked by several different medications. Medications that exacerbate myasthenia gravis impair neuromuscular transmission through a direct effect. Some medications (penicillamine, chloroquine, and trimethadione) cause neuromuscular dysfunction by causing an immune response. Many poisons, snake venom, and some spider bites also have an effect on the neuromuscular junction.

MOTOR NEURON DISEASE

A 52-year-old man reports that his right footdrop has developed gradually over the last several months. He denies having any pain, sensory symptoms, or bowel or bladder difficulty. Examination demonstrated weakness in the right foot and toe extensors, mild weakness in the interosseous muscles of the finger, and minimal atrophy of the anterior tibial and interosseous muscles. Sensory examination findings were normal. Muscle stretch reflexes were increased, and plantar reflexes were extensor (Babinski sign). Fasciculations were observed in the calf muscles bilaterally. Magnetic resonance imaging of the lumbar spine was performed because of a previous history of low back pain. The study revealed a mild central disk bulge at L5. What is the cause of the footdrop? What further investigation would you recommend?

The differential diagnosis of footdrop emphasizes the importance of all components of the neurologic examination. Footdrop due to peripheral neuropathy or L5 radiculopathy would be associated with sensory findings and decreased muscle stretch reflexes. Although the patient has protrusion of the L5 disk, the absence of pain and sensory findings suggests that this is asymptomatic. Muscle atrophy and fasciculations in the presence of weakness suggest lower motor neuron dysfunction. In addition, hyperactive reflexes (or increased muscle stretch reflexes) indicate an upper motor neuron problem. The clinical presentation of this patient is consistent with motor neuron disease or ALS.

There are several types of motor neuron disease. The most common disorder of the motor neurons is ALS, or Lou Gehrig disease, which affects both upper and lower motor neurons. In *progressive bulbar palsy*, primarily the bulbar muscles are affected. Progressive bulbar palsy is characterized by speech and swallowing dysfunction and may be the initial manifestation of motor neuron disease. *Spinal muscular atrophy* is a motor neuron disease with predominantly lower motor neuron involvement. Several inherited disorders, based on age at onset, are included in the category of spinal muscular atrophy. *Primary lateral sclerosis* is a disorder of upper motor neuron dysfunction. Spinal muscular atrophy and primary lateral sclerosis are both rare forms of motor neuron disease.

If both upper and lower motor neurons are involved, the differential diagnosis is limited. Cervical spondylosis can cause weakness, atrophy, and fasciculations in the upper extremities because of nerve root involvement and hyperreflexia in the lower extremities because of spinal cord compression. Hyperthyroidism causes muscle wasting and weight loss and may resemble ALS. If lower motor neurons are predominantly involved, consider inclusion body myositis and multifocal motor neuropathy. Multifocal motor neuropathy responds to immunosuppressive treatment. Lymphoma (through its remote effect), radiation exposure, hyperparathyroidism, and adult-onset hexosaminidase A deficiency can mimic ALS. Diagnostic tests used to confirm and to exclude other causes of ALS are summarized in Table 7–3.

A multidisciplinary approach should be taken in treating ALS. Although the prognosis is poor, much can be done to care for patients. Active participants in this care should include neurologists; nurses; physical, occupational, and speech therapists; dietitians; home health aides; mental health workers; and other medical specialists. Currently, riluzole, an inhibitor of glutamate metabolism, is the only medicine available that slows the progression of the disease. Tertiary medical care centers should be contacted about the availability of other drug treatments being used in clinical trials.

TABLE 7–3. DIAGNOSTIC TESTS IN AMYOTROPHIC LATERAL SCLEROSIS (ALS)

Diagnostic Test	Findings in ALS	Other Diagnoses the Test Will Exclude
Electromyography	Large, polyphasic motor unit potentials with fibrillation potentials	Multifocal motor neuropathy Inclusion body myositis Myasthenia gravis
Cervical cord imaging	Normal or asymptomatic degenerative changes	Cervical spondylosis with cord compression
Creatine kinase	< 1,000 IU/L	Inclusion body myositis
Muscle biopsy	Neurogenic changes	Inclusion body myositis
Serum protein electrophoresis	Normal	Lymphoma Multifocal motor neuropathy
Anti-GM$_1$ ganglioside antibody	Negative	Multifocal motor neuropathy
Thyroid-stimulating hormone	Normal	Hyperthyroidism
Blood levels of calcium, phosphorus, alkaline phosphatase	Normal	Hyperparathyroidism
Hexosaminidase A	Normal	Hexosaminidase A deficiency

POLIOMYELITIS

Poliomyelitis was a common disorder of motor neurons until vaccination became available. Patients who had polio early in life are at risk for postpolio syndrome. The clinical features of this syndrome include fatigue, myalgias, arthralgias, weakness, cold intolerance, sleep apnea syndrome, and depression. The cause has not been established; two suggestions are that it is caused by a gradual loss of motor units, as a result of aging, or it is due to increased metabolic demand on reinnervated muscle motor units. Treatment guidelines for postpolio syndrome include assessment for and treatment of sleep apnea, depression, pulmonary function, and any other medical disorder. Patients should avoid exhausting activities and maintain an ideal body weight. Individualized physical therapy, with stretching, range-of-motion, and nonfatiguing exercises, is helpful. Joint and muscle pain can be reduced with heat, massage, and anti-inflammatory medication.

CRAMPS AND FASCICULATIONS

Muscle cramps and fasciculations are often considered manifestations of motor neuron disease, and although they can represent serious disease, most of the time patients need only to be reassured that these are normal phenomena. Fasciculations are the visible, spontaneous contractions of muscle fibers and the only sign of lower motor neuron dysfunction in the presence of weakness. A cramp is a painful muscle spasm, usually occurring in the muscles of the calf and feet. Dehydration from exercise, diuretics, or hemodialysis is frequently associated with muscle cramps. Metabolic abnormalities associated with muscle cramps include hyponatremia, hypomagnesemia, hypocalcemia, and hypoglycemia. Other conditions associated with muscle cramps are thyroid disease, adrenal insufficiency, and pregnancy. Medications that can cause cramps include terbutaline, albuterol, labetalol, nifedipine, clofibrate, and cyclosporine. The neurologic causes of cramps are motor neuron disease and peripheral neuropathies. There is a rare familial cramp syndrome.

The treatment of cramps involves eliminating any underlying metabolic or medical condition that could be associated with them. Quinine sulfate (260 mg at bedtime) has been prescribed to prevent and to treat painful muscle spasm, but it has several adverse effects. Carbamazepine, phenytoin, tocainide, and verapamil have also been used to treat this painful condition.

SUGGESTED READING

Dalakas, MC: Polymyositis, dermatomyositis and inclusion-body myositis. N Engl J Med 325:1487–1498, 1991.

Engel, AG: The muscle biopsy. In Engel, AG, and Franzini-Armstrong, C (eds): Myology. Vol 2, ed 2. McGraw-Hill, New York, 1994, pp 822–831.

Engel, AG, Hohlfeld, R, and Banker, BQ: The polymyositis and dermatomyositis syndromes. In Engle, AG, and Franzini-Armstrong, C (eds): Myology. Vol 2. ed 2. McGraw-Hill, New York, 1994, pp 1335–1383.

Harper, PS, and Rüdel, R: Myotonic dystrophy. In Engle, AG, and Franzini-Armstrong, C (eds): Myology. Vol 2, ed 2. McGraw-Hill, New York, 1994, pp 1192–1219.

Hopkins, LC: Clinical features of myasthenia gravis. Neurol Clin 12:243–261, 1994.

Jones, HR, Jr: Lambert-Eaton myasthenic syndrome. In Samuels, MA, and Feske, S (eds): Office Practice of Neurology. Churchill Livingstone, New York, 1996, pp 567–571.

Kaminski, HJ, and Ruff, RL: Endocrine myopathies (hyper- and hypofunction of adrenal, thyroid, pituitary, and parathyroid glands and iatrogenic corticosteroid myopathy). In Engle, AG, and Franzini-Armstrong, C (eds): Myology. Vol 2, ed 2. McGraw-Hill, New York, 1994, pp 1726–1753.

Massey, JM: Treatment of acquired myasthenia gravis. Neurology 48(Suppl 5):S46–S51, 1997.

Mitsumoto, H, et al: Motor neuron disease. Continuum 3:8–127, 1997.

Pickett, J: Toxic and metabolic disorders of the neuromuscular junction. In Samuels, MA, and Feske, S (eds): Office Practice of Neurology. Churchill Livingstone, New York, 1996, pp 571–577.

Preston, DC: Myasthenia gravis. In Samuels, MA, and Feske, S (eds): Office Practice of Neurology. Churchill Livingstone, New York, 1996, pp 562–567.

Victor, M, and Sieb, JP: Myopathies due to drugs, toxins, and nutritional deficiency. In Engle, AG, and Franzini-Armstrong, C (eds): Myology. Vol 2, ed 2. McGraw-Hill, New York, 1994, pp 1697–1725.

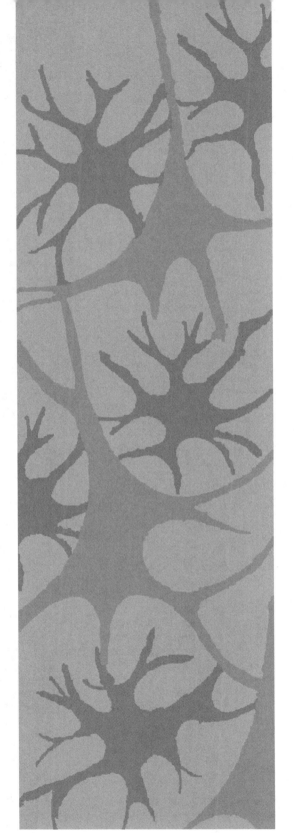

CHAPTER 8

Memory Loss

CHAPTER OUTLINE

Diagnostic Approach
 History
 Neurologic Examination
 Mental Status Examination
 Laboratory Investigation
Forms of Dementia
 Alzheimer Dementia
 Dementia With Lewy Bodies
 Vascular Dementia
 Normal-Pressure Hydrocephalus
 Frontotemporal Dementia

A 75-year-old woman is brought in for evaluation of memory loss and confusion. She denies that she has any difficulty other than the "normal forgetfulness" for age. Over the last 1 or 2 years, she has had increasing difficulty remembering names and items she needs from the grocery store. Her husband started managing the checkbook 6 months ago because she forgot to pay some of the bills. She was involved in a minor motor vehicle accident several months ago, and now her husband accompanies her when she goes shopping. The patient's family insisted on an evaluation because at a recent family party she did not remember her grandchildren and the smoke alarm went off because she forgot she had cookies in the oven. How do you proceed to evaluate this patient? What do you tell the family when they ask you questions about driving and safety issues and about whether they are at risk for dementia?

The brief history of the woman is consistent with dementia, which is defined as significant loss of cognitive function involving multiple cognitive areas and the absence of clouded consciousness. Memory, the ability to learn new information or to recall previously learned information, is impaired. The diagnostic criteria for dementia include at least one of the following: language disturbance (aphasia), impaired ability to carry out motor activities despite intact motor function (apraxia), failure to recognize or to identify objects despite intact sensory function (agnosia), personality change, constructional difficulties, and a disturbance in executive functioning. Executive functioning includes planning, organizing, sequencing, or abstracting. The loss of intellectual abilities needs to be sufficiently severe to interfere with social or occupational functions.

The most common cause of dementia is Alzheimer disease (Table 8–1). Accurate diagnosis is important, to exclude reversible causes of dementia (new treatment options are available for the treatment of degenerative dementias). Early diagnosis is advantageous not only for treatment but also so the patient can be more involved in making important decisions before the disease progresses to the point where this is not possible. Family members can be educated about the disease process, and proactive measures can be taken with regard to financial affairs, legal matters, driving, living arrangements, and safety. The inherited nature of some dementing illnesses makes the correct diagnosis of dementia significant to family members.

The incidence and prevalence of dementia increases with increasing age, with prevalence doubling every 5 years. Of persons 65 years old, 1% have dementia, and 50% of those older than 90 years are demented. As the population ages, prompt recognition and intervention will become increasingly important. Failure to diagnose dementia correctly has been attributed to lack of attention to cognitive functioning in routine medical examinations and to misperceptions about the normal aging process.

DIAGNOSTIC APPROACH

From 50% to 75% of patients with dementia have Alzheimer dementia. When a patient complains of cognitive impairment, the initial focus is to determine whether the symptoms suggest dementia, delirium, or depression. The characteristic feature of a patient with delirium or an acute confusional state is inattention and an impaired and fluctuating level of consciousness. This is uncommon in an outpatient setting.

HISTORY

The history of a patient with memory loss or cognitive dysfunction is critical. However,

TABLE 8–1. CAUSES OF DEMENTIA

Degenerative

Alzheimer disease
Parkinson disease
Frontotemporal dementia
Pick disease
Huntington disease
Progressive supranuclear palsy
Diffuse cortical Lewy body disease
Multisystem atrophy
Olivopontocerebellar degeneration
Focal cortical degeneration
Corticobasal degeneration
Wilson disease
Hallervorden-Spatz disease

Vascular

Multi-infarct dementia
Binswanger encephalopathy
Amyloid dementia
Vasculitis
Specific vascular syndrome (thalamic, inferotemporal, bifrontal)
Diffuse hypoxic/ischemic injury
Mitochondrial disease
CADASIL

Trauma

Subdural hematoma
Postconcussion syndrome
Dementia pugilistica
Anoxic brain injury

Inflammation/Infection

HIV dementia, opportunistic organisms
Chronic meningitis (tuberculosis, cryptococcosis, cysticercosis)
Syphilis
Lyme encephalopathy
Creutzfeldt-Jakob disease
Post–herpes simplex encephalitis
Progressive multifocal leukoencephalopathy
Sarcoidosis
Whipple disease of the brain
Subacute sclerosing panencephalitis

Neoplastic

Primary brain tumors
Metastatic tumors
Lymphoma
Paraneoplastic limbic encephalitis

Drugs/Toxins

Medications: β-blockers, neuroleptics, antidepressants, anticonvulsants, histamine receptor blockers, dopamine blockade
Alcohol abuse
Recreational drug abuse
Lead
Mercury
Arsenic

Psychiatric

Depression
Personality disorder
Anxiety disorder

Metabolic

Thyroid deficiency
Vitamin B_{12} deficiency (pernicious anemia)
Vitamin B_1 (thiamine) deficiency (Wernicke-Korsakoff)
Uremia/dialysis dementia
Chronic hepatic encephalopathy
Chronic hypoglycemic encephalopathy
Chronic hypercapnia/hypoxemia
Chronic hypercalcemia/electrolyte imbalance
Addison disease
Cushing disease
Hartnup disease

Autoimmune

Systemic lupus erythematosus
Polyarteritis nodosa
Temporal arteritis
Isolated angiitis of the central nervous system
Wegener granulomatosis

Demyelinating

Multiple sclerosis
Adrenoleukodystrophy
Metachromatic leukodystrophy

Obstructive

Normal-pressure hydrocephalus
Obstructive hydrocephalus

CADASIL, cerebral autosomal dominant arteriopathy with subcortical infarcts and leukoencephalopathy; HIV, human immunodeficiency virus.

the patient may not be able to provide sufficient information, and a corroborative history is needed from family or friends or both. It is more meaningful when a relative complains that the patient has impaired memory than when the patient complains of memory difficulty. Studies have shown that when a family member complains that the patient's memory is impaired, the likely diagnosis is dementia; however, when the patient complains of memory difficulty, it likely is depression, not dementia.

The history should document the temporal profile, including the onset, duration, and progression of symptoms. A gradual onset and slow insidious progression of symptoms characterize degenerative dementias such as Alzheimer disease. Information about any changes in the patient's activities, and when these changes occurred and why, may help to clarify the onset of symptoms. For example, the husband of the confused woman in the case above started managing the checkbook 6 months earlier because his wife forgot to write checks for bills. This indicates that the symptoms started at least 6 months ago. Inquiring about instrumental activities of daily living is very useful. These include questions about money management, meal preparation, shopping, traveling, housework, using the telephone, and taking medications. In a hospital setting, a patient with an unrecognized mild dementia may have an acute onset of dementia. A change in familiar surroundings, medications, and anesthesia and the greater risk for an acute confusional state in demented patients are all factors for the "sudden" onset of dementia.

Vascular, traumatic, and toxic causes of dementia can have an acute onset. The onset of multi-infarct dementia can be sudden, with a stepwise deterioration in the patient's mental status. The progression of symptoms is important. Viral or prion diseases (e.g., Creutzfeldt-Jakob disease) are rapidly progressive illnesses that occur over several months. Is the problem one of memory loss or memory lapse? Transient symptoms may suggest partial seizure activity, transient global amnesia, or complicated migraine.

In this case study, the woman attributed her problem to normal aging. The distinction between mild dementia and normal cognitive aging can be difficult to make. Complicating this is the marked increase in the incidence of dementia with advancing age. Cognitive functions that demonstrate decline with age include sustained attention, mental flexibility, response speed, and visual memory recall. Preserved function includes immediate attention, vocabulary, temporal orientation, and certain visuospatial skills. A normal 90-year-old person is able to live independently.

Any history of personality changes is significant. Depression can complicate the diagnosis of dementia. Depression is frequently associated with degenerative dementias, and severe depression can mimic dementia. On mental status examination, patients with depression demonstrate diminished attention, memory impairment, apathy, and social withdrawal. Historical points that may lead to the diagnosis of depression include a previous history or family history of depression, sleep difficulty, and the vegetative signs of depression. The onset of symptoms may follow a major event such as the death of a spouse. Cognitive testing in depression demonstrates impaired attention and performance variability. Patients frequently respond to questions with "I don't know." Some features that distinguish between dementia and depression are listed in Table 8–2.

In addition to depression, prominent changes in personality early in the course of a dementing illness may suggest a frontal lobe process, for example, tumor, frontotemporal dementia, or Pick disease. Any change in behavior needs to be interpreted with respect to the patient's previous personality, occupation, and standing in the community. Previous psychiatric illness, such as bipolar affective disorder or schizophrenia, is relevant.

The medical history may suggest the cause of dementia. A history of vascular disease and vascular risk factors are consistent with multi-infarct dementia. A history of thyroidectomy suggests hypothyroidism, and a history of gastrectomy suggests vitamin B_{12} deficiency. Historical information on head trauma, exposure to toxins, systemic illness, risk factors for human immunodeficiency virus (HIV), and alcohol intake and smoking

TABLE 8–2. COMPARISON OF THE FEATURES OF DEPRESSION AND DEMENTIA

Depression	Dementia
Patient complains of memory problems	Patient minimizes memory problems
Relatives concerned about depression	Relatives concerned about memory problems
Vegetative symptoms, anxiety	No or few symptoms of depression
Subacute onset of cognitive symptoms; symptoms follow traumatic event	Insidious onset of cognitive symptoms
History of depression common	History of depression less common
Orientation intact	Orientation impaired
Concentration impaired	Recent memory impaired
Variable results on mental status testing	Consistent results on mental status testing
Poor effort on testing	Good effort on testing
Aphasia and apraxia absent	Aphasia and apraxia present

habits is important. Information needs to be obtained also about what medications the patient is taking, because medications frequently cause cognitive impairment. Some of the agents that can cause cognitive side effects are β-blockers, antidepressants, psychotropic drugs, anticonvulsants, H_2-receptor blockers, and dopamine blockers.

The family history is important. Evidence indicates that mutations in at least four genes can cause Alzheimer dementia. Other inherited degenerative dementias include Huntington disease, Pick disease, frontotemporal lobe dementia, Parkinson disease, and prion disease. Advanced age and a positive family history of dementia are major risk factors for dementia.

NEUROLOGIC EXAMINATION

When examining a patient who has memory loss, look carefully for neurologic signs. Evidence of any focal neurologic deficit may indicate a previous stroke. Abnormal gait is usually seen in Parkinson disease, normal-pressure hydrocephalus, and vascular dementias. Hyperkinetic movement in association with dementia suggests Huntington disease. If there is evidence of peripheral

neuropathy, investigate whether the patient abuses alcohol or has vitamin B_{12} deficiency, hypothyroidism, or an infectious or inflammatory condition (see Table 8–1).

MENTAL STATUS EXAMINATION

The mental status examination is crucial in the evaluation of memory loss and cognitive impairment. A mild cognitive deficit may not be noticed during superficial conversation or when the history is being taken for an unrelated problem. Major deficits in the history or non sequiturs are reasons to perform a more thorough cognitive evaluation. The mental status examination should determine whether dementia is present or it should establish a baseline status that can be followed at subsequent evaluations. Refer the patient for additional neuropsychologic testing if the results of mental status screening are equivocal.

Important factors to be aware of before testing mental status are the patient's mood and motivation. Depression has a significant impact on mental status functioning. Poor motivation also affects performance on tests of cognition. Areas of cognitive function that you should test are attention, recent and remote memory, language, praxis, visuospatial relationships, judgment, and calculations. The short screening tests for cognitive impairment such as the Short Test of Mental Status or the Mini-Mental State Exam (Table 8–3) are very useful, despite the criticism that they are time-consuming and insensitive to mild dementia. However, these standardized tests are in widespread use, and the normal values for age and education level are known. The interpretation of results must be placed in the context of the patient's age and education (Table 8–4). A score of 23 or less on the Mini-Mental State Exam or a score of 29 on the Short Test of Mental Status suggests cognitive impairment. These tests are screening tests only. False-positive results can be obtained for patients with depression and false-negative results for patients with high intelligence and mild dementia. Mental status screening tests are valuable for longitudinal screening

and should aid in decisions about additional testing.

First, test attention on the mental status examination, because inattention can degrade all other mental state functions. Disruption in attention is the defining feature of an acute confusional state. Attention can be tested in several ways, including the use of digit span, as in the Short Test of Mental Status, or spelling "world" backwards, as on the Mini-Mental State Exam. Problems with attention may indicate diffuse brain dysfunction that can occur in a toxic encephalopathy or in frontal lobe dysfunction, as in the frontotemporal dementias. Tests of language, including reading and writing, evaluate left hemisphere function. Calculations, right-left orientation, and finger recognition ("show me your left index finger") test left parietal lobe function. Test right parietal lobe function, which includes complex perceptual

---

TABLE 8–3. MINI-MENTAL STATE EXAM

1. Orientation
   What is the day? date? month? year? season?
   What is the city? state? county? building? floor?
   (Give one point for each correct answer.)
2. Registration
   Name three objects and take 3 seconds to say each. Then ask the patient to repeat the names of the three objects. (Give one point for each correct answer. Repeat until the patient can name all three objects.)
3. Attention and calculation
   Serial 7s: Ask the patient to count backwards by 7 from 100. (Stop after five answers. Give one point for each answer.) Alternate: Spell "world" backwards. (Give one point for each correct answer.)
4. Recall
   After 2 minutes, ask the name of the three objects in question 2. (Give one point for each correct answer.)
5. Language
   Point to a pencil and a watch. Ask the patient to name each as you point. (Give one point for each correct answer.)
   Ask the patient to repeat the following phrase: No ifs, ands, or buts. (Give one point for each correct answer.)
   Ask the patient to perform the following three-stage command: Take this piece of paper in your left hand, fold it in half, and lay it on the table. (Give one point for each correct step.)
   Ask the patient to read and carry out the following written command: Close your eyes. (Give one point for each correct response.)
   Ask the patient to write a sentence. It must contain a noun and a verb and make sense. Ignore spelling errors. (Give one point for each correct answer.)
   Ask the patient to draw two interlocking pentagons. There must be five sides to each pentagon and four interlocking sides. (Give one point for each correct answer.)
Maximum Total = 30 points

Modified from Folstein, MF, et al: "Mini-mental state." A practical method for grading the cognitive state of patients for the clinician. J Psychiatr Res 12:189–198, 1975. By permission of MiniMental LLC.

TABLE 8–4. MINI-MENTAL STATE EXAM SCORES: REVISED CUTOFF SCORES FOR THE MINI-MENTAL STATE EXAM, STRATIFIED BY AGE AND EDUCATION*

Age (Years)	Education (Number of Years)					
	6–8	9–11	12	13–16	17–18	≥19
60–64	26	27	27	28	29	29
65–69	25	26	27	27	28	29
70–74	24	25	26	27	27	28
75–79	23	24	25	26	27	27
80–84	23	23	24	24	25	26
85–89	23	23	23	24	25	26
90–95	23	23	23	23	24	25

*Scores less than or equal to those shown suggest that further evaluation for dementia is needed. Scores greater than 23 are based on being one standard deviation below the age- and education-appropriate mean (23 was adopted as a minimal cutoff score on the basis of sensitivity and specificity analyses).

From Tangalos, EG, et al: The Mini-Mental State Examination in general medical practice: Clinical utility and acceptance. Mayo Clin Proc 71:829–837, 1996. By permission of Mayo Foundation for Medical Education and Research.

functions, by asking the patient to draw a cube or clock, as in the Short Test of Mental Status. Testing memory and the "localization" of memory is more complicated. Working memory (for example, remembering a telephone number for a short time) is a function primarily of the frontal lobes. The ability to learn, store, and retrieve information (i.e., declarative memory) involves the medial temporal lobes and limbic structures. On both the Mini-Mental State Exam and the Short Test of Mental Status, recall is used to test declarative memory. Remote memories are represented diffusely throughout the cerebral hemispheres (association cortex) and are the memories most resistant to pathologic changes. The different components of the mental status examination provide localizing information (Fig. 8–1).

The evaluation of mental status is dependent on the patient's use of language. Memory complaints may actually represent aphasia or a language problem. Pay attention to the patient's speech during the interview. Fluency of speech is usually normal if the patient uses sentences with seven or more words. Phonemic ("the sky is glue") or paraphasic ("the sky is cheese") errors indicate a language problem. The Mini-Mental State Exam assesses language by having the patient name objects, repeat a phrase, and read and write a sentence. To test for comprehension, ask the patient to perform a three-stage command, for example, "Look up, raise your hand, and point to the door."

Further neuropsychologic testing may be indicated if the initial evaluation of the patient is borderline or suspicious for dementia. Neuropsychologic tests are very helpful in identifying dementia in highly intelligent persons who may have normal results on mental status screening examinations. These tests may be needed for patients with limited educational background or mentally retarded persons, because of the limitations of mental status screening tests. Neuropsychologic tests are recommended for making the distinction between dementia and depression, in determining competency for legal purposes, and for determining disability. As with screening tests, a baseline study with follow-up evaluation may be necessary to make the diagnosis of dementia.

LABORATORY INVESTIGATION

The laboratory work-up in the evaluation of dementia is dictated by the findings obtained with the history and physical

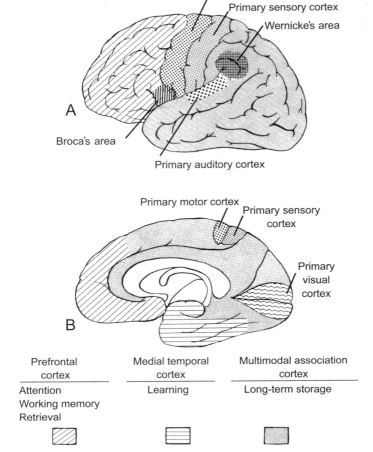

FIG. 8–1. Functional areas of the cerebral cortex. (A) Lateral and (B) medial surfaces of the cerebral hemisphere.

examination. Laboratory tests are performed to exclude metabolic and structural causes of dementia that may be amenable to specific treatment. The routine tests recommended by the American Academy of Neurology include a complete blood count; serum level of electrolytes, calcium, and glucose; blood urea nitrogen, creatinine, and vitamin B_{12}; liver function tests; free thyroid index and thyroid-stimulating hormone; and syphilis serology. Optional studies include erythrocyte sedimentation rate, serum folate level, human immunodeficiency virus testing, chest radiography, urinalysis, 24-hour urine collection for heavy metals, toxicology screen, neuroimaging study (computed tomography [CT] or magnetic resonance imaging [MRI]), neuropsychologic testing, lumbar puncture, electroencephalography (EEG), positron emission tomography (PET), and single-photon emission computed tomography (SPECT).

Cerebrospinal fluid (CSF) analysis is recommended in the evaluation of dementia if there is a possibility of a central nervous system infection, metastatic cancer, or suspicion of central nervous system vasculitis. Consider performing a CSF analysis if there are atypical features such as the onset of symptoms before age 55 years or rapid progression of symptoms. Before performing a lumbar puncture for CSF analysis, review the indications and contraindications for the procedure (see Chapter 2). Lumbar puncture and removal of CSF are useful in patients who have normal-pressure hydrocephalus. The clinical features of normal-pressure hydrocephalus include dementia, gait disturbance, and incontinence. Brain imaging demonstrates ventricular enlargement out of proportion to cortical atrophy. Ventricular shunting may be reasonable to consider if the patient's gait improves after CSF has been removed (see below).

EEG is an optional study that may have some value in investigating possible dementia. Patients who have cognitive impairment and seizures should be evaluated with EEG. This test may be valuable in distinguishing between delirium and dementia or in evaluating any patient who has a fluctuating level of consciousness. EEG may also be useful in distinguishing between dementia and depression. If a patient has depression, you would expect the EEG to be normal, compared with the slow pattern likely to be seen if the patient has dementia. The EEG of a patient who has a rapid decline in cognitive function over a 3-month period or less and early neurologic findings may suggest prion disease. Creutzfeldt-Jakob disease often shows characteristic sharp waves on EEG.

Neuroimaging is optional because there is no consensus about the need for these studies when patients have the insidious onset of dementia after age 60 years without focal signs or symptoms, seizures, or gait abnormalities. A study on the usefulness of the practice parameters of the American Academy of Neurology indicated that the guidelines represented a first step toward improving the cost-effectiveness of a dementia work-up. However, a small percentage (5%) of clinically meaningful information may be missed if these guidelines are followed. Neuroimaging is reasonable at least once in the evaluation of a patient with dementia. CT can detect all the potentially treatable causes of dementia, including tumor, subdural hematoma, hydrocephalus, and stroke. MRI is more sensitive in detecting vascular and demyelinating diseases, and it often detects nonspecific white matter changes. *Leukoaraiosis*, a term used to describe periventricular white matter abnormalities, occurs in multiple sclerosis, in certain infections, after cardiac arrest, and in elderly pa-

tients. Leukoaraiosis is recognized as a risk factor for dementia. On CT, leukoaraiosis appears as periventricular low attenuation.

The role of MRI in the evaluation of dementia is likely to expand in the future. For example, it has been shown that quantitative measurements of brain structure and size made with MRI have some predictive value in the diagnosis of Alzheimer dementia.

PET and SPECT measure glucose metabolism and regional blood flow and may also be used in the evaluation of dementia. Patients with Alzheimer dementia have decreased glucose metabolism and cerebral blood flow in the temporoparietal regions compared with normal controls. Although cerebral blood flow patterns are not specific for a given disease, they may be useful for distinguishing Alzheimer disease from vascular or frontotemporal dementia. However, the clinical usefulness of these tests has not been established. The indications for optional laboratory tests used in the evaluation of memory loss are summarized in Table 8–5. The laboratory tests and the rationale for each of them are summarized in Table 8–6.

FORMS OF DEMENTIA

ALZHEIMER DEMENTIA

Alzheimer disease is the most common form of dementia. The definitive diagnosis is made at autopsy, with the demonstration of neuronal loss, neurofibrillary tangles, neuritic plaques, and amyloid angiopathy. Autopsy studies have confirmed that the clinical diagnosis of Alzheimer disease has a high rate of accuracy.

Alzheimer disease is a complex and heterogeneous disorder, and many genes have been identified in its development. It has been divided on the basis of genetic studies into "early-onset disease" (before age 60) and "late-onset disease." Genes associated with the early-onset form include the amyloid β-protein precursor on chromosome 21, *presenilin* 1 on chromosome 14, and *presenilin* 2 on chromosome 1. The genetic risk factor identified with the late-onset form is apolipoprotein E-4 (APOE-4). APOE is on chromosome 19, with three alleles (2, 3, and 4). APOE-4

TABLE 8–5. DIAGNOSTIC TESTS AND THEIR INDICATIONS FOR EVALUATION OF DEMENTIA

Indication for Test	Test
Routine dementia screen	Complete blood count Electrolytes, glucose, calcium, BUN, creatinine Liver function tests Thyroid function test Vitamin B_{12} Syphilis serology
Duration of symptoms < 6 mo Age at symptom onset < 60 yr Focal signs or symptoms Seizure Ataxic or apraxic gait	Head CT or MRI
CNS infection CNS vasculitis Metastatic cancer Rapidly progressive dementia Early age at symptom onset	CSF analysis
Normal-pressure hydrocephalus	Lumbar puncture
Dementia versus delirium Dementia versus depression Seizures	EEG
Suspicious or borderline mental status screening test results Dementia versus depression Legal competency determination Disability determination Baseline	Neuropsychologic tests

BUN, blood urea nitrogen; CNS, central nervous system; CSF, cerebrospinal fluid; CT, computed tomography; EEG, electroencephalography; MRI, magnetic resonance imaging.

has been called a "susceptibility gene"; it does not cause the disease but may modulate the age at onset and increase the probability of the disease developing. Apolipoprotein is a plasma protein produced in the brain by astrocytes. It is involved with cholesterol transport and is found in neuritic plaques, neurofibrillary tangles, and vascular amyloid. Apolipoprotein binds strongly to the amyloid protein. A patient with dementia who has the APOE-4 genotype is more likely to have Alzheimer disease than any other dementing illness. The use of APOE-4 as a predictive test for Alzheimer disease has been suggested, but the genotype is not necessary or sufficient for the diagnosis. Currently, APOE-4 testing is not recommended for diagnosing or predicting Alzheimer disease. Testing for amyloid β-protein precursor, *presenilin* 1, and *presenilin* 2 may be appropriate in families with an autosomal dominant pattern of inheritance of dementia. Appropriate genetic counseling should also be part of the genetic testing.

When discussing with family members the risk of developing Alzheimer disease, emphasize that it is an age-related disease. Although the risk of developing the disorder increases with age, patients in whom it develops live a substantial portion of their lives without the

TABLE 8–6. LABORATORY TESTS USED IN THE DIFFERENTIAL DIAGNOSIS OF DEMENTIA

Test	Evaluation for
Complete blood count	Anemia, infection
Electrolytes, calcium, glucose	Metabolic dysfunction
Glucose	Endocrine dysfunction
BUN, creatinine	Renal dysfunction
Liver function tests	Liver dysfunction
Thyroid function	Hypothyroidism
Vitamin B_{12}	Vitamin B_{12} deficiency
Syphilis serology	Syphilis
CT/MRI scan	Vascular disease, mass lesion, hydrocephalus, demyelinating disease, focal or diffuse atrophy
CSF analysis	Chronic meningitis, syphilis, vasculitis, meningeal carcinomatosis
EEG	Seizures, Creutzfeldt-Jakob disease, metabolic disturbances
Heavy metal screen	Lead, mercury, arsenic intoxication
Erythrocyte sedimentation rate	Inflammatory disease
Antinuclear antibody	Inflammatory disease
Anti-extractable nuclear antibodies	Inflammatory disease
HIV	HIV dementia
Chest radiography	Cardiopulmonary disease, lung tumor
ECG	Cardiopulmonary disease
SPECT	Focal cortical atrophy, frontotemporal dementia, Pick disease
Long-chain fatty acids	Adrenoleukodystrophy
Arylsulfatase A	Metachromatic leukodystrophy
Ceruloplasmin, copper level	Wilson disease
Angiography	Arteritis
Cerebral biopsy	Inflammatory disease
Paraneoplastic antibodies	Cancer

BUN, blood urea nitrogen; CSF, cerebrospinal fluid; CT, computed tomography; ECG, electrocardiography; EEG, electroencephalography; HIV, human immunodeficiency virus; MRI, magnetic resonance imaging; SPECT, single-photon emission computed tomography.

disease. The risk of the disease in the population with a negative family history is about 8% per decade starting at age 70. In persons with a first-degree family member with the disorder, the risk doubles. The age at onset of dementia is also correlated in families. Despite all this, the chances are greater that first-degree relatives will not develop the disease.

Many risk factors have been identified for Alzheimer disease. In addition to advanced age and a positive family history, female gender, history of head trauma, small head circumference, and lower intelligence are risk factors. Although women live longer than men, the risk for Alzheimer disease is still higher even after adjusting for survival. The increased risk associated with head in-

jury is thought to be related to an increase in amyloid deposition, neuronal injury, and synaptic disruption. Patients with smaller brains and lower intelligence are thought to have smaller cognitive reserves and, thus, be at greater risk for developing the disease. The APOE-4 genotype is another risk factor.

Factors that may help prevent or delay the onset of Alzheimer disease are being investigated for potential therapies. Use of nonsteroidal anti-inflammatory drugs (NSAIDs) has been associated with a lower risk for the disease and a slower rate of cognitive decline. Estrogen replacement therapy in postmenopausal women has been shown to be a protective factor against the disease. Estrogen increases cerebral blood flow and may have some neurotrophic and neuroprotective effects. Other identified protective factors are APOE-2 genotype, level of formal education, and challenging occupations.

The diagnosis of Alzheimer disease is understandably devastating to the patient and family. The diagnosis is a "family" diagnosis, because of the significant effect the disease will have on the patient's caregiver. The patient and caregiver need to know that the disease is progressive and that cognition and function will continuously decline. Changes in the patient's behavior and personality are common and part of the dementing process. Although there is no cure for the disease, many of the common symptoms can be treated. The clinician often needs to attend to the caregiver as much as to the patient. In addition to the medical management of the disease, clinicians play an important part in addressing issues of living arrangements, legal matters, and driving.

The strategy in the treatment of patients with Alzheimer disease is to improve the quality of life and to maximize function. Several pharmacologic treatments are based on the neurodegenerative mechanisms involved in the disease. For example, the observation of a cholinergic deficit in the brains of patients with Alzheimer disease led to the development of tacrine (a cholinesterase inhibitor), the first drug approved for the treatment of the disease. Clinical studies have demonstrated that cholinesterase inhibitors have a modest benefit in treating the clinical symptoms of mild-to-moderate Alzheimer disease. However, liver toxicity and cholinergic side effects (nausea, vomiting, diarrhea) have limited the use of tacrine. Donepezil, another available cholinesterase inhibitor, has fewer side effects and is better tolerated. Also, it has a longer duration of action than tacrine and can be given only once a day instead of four times per day as with tacrine. Other cholinesterase inhibitors are awaiting approval for use in treating Alzheimer disease.

Antioxidant agents are being investigated for treating Alzheimer disease. Free radicals, byproducts of oxidative metabolism, damage cell membranes and tissues. According to the oxidative stress hypothesis of neuronal death, antioxidants should prevent this cytotoxic injury. Selegiline, a monoamine oxidase inhibitor, may act as an antioxidant and reduce neuronal damage. It also may improve cognitive deficits by increasing levels of catecholamines. Vitamin E, or α-tocopherol, is another antioxidant. Preliminary evidence suggests that selegiline and vitamin E may slow the progression of Alzheimer disease. Currently, selegiline is not recommended, because of its adverse effects and cost; however, vitamin E is reasonable to use, based on its high safety profile and low cost.

Estrogen may also act as an antioxidant. Other actions of estrogen that may be effective in treating Alzheimer disease include improved glucose transport in the hippocampus, promotion of neuronal viability and synaptic integrity, enhanced choline uptake, and increased cerebral blood flow. Estrogen may reduce neuronal injury by decreasing the amount of amyloid formation. Studies evaluating the use of estrogen in Alzheimer disease have not been completed, and no recommendation can be made about it for treating the disease. However, the favorable information about estrogen replacement therapy and cognition should be considered when reviewing the risks versus benefits of estrogen therapy for other conditions.

NSAIDs may delay the onset or slow the progression of Alzheimer disease by decreasing the inflammatory processes that contribute to neuronal destruction. Prospective clinical trials are under way to determine whether NSAIDs should be used to treat this disease. In one study, the group taking indomethacin had a high dropout rate because of gastrointestinal side effects. Other anti-inflammatory drugs, cyclooxygenase inhibitors, are also being investigated for treating dementia.

An herbal remedy extracted from the leaves of the ginkgo tree, *Ginkgo biloba*, is claimed to be effective in treating memory deficits. Its mechanism of action is not known, but it may be an antioxidant. Although a randomized trial reported the extract had a slight positive effect on dementia, several flaws have been cited in the study, limiting its usefulness. Ginkgo has platelet-inhibitory effects, but bleeding is not a common side effect. Reported adverse effects include mild gastrointestinal symptoms, headache, and allergic reactions. The purity and potency of the extract are not known. Further study is needed before treatment with *Ginkgo biloba* can be recommended.

Dementia-related behavioral symptoms are common. Problems include sleep disruption, agitation, depression, hallucinations, and delusions. Before initiating treatment with a psychoactive drug, document the specific behavior and investigate its cause or any contributing factors. Some of the causes of abnormal behavior are pain, depression, medication effect, infection, physical limitations, and hospitalization. Intervention may not be needed if safety is not an issue, if the patient is not distressed, or if the living situation is not compromised. Often, nonpharmacologic approaches can be used.

When psychoactive drugs are prescribed, they should be prescribed on a scheduled basis instead of an "as needed" basis. One drug should be prescribed and started at a very low dose and advanced slowly until the desired therapeutic effect occurs. Monitor the patient's condition regularly to assess response and adverse effects to the medication. Attempt periodic removal of the treatment. Some pharmacologic and nonpharmacologic options for the symptomatic treatment of dementia are summarized in Table 8–7.

DEMENTIA WITH LEWY BODIES

Dementia with Lewy bodies is a distinct clinical and neuropathologic dementia syndrome. It is the second most common dementing disorder, accounting for 15% to 25% of all cases of dementia. Lewy bodies are eosinophilic neuronal inclusion bodies; when present in subcortical nuclei, they are the pathologic hallmark of idiopathic Parkinson disease. Lewy bodies are present in the brainstem and cerebral cortex of patients who have dementia with Lewy bodies.

Similar to Alzheimer disease, the clinical criteria for dementia with Lewy bodies include progressive cognitive decline that interferes with normal social and occupational functions. Memory impairment occurs in the later stages of the disease. Prominent deficits are apparent on tests of attention and executive and visuospatial ability. The core features of dementia with Lewy bodies are fluctuating cognition with pronounced variation in attention and alertness, recurrent visual hallucinations that are particularly well-formed and detailed, and spontaneous motor features of parkinsonism (i.e., bradykinesia, resting tremor, rigidity, and loss of postural reflexes). The consensus criteria for "probable dementia with Lewy bodies" include dementia plus two of the core features, and "possible dementia with Lewy bodies" includes dementia and one core feature. Clinical features that support the diagnosis are repeated falls, syncope, delusions, transient loss of consciousness, and other hallucinations (auditory, olfactory, tactile). Neuroleptic sensitivity also supports the diagnosis and greatly affects medical management of the disease.

The differential diagnosis of dementia with Lewy bodies includes Alzheimer disease and Parkinson disease. All three disorders occur in higher frequency in older age groups. Both dementia with Lewy bodies and Parkinson disease show a male predominance. Unlike Alzheimer disease and Parkinson disease, dementia with Lewy bodies can have an abrupt onset and a fluctuating and rapid progression, a feature that may cause this disease to be confused with delirium. Visual hallucinations and other psychotic symptoms are prominent features of dementia with Lewy bodies, and although hallucinations occur in Alzheimer disease, they usually are a late feature. Drug-induced hallucinations occur in Parkinson disease. The clinical features of these three disorders are summarized in Table 8–8.

The treatment of dementia with Lewy bodies is the same as for Alzheimer disease. Cholinesterase inhibitors are reasonable for symptomatic treatment. It is difficult to treat the symptoms of parkinsonism in patients with dementia with Lewy bodies because the condition is resistant to dopaminergic medication, and the medication exacerbates the psychosis and confusion. Avoid neuroleptic agents.

VASCULAR DEMENTIA

Vascular disease is an important cause of dementia. Vascular dementia includes dementia that results from multi-infarct, strategic infarct, small-vessel disease, hypoperfusion, or hemorrhage. Among its features is a tem-

TABLE 8–7. SYMPTOMATIC TREATMENT OF DEMENTIA

Symptom	Nonpharmacologic Therapy	Pharmacologic Therapy, Initial Dose	Adverse Effects
Cognitive impairment	Compensatory strategies: notes, pillbox, calendar, signs	Cholinesterase inhibitors: Tacrine (Cognex), 10 mg 4 times daily	Nausea, vomiting, liver toxicity
		Donepezil (Aricept), 5 mg daily	Nausea, diarrhea, insomnia, muscle cramps
Agitation, hallucinations, delusions	Redirect patient, reassure patient and caregiver	Haloperidol (Haldol), 0.25 mg daily	Parkinsonism, tardive dyskinesia, postural hypotension
		Thioridazine (Mellaril), 10 mg 1–2 times daily	As above, more sedating, anticholinergic side effects
		Risperidone (Risperdal), 0.5 mg twice daily	Nausea, insomnia, less parkinsonism
Depression	Modify environment, reduce demands on patient	SSRIs: Sertraline (Zoloft), 50 mg daily	Nausea, diarrhea, insomnia
		Paroxetine (Paxil), 10 mg every morning	Somnolence, insomnia
Insomnia	Improve sleep hygiene, eliminate or limit naps, daytime exercise, avoid caffeine and night lights	Trazodone (Desyrel), 25 mg at bedtime	Oversedation, hypotension
		Chloral hydrate (Noctec), 250 mg at bedtime	Confusion, rash, leukopenia
Anxiety, agitation	Reassurance, lessen demands on memory, reduce noise	Lorazepam (Ativan), 0.5 mg 1–2 times daily	Sedation, confusion, falls, dependency

SSRIs, selective serotonin reuptake inhibitors.

poral relation between the clinical characteristics of dementia and cerebrovascular disease. Evidence of cerebrovascular disease can be demonstrated by history (sudden onset dementia, fluctuating course), clinical examination, and brain imaging (CT or MRI).

Multi-infarct dementia is the most frequent subtype of vascular dementia. The dementia results from multiple, bilateral cortical and subcortical infarcts. Multi-infarct dementia occurs more often in men than in women. Hypertension and peripheral vascular disease are often associated with this dementia. The cognitive and neurologic findings vary depending on the location of the infarcts; however, gait disturbances, urinary incontinence, and pseudobulbar palsy are common. Pseudobulbar palsy is a syndrome characterized by emotional incontinence and slow, strained speech.

Vascular dementia can also result from a single infarct in a functionally important cortical or subcortical area. For example, a thalamic infarct can produce disturbances in attention, memory, language, and abstract thinking. An infarct in the left angular gyrus

TABLE 8–8. COMPARISON OF THE CLINICAL FEATURES OF DEMENTIA WITH LEWY BODIES, ALZHEIMER DEMENTIA, AND PARKINSON DISEASE

Clinical Feature	Dementia With Lewy Bodies	Alzheimer Dementia	Parkinson Disease
Initial symptom	Confusional state	Memory impairment	Tremor, bradykinesia, rigidity
Onset	Abrupt or insidious	Insidious	Insidious
Progression	Fluctuating, rapid	Gradual	Gradual
Gender distribution	Male	Female	Male
Prominent feature	Visual hallucinations	Dementia	Tremor, bradykinesia, rigidity

or left frontal lobe can impair memory. If dementia occurs acutely, consider vascular dementia due to a strategic single infarct.

Another cause of vascular dementia is small-vessel disease. Hypertension and diabetes mellitus are frequently associated with small-vessel cerebrovascular disease. Binswanger encephalopathy, or subcortical arteriosclerotic encephalopathy, is a dementing syndrome caused by small-vessel ischemic disease. Chronic ischemia due to hypertension and arteriolar sclerosis produces central white matter demyelination, and leukoaraiosis is seen on brain imaging studies (Fig. 8–2). Diffuse brain ischemia due to cardiac arrest or severe hypotension can also cause vascular dementia.

Chronic subdural hematomas, subarachnoid hemorrhage, and cerebral hemorrhage all can impair cognition, causing "hemorrhagic dementia," another form of vascular dementia.

Vascular dementia is treated by reducing cerebrovascular risk factors and preventing additional strokes (see Chapter 11). Also, consider treatment with cholinesterase inhibitors for patients with either vascular or degenerative dementia. The treatment of the symptoms of vascular dementia is the same as that for Alzheimer disease.

NORMAL-PRESSURE HYDROCEPHALUS

Normal-pressure hydrocephalus is characterized by the triad of dementia, gait disturbance, and urinary incontinence. It is impor-

tant that you recognize this disorder early in its course because it potentially can be treated with shunting. The cause of normal-pressure hydrocephalus is not known, but it occurs in conditions that can interfere with CSF absorption, such as subarachnoid hemorrhage, infection, and trauma.

Despite normal CSF pressure, as determined by lumbar puncture, normal-pressure hydrocephalus causes enlargement of the

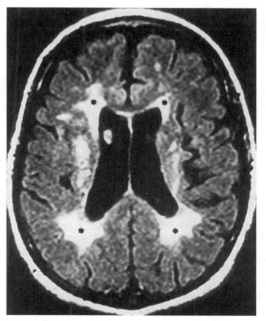

FIG. 8–2. Magnetic resonance image demonstrating leukoaraiosis (*).

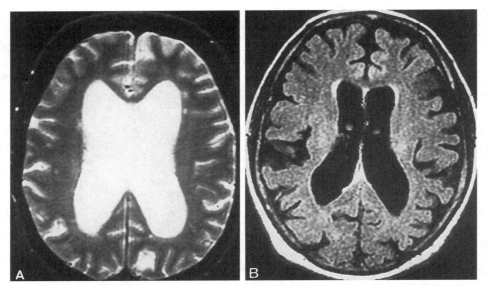

FIG. 8–3. Magnetic resonance images. (A) Normal pressure hydrocephalus; **(B)** Alzheimer dementia. In **B,** note ventricular enlargement with cortical atrophy.

lateral ventricles and, thus, compression of adjacent structures. The dementia is thought to be caused by compression of the cerebral cortex and is difficult to distinguish from that of Alzheimer disease. The radiographic feature of this disorder is enlarged ventricles disproportionate to cortical atrophy (Fig. 8–3).

The gait disorder in normal-pressure hydrocephalus is characterized by slow short steps, reduced step height, and a widened base and is often described by the terms *magnetic* and *lower half Parkinson*. *Magnetic* refers to the shuffling nature of the steps. *Parkinson* refers to the slowness and stiffness of the gait and the tendency of the patient to move en bloc. However, the arm swing is normal, unlike that in Parkinson disease. The incontinence in normal-pressure hydrocephalus results from an uninhibited bladder (see Table 4-4).

The earlier the diagnosis of normal-pressure hydrocephalus, the greater the chance of reducing the symptoms with a shunt. A useful test to determine the potential benefit from shunting is to remove 30 to 50 mL of CSF and see if the clinical symptoms improve.

FRONTOTEMPORAL DEMENTIA

The term *frontotemporal dementia* includes focal degenerative dementias of the frontal and temporal lobes. The clinical features include behavioral and language problems. Patients may become disinhibited and exhibit inappropriate social behavior or they may be apathetic, lack motivation, and show little response to stimuli. One of the more common examples, Pick disease, is characterized by argyrophilic neuronal inclusions (Pick bodies). *Pick complex* is a large group of dementia syndromes that include Pick disease, lobar atrophy, corticobasal degeneration, frontal lobe dementia, and others.

SUGGESTED READING

Blacker, D, and Tanzi, RE: The genetics of Alzheimer disease: Current status and future prospects. Arch Neurol 55:294–296, 1998.

Chui, H, and Zhang, Q: Evaluation of dementia: A systematic study of the usefulness of the American Academy of Neurology's practice parameters. Neurology 49:925–935, 1997.

Cummings, JL, et al: Alzheimer's disease: Etiologies, pathophysiology, cognitive reserve, and treatment opportunities. Neurology 51(Suppl 1):S2–S17, 1998.

Diagnostic and Statistical Manual of Mental Disorders: DSM-IV, ed 4. American Psychiatric Association, Washington, DC, 1994.

Eccles, M, et al: North of England Evidence Based Guidelines Development Project: Guideline for the primary care management of dementia. Br Med J 317: 802–808, 1998.

Fleming, KC, and Evans, JM: Pharmacologic therapies in dementia. Mayo Clin Proc 70:1116–1123, 1995.

Folstein, MF, Folstein, SE, and McHugh, PR: "Mini-mental state." A practical method for grading the cognitive state of patients for the clinician. J Psychiatr Res 12:189–198, 1975.

Kaye, JA: Diagnostic challenges in dementia. Neurology 51(Suppl 1):S45–S52, 1998.

Kertesz, A, and Munoz, D: Pick's disease, frontotemporal dementia, and Pick complex: Emerging concepts. Arch Neurol 55:302–304, 1998.

Knopman, DS, and Morris, JC: An update on primary drug therapies for Alzheimer disease. Arch Neurol 54:1406–1409, 1997.

Kosik, KS, et al: Dementia care. Continuum 16:11–185, 1996.

Le Bars, PL, et al: A placebo-controlled, double-blind, randomized trial of an extract of *Ginkgo biloba* for dementia. North American EGb Study Group. JAMA 278:1327–1332, 1997.

McKeith, IG, et al: Consensus guidelines for the clinical and pathologic diagnosis of dementia with Lewy bodies (DLB): Report of the Consortium on DLB International Workshop. Neurology 47:1113–1124, 1996.

Price, BH: Differential diagnosis of dementia. In Samuels, MA, and Feske, S (eds): Office Practice of Neurology. Churchill Livingstone, New York, 1996, pp 705–710.

Report of the Quality Standards Subcommittee of the American Academy of Neurology: Practice parameter for diagnosis and evaluation of dementia. (Summary statement.) Neurology 44:2203–2206, 1994.

Román, GC, et al: Vascular dementia: Diagnostic criteria for research studies. Report of the NINDS-AIREN International Workshop. Neurology 43:250–260, 1993.

Sano, M, et al: A controlled trial of selegiline, alpha-tocopherol, or both as treatment for Alzheimer's disease. The Alzheimer's Disease Cooperative Study. N Engl J Med 336:1216–1222, 1997.

Small, GW, et al: Diagnosis and treatment of Alzheimer disease and related disorders. Consensus statement of the American Association for Geriatric Psychiatry, the Alzheimer's Association, and the American Geriatrics Society. JAMA 278:1363–1371, 1997.

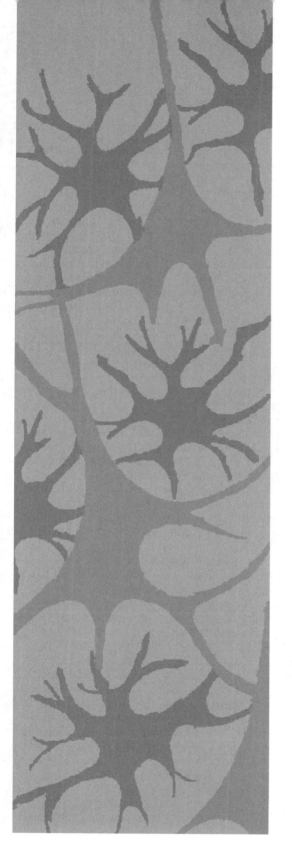

CHAPTER 9

Spells, Seizures, and Sleep Disorders

CHAPTER OUTLINE

Spells
Seizures
    Diagnostic Approach to a First Seizure
    Treatment of Seizure Disorder
    Epilepsy in Women
Sleep Disorders
    Excessive Daytime Somnolence
    Insomnia
    Parasomnias

A 35-year-old woman comes to you for evaluation of "spells." For the last year, she has experienced episodes in which she is reminded of a past event and has a sensation of apprehension and fear. She becomes diaphoretic, her heart races, and she feels as if she might pass out. Initially, the spells occurred only at night and lasted less than a few minutes. Within the last month, the spells have occurred during the day, last up to 10 minutes, and are associated with "lost time," sleepiness, and headache. Coworkers have expressed concern because her work has become less reliable than previously. Her sister has migraines and a maternal cousin has epilepsy. She is worried that she may be losing her mind. Findings on neurologic examination are normal. How do you proceed to evaluate this patient? What are the diagnostic considerations?

SPELLS

This young woman is experiencing "spells." Spells are transient disorders that indicate reversible alterations in neuronal excitability. Transient disorders can affect the central or peripheral nervous system and can be focal or generalized. Examples of generalized transient disorders are generalized seizures, syncope, concussion, and cataplexy. Examples of focal transient disorders are partial seizure disorders, transient ischemic attacks, migraine, transient mononeuropathies, paresthesias, muscle cramps, and tonic spasms.

The results of a neurologic examination of a patient with a transient disorder are frequently normal because the disorder is caused by a physiologic rather than an anatomical mechanism. The nervous system transmits, stores, and processes information through electrical activity and the action of neurotransmitters. Alterations in neuronal excitability, either excess activity or a loss of activity, can cause a transient disorder. Transient disorders can be caused by many mechanisms, including hypoxia, ischemia, seizures, electrolyte imbalances, drugs, and toxins. The absence of physical findings emphasizes the importance of taking a careful history. As in the case above, accurate diagnosis may depend on additional information from the patient's family, friends, and coworkers. In this case, the diagnostic possibilities include complex partial seizure, migraine, and psychiatric illness.

Syncope, a nonepileptic loss of consciousness, indicates global diminution in brain metabolism. It has many causes. Ones well known to primary care clinicians are brain hypoperfusion from volume loss, inadequate postural reflexes, increased vagal tone, and cardiac causes. Situational causes of syncope, such as micturition and cough syncope, are due to a combination of mechanisms. Syncope can result from metabolic impairment despite adequate perfusion, as in hypoxia, carbon monoxide poisoning, anemia, and hypoglycemia. Syncope caused by acute intracranial hypertension, which may be due to a mass, hemorrhage, or cerebrospinal fluid obstruction, is less frequent.

The differential diagnosis of spells is extensive. Determining whether the spell has focal signs or symptoms is key to making an accurate diagnosis. The common causes of focal spells are transient ischemic attacks, migraine, and partial seizures. Spells without focal signs or symptoms can include confusional states in which the patient's reactions to environmental stimuli are inappropriate. Confusional states occur in complex partial and absence seizures, toxic encephalopathies, confusional migraine, and psychiatric illnesses. Transient episodes of memory loss, as in transient global amnesia, are spells without focal symptoms. Patients with transient global anemia have anterograde amnesia that can last several hours. Drop attacks, which are episodes of sudden loss of postural tone without impairment of consciousness, also can cause spells without focal symptoms. Other spells without focal features include dizziness, psychiatric illness, sleep disorders, and pseudoseizures (Table 9–1).

The accurate diagnosis of spells depends on a careful medical history. As noted above, it is important to obtain additional information from others who have witnessed the spell or transient event. The patient's medical history, family history, and social history are necessary in differentiating the features of various spells. Laboratory studies, neu-

TABLE 9–1. DIFFERENTIAL DIAGNOSIS OF SPELLS

Spells Without Focal Symptoms

Confusional states
  Complex partial seizures
  Absence seizures
  Migraine
  Metabolic, toxic encephalopathies
  Psychiatric disease
Memory loss
  Transient global amnesia
  Drug effect
  Fugue states
Drop attacks
  Vertebrobasilar ischemia
  Anterior cerebral artery ischemia
  Foramen magnum and upper cord lesions
  Cataplexy
  Acute vestibulopathies
Sleep disorders
  Narcolepsy
  Parasomnias
Dizziness
  Vertigo
Psychiatric
  Panic attacks, anxiety disorders
  Episodic dyscontrol
  Pseudoseizures

Spells With Focal Symptoms

Transient ischemic attacks
Partial seizures
Migraine
Multiple sclerosis
Movement disorders

Modified from Drislane, FW: Transient events. In Samuels, MA, and Feske, S (eds): Office Practice of Neurology. Churchill Livingstone, New York, 1996, pp 111–121. By permission of the publisher.

roimaging, electroencephalography (EEG), and prolonged EEG monitoring may be needed to establish the diagnosis. Despite the many diagnostic tests available, time and continued clinical observation may be necessary for an accurate diagnosis. Some important differentiating features of various spells are summarized in Table 9–2.

This chapter discusses common neurologic transient disorders, including seizures and sleep disorders, seen in a primary care practice. Other causes of spells such as syncope, migraine, paroxysmal vertigo, and transient ischemic attacks are discussed in other chapters.

SEIZURES

A 26-year-old woman was brought to the emergency room because her husband thought she had a seizure. He was awakened at night by a cry from his wife. He said, "First, she got stiff, and then her arms and legs began to jerk." He was unable to arouse her, but when the paramedics arrived she was conscious but confused. By the time she reached the hospital, she was alert but could only remember going to bed that evening. She had lost control of her bladder and had bitten her tongue. Neurologic examination, complete blood count, electrolytes, chemistry screen, drug and toxin screen, and computed tomography (CT) of the head did not show any abnormality. Arrangements are made for her to be evaluated by you in follow-up. How do you manage this patient?

DIAGNOSTIC APPROACH TO A FIRST SEIZURE

The first diagnostic consideration in a patient with a spell is to determine whether the episode was an epileptic seizure or a nonepileptic event. This woman has a history consistent with a convulsive epileptic seizure. This event, or ictus, is the result of

TABLE 9–2. DIFFERENTIATING FEATURES OF SPELLS WITHOUT FOCAL SYMPTOMS

Confusional Spells

Complex partial seizures—stereotyped spells with automatisms (e.g., lip smacking), EEG is helpful
Absence seizures—may have previous history of seizures, EEG confirms diagnosis
Migraine—headache-associated, family history of migraine
Psychiatric—complex and variable behavior with spell, previous history of psychiatric illness
Toxic encephalopathies—history of chronic illness, medications, infections

Spells Associated With Memory Loss

Transient global amnesia—sudden anterograde amnesia lasting hours, patient repeats same questions during spell, patient usually older than 50 years, correlation with cerebrovascular risk factors
Drug effect—use of benzodiazepines or anticholinergic drugs
Fugue state—prolonged episode of purposeful behavior, history of psychiatric illness

Drop Attacks

Vertebrobasilar ischemia—older patients, other symptoms of brainstem ischemia
Anterior cerebral artery ischemia—rare, cerebrovascular risk factors
Foramen magnum and upper cord lesions—brainstem or myelopathic features
Cataplexy—precipitated by emotion, associated with narcolepsy

Sleep Disorders

Narcolepsy—excessive daytime somnolence, cataplexy, hypnagogic hallucinations, sleep paralysis
Parasomnias—sleepwalking, night terrors

Dizziness

Vertigo—benign positional vertigo, Ménierè disease

Psychiatric

Panic attacks—discrete episodes of apprehension and fear and autonomic symptoms
Episodic dyscontrol—associated with head injury, well-identified precipitant
Pseudoseizures—bizarre spells, high frequency in epileptics

EEG, electroencephalography.

abnormal and excessive discharge of nerve cells and can be caused by many factors. Remind the patient that a seizure is only a symptom, not a condition. The features consistent with an epileptic seizure include the loss of consciousness, tonic (continuous muscle contraction) and clonic (alternating contraction and relaxation of muscle) motor activity, injury, bladder incontinence, and postictal confusion. Syncope can be distinguished from seizure activity clinically by its relation to posture, usual occurrence during the day, and associated cardiovascular features. Convulsive activity, injury (e.g., a bitten tongue), postictal confusion, amnesia, and incontinence rarely occur in syncope.

The second step in the evaluation is to determine whether the seizure was provoked or unprovoked. Provoked seizures are caused by factors that can disrupt cerebral function. Possible precipitating factors are drug ingestion or withdrawal, structural lesions of the brain, physical injuries, vascular insults, infections, and metabolic or toxic abnormalities. Some frequent causes of provoked seizures and investigative factors that may help elicit the cause are listed in Table 9–3. If the seizure occurs within 1 week after a precipitating factor, it is classified as an "acute symptomatic seizure." The term "remote symptomatic seizure" is used if the known provoking factor occurred more than 1 week before the seizure, for example, a seizure that occurs several years after a skull fracture. A seizure that occurs in the absence of

any identifiable factor is an "unprovoked seizure." The terms "idiopathic" or "cryptogenic" are used to describe seizures with no

TABLE 9–3. CAUSES OF PROVOKED SEIZURES AND INVESTIGATIVE EVALUATION

Cause	Evaluation
Genetic and Birth Factors	History regarding pregnancy, birth, and delivery
Genetic influence Congenital abnormalities Antenatal factors—infections, drugs, anoxia Perinatal factors—birth trauma, infections	
Infectious Disorders	History—infections, HIV risk factors
Meningitis, encephalitis Brain, epidural, or subdural abscess	Exam—nuchal rigidity, increased temperature Lab—elevated leukocyte count and ESR, positive serologic tests, CSF pleocytosis CT or MRI: mass or abscess
Toxic and Metabolic	
Hypoglycemia, nonketotic hyperglycemia Hypoxia Hyponatremia, hypomagnesemia, hypocalcemia Uremia Liver failure	Serum glucose level Blood gas Sodium, magnesium, calcium Creatinine, blood urea nitrogen Liver function tests
Drugs and Drug Withdrawal, Alcohol	Toxic screen—cocaine, amphetamines, phencyclidine, hypnotic agents Alcohol level
Neoplasms	MRI
Primary intracranial Metastatic Lymphoma and leukemia	
Trauma	History and examination of trauma
Acute craniocerebral injury Subdural or epidural hematoma	CT or MRI CT or MRI
Vascular insult	Cerebrovascular risk factors
Ischemic stroke Hemorrhagic stroke	CT or MRI CT or MRI
Heredofamilial	Characteristic clinical features on exam
Neurofibromatosis, tuberous sclerosis, Sturge-Weber syndrome	
Degenerative Disease	History of dementia
Alzheimer dementia	

CSF, cerebrospinal fluid; CT, computed tomography; ESR, erythrocyte sedimentation rate; HIV, human immunodeficiency virus; MRI, magnetic resonance imaging.

identifiable cause. If the seizure is caused by a specific provoking factor and that factor can be corrected, no further treatment is required. For example, if a patient has a seizure after an episode of excessive alcohol consumption, the avoidance of alcohol is preferred to treatment with anticonvulsants. Management of unprovoked seizures is more complicated, and the risks of recurrent seizure need to be assessed and discussed with the patient and family.

The third step is to determine whether the seizure was generalized or partial. Partial seizures can become generalized seizures. For appropriate classification, prognosis, and treatment, you need to distinguish between secondary generalized partial seizures and primary generalized seizures. Partial seizures are associated with a focal brain lesion and require a thorough investigation with imaging studies. Partial seizures are also a risk factor for recurrent seizure activity. The history of a patient with a seizure should include information from anyone who witnessed the event.

Warning signs and symptoms that precede the convulsion and indicate partial seizure activity include automatisms (e.g., lip smacking, chewing, and complex pattern movements such as repetitive buttoning and unbuttoning of clothing) and an aura. Examples of a preceding aura are an epigastric or abdominal "rising" sensation, a sense of fear or apprehension, and other sensory symptoms (taste, smell, visual, or auditory hallucinations). A period of unresponsiveness and focal or asymmetric motor activity are also common in partial seizure activity. Persistent weakness less than 24 hours after a seizure is called *Todd paralysis* and is evidence of a focal seizure disorder.

A common partial seizure disorder of childhood, called "benign childhood epilepsy with centrotemporal spikes" or "benign rolandic epilepsy," is not associated with an underlying focal brain lesion. The onset is between the ages of 3 and 13 years. The child often awakens from sleep with motor and sensory symptoms of the face and hand. Drooling and arrest of speech are common. This benign disorder has a characteristic EEG pattern. Neurologic examination findings are normal, and the disorder usually remits in adolescence.

For determining prognosis, it is crucial to know whether the event truly was the patient's first seizure. The patient should be asked if he or she ever had a seizure, a fit, or a convulsion with a fever as a young child. The risk for recurrent seizure after a second seizure is high, and most neurologists begin treatment after a second seizure. Information about the patient's gestation, birth, delivery, and childhood development is important with regard to complications associated with seizures (Table 9–3). A history of head trauma or serious infection may also indicate the possibility of remote symptomatic seizure. Any information about drug use is important. Central nervous system stimulants such as amphetamines, cocaine, and phencyclidine can induce seizure activity. Phenothiazines, some new atypical neuroleptics, penicillin, theophylline, and some tricyclic antidepressants reduce seizure threshold in susceptible persons. The family history is extremely important because a positive family history of epilepsy is a risk factor for recurrent seizure.

Focus the physical examination on detecting any underlying medical illness that would suggest a symptomatic seizure. Focal neurologic signs indicate partial seizure activity and increase the risk of recurrent seizure activity. Skin abnormalities may provide clues to an underlying neuroectodermal disorder, for example, café-au-lait spots in neurofibromatosis or angiofibromas on the bridge of the nose in patients with tuberous sclerosis.

EEG is indispensable in the evaluation of a patient with seizures. EEG findings help determine the prognosis for recurrent seizure and help in classifying the seizure type as partial or generalized. EEG abnormalities, including focal and generalized epileptiform discharges and focal slowing, are associated with a higher risk of seizure recurrence. EEG should be performed as soon after the seizure as possible and should include a sleep recording to maximize the chance of finding epileptiform abnormalities. Remember that normal EEG findings do not exclude the possibility of epilepsy, and repeat studies may be needed in certain clinical situations.

Magnetic resonance imaging (MRI) is the imaging study preferred for evaluating a patient with seizures. Compared with CT, MRI is more sensitive and accurate because of better soft tissue contrast, multiplanar imaging capability, and the absence of beam-hardening artifacts. The major structural causes of seizures, including tumors or any mass lesion, disorders of neuronal migration and cortical organization, vascular malformations, and mesial temporal sclerosis, are visualized best with MRI. MRI can also detect evidence of previous brain injury from trauma, infection, inflammation, or infarction. Any structural abnormality seen on an imaging study increases the risk of recurrent seizures.

MRI is recommended for almost all patients with seizures. However, imaging may not be necessary for patients with the characteristic features of primary generalized epilepsy or primary partial epilepsy. In the preceding case, the emergent CT did not provide all the necessary information needed from an imaging study. Unless the findings on the emergent CT are expected to alter management, it may be best to perform MRI instead to avoid added cost.

After the diagnostic evaluation, decide about treatment. The purpose of treatment is to prevent recurrent seizures and the associated complications. Although antiepileptic drugs reduce the risk for recurrent seizures, there is no evidence that treatment affects long-term prognosis. Several complications are associated with antiepileptic drugs. Up to 10% of patients who take these drugs develop a skin rash, and almost 25% of newly treated patients have unacceptable side effects. The cost of the drugs, laboratory evaluations, and follow-up visits needs to be considered. Treatment also has implications for employment, insurance eligibility, and the social stigma of being labeled "epileptic."

The risk for recurrent seizures after a single unprovoked seizure is approximately 35% for the subsequent 5 years. The range varies from less than 20% to 100%, depending on the presence or absence of risk factors. Risk factors for recurrent seizure include a previous provoked seizure, a focal seizure, abnormal results on neurologic examination, a family history of epilepsy, and abnormal EEG findings.

The decision about whether to treat an adult with an anticonvulsant medication depends on the estimate of recurrent risk. Also, an assessment should be made of the consequences of a recurrent seizure, including the potential impact on the patient's social, occupational, and psychologic status. The patient and family should participate in the decision-making process, and the patient's preferences should be considered. For a child, antiepileptic drug treatment is not initiated after a first unprovoked seizure unless there are serious consequences associated with recurrent seizure activity.

Treatment with antiepileptic drugs is usually considered for provoked seizures when the provoking factor cannot be corrected. Treatment is recommended after a second unprovoked seizure, because the risk of recurrent seizure increases to approximately 75%. Some seizure types, like absence and myoclonic seizures, are recurrent and are usually treated. The decision-making steps for treating a patient who has a first-time seizure are shown in Figure 9–1.

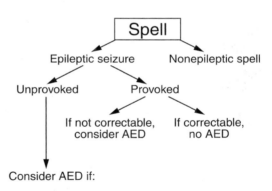

Consider AED if:

1) Recurrent seizure risk factor present
    Previous seizure
    Remote symptomatic cause
    Focal seizure by history or exam
    Family history of epilepsy
    Abnormal EEG
    Abnormal imaging findings

2) Consequences with recurrent seizure are significant

3) Recurrent seizure type
    Absence
    Myoclonic

FIG. 9–1. Algorithm for evaluating spells. AED, antiepileptic drug; **EEG,** electroencephalography.

After a patient has a seizure, several important safety issues need to be discussed. Patients should not engage in any situation in which they would injure themselves or others if they had a recurrent seizure. Driving regulations must be discussed and the conversation documented in the medical record. You should know the current driving regulations of the state in which you practice. Some states require that the physician report seizures or any episode of loss of consciousness. Most states require the patient to have a seizure-free period (30 days to 1 year) before being allowed to drive. Exceptions vary by state. Periodic medical updates are required in many states. Consult the Department of Motor Vehicles for this information.

TREATMENT OF SEIZURE DISORDER

After the decision has been made to treat a seizure disorder, many factors determine which antiepileptic drug is prescribed. These factors include the effectiveness of the drug in controlling seizures, tolerability of side effects, pharmacokinetic properties, patient characteristics, drug interactions, and cost of therapy. The best antiepileptic drug is the one that controls seizures without causing unacceptable side effects. Therapy needs to be individualized. The dose of one antiepileptic drug should be increased gradually until seizure control is achieved without provoking unacceptable adverse effects. If monotherapy is not effective, consider neurologic consultation. Antiepilep-

TABLE 9–4. ANTIEPILEPTIC DRUGS

Drug	Seizure Type	Dose—Initial Adult Dose	Time to Steady State
Carbamazepine (Tegretol)	Partial seizures with complex symptoms, generalized	10–20 mg/kg daily in divided doses—200 mg 2 times daily	4–6 wk; after induction 2–4 days
Clonazepam (Klonopin)	Generalized, absence, myoclonic, akinetic, absence variant	0.01–0.03 mg/kg daily in divided doses—0.5 mg 3 times daily	4–10 days
Ethosuximide (Zarontin)	Absence	15 mg/kg daily in 2 divided doses—250 mg 2 times daily	7–14 days
Felbamate (Felbatol)	Partial seizures with or without secondary generalization, Lennox-Gastaut	15 mg/kg—300 mg 4 times daily	5–7 days
Gabapentin (Neurontin)	Adjunctive therapy for partial seizures	300 mg 3 times daily	12 days with normal renal function
Lamotrigine (Lamictal)	Adjunctive therapy for partial seizures	50 mg daily	3–15 days
Phenobarbital	Generalized and partial seizures	1–3 mg/kg daily	1–4 wk
Phenytoin (Dilantin)	Partial seizures with and without secondary generalization	5 mg/kg daily—300 mg daily	1–3 wk
Primidone (Mysoline)	Partial seizures with and without secondary generalization	10–25 mg/kg—125 mg at bedtime	3–7 days for primidone, 1–4 wk for phenobarbital metabolite
Topiramate (Topamax)	Adjunctive therapy for partial seizures	200 mg 2 times daily	5–10 days
Valproate (Depakote)	Generalized and partial seizures	10–15 mg/kg daily—250 mg 2 times daily	5–10 days

tic drugs and the indication by seizure type, dose, and time to steady state (5 to 7.5 times the half-life) are listed in Table 9–4.

One of the first steps in selecting an antiepileptic drug is to determine whether the seizure is generalized or partial. Valproate (Depakote) is the most effective drug for controlling generalized seizures, including absence seizures, myoclonic seizures, and primary generalized tonic-clonic seizures. Ethosuximide (Zarontin) is equally efficacious for absence seizures but is not effective for generalized tonic-clonic seizures. Valproate may be preferred for patients with both absence and generalized tonic-clonic seizures. Clonazepam (Klonopin) is effective for myoclonic seizures but is usually the second choice after valproate.

Antiepileptic drugs effective for partial seizures or secondary generalized tonic-clonic seizures include valproate, phenytoin (Dilantin), carbamazepine (Tegretol), and phenobarbital. Although felbamate (Felbatol) is effective in treating partial seizures, its use is restricted for catastrophic seizures, because of the risk of aplastic anemia and liver failure. Lamotrigine (Lamictal), gabapentin (Neurontin), topiramate (Topamax), and tiagabine (Gabitril) have been approved as adjunct agents for the treatment of partial seizures. The use of these newer drugs as monotherapy in the treatment of partial seizures is being investigated.

All antiepileptic drugs are associated with adverse side effects. Many of the side effects a patient experiences at the initiation of therapy can be avoided by starting treatment at a low dose and gradually increasing it. Unless the clinical situation dictates prompt protection against seizure recurrence, avoid full or loading doses to minimize the chance of adverse effects. Common side effects associated with all antiepileptic drugs are nausea and other gastrointestinal symptoms, sedation, dizziness, and incoordination. Before a patient drives a motor vehicle or operates dangerous equipment, he or she should find out whether the drug causes adverse effects that impair mental or motor performance. Within 6 weeks after starting treatment, approximately 10% of patients develop a rash. Rash is less likely with valproate or gabapentin (2% of patients) than with phenytoin, carbamazepine, or lamotrigine (10% of patients).

Liver dysfunction is rare but has been associated with valproate, which should be avoided or prescribed with caution in patients with a metabolic disorder, poor nutritional status, mental retardation, congenital neurologic illnesses, or use of multiple antiepileptic drugs and in infants. Weight gain is an important side effect associated with valproate. Alternate antiepileptic drugs should be considered for patients with a problem with obesity. The tremor associated with valproate may limit its use for patients whose employment requires fine motor skills, for example, a jeweler.

The risk of bone marrow suppression with antiepileptic drug treatment is low; however, this side effect is associated with carbamazepine more than with the other drugs. Avoid treatment with carbamazepine if the patient has a hematologic illness. Inform the patient or the patient's caregiver about the symptoms of early bone marrow suppression. Symptoms of fatigue, postural dizziness, bruises, fever, and sore throat may indicate anemia, coagulopathy, or infection before changes are detected with laboratory tests. Also, avoid treatment with carbamazepine if the patient has a demonstrated hypersensitivity to tricyclic antidepressants or is also taking a monoamine oxidase inhibitor.

Barbiturates, including phenobarbital and primidone (Mysoline), are commonly associated with behavioral and cognitive disturbances, and in elderly patients, phenobarbital is associated with an increased risk of falls and fractures. In addition to cognitive disturbances, barbiturates are known to cause paradoxical hyperactivity in children. Barbiturates also have been associated with Dupuytren contractures, frozen shoulder, decreased libido, and impotence. They should be prescribed with extreme caution in patients who are mentally depressed, have suicidal tendencies, have a history of drug abuse, or are receiving other central nervous system depressants. Because of the undesirable side effects of barbiturates, avoid treatment with these drugs. The adverse effects associated with different antiepileptic drugs are listed in Table 9–5.

The use of an antiepileptic drug may depend on its pharmacokinetic properties. The longer serum half-life of a drug may be significant for dosage schedule and patient

TABLE 9–5. ADVERSE EFFECTS OF ANTIEPILEPTIC DRUGS

Drug	Warnings and Precautions	Common Side Effects	Other Side Effects to Consider	Idiosyncratic Side Effects
Carbamazepine (Tegretol)	Use with care in patients with mixed seizure disorder that includes atypical absence	Dizziness, diplopia	Hyponatremia, neural tube defects in pregnancy, atrioventricular conduction defect and ventricular automaticity	Leukopenia
Clonazepam (Klonopin)	CNS depression Can cause generalized tonic-clonic seizures in patients with mixed seizure disorder Contraindicated in acute narrow-angle glaucoma	Sedation, ataxia	Tolerance to anticonvulsant activity may develop	Confusion, depression
Ethosuximide (Zarontin)	Caution in kidney and liver dysfunction Abrupt withdrawal can precipitate absence status May increase generalized tonic-clonic convulsions when used in mixed seizure disorders	Nausa, vomiting	Aggressiveness, psychosis	Blood dyscrasias, rash
Felbamate (Felbatol)	Need informed consent Aplastic anemia Liver failure	Anorexia, vomiting, nausea	Headache, insomnia, weight loss	Aplastic anemia Liver failure
Gabapentin (Neurontin)	CNS depression	Fatigue, somnolence, dizziness, ataxia		Not established
Lamotrigine (Lamictal)	CNS depression Liver dysfunction Platelet and coagulation tests should be performed periodically	Abnormal thinking, dizziness, ataxia, diplopia, nausea, weight gain	Rash	Rash

TABLE 9–5. ADVERSE EFFECTS OF ANTIEPILEPTIC DRUGS *(continued)*

Drug	Warnings and Precautions	Common Side Effects	Other Side Effects to Consider	Idiosyncratic Side Effects
Phenobarbital	CNS depression May be habit-forming Use with care in depressed patients	Sedation	Behavioral and cognitive disturbance Painful shoulder-hand syndromes	May cause paradoxical hyperactivity
Phenytoin (Dilantin)	Abrupt withdrawal may cause status epilepticus Lymphadenopathy Hyperglycemia	Nystagmus, ataxia	Gingival hyperplasia Hirsutism Coarsening of facial features Atrioventricular conduction defect and ventricular automaticity	
Primidone (Mysoline)	CNS depression May be habit-forming Use with care in depressed patients	Sedation, dizziness, ataxia	Behavioral and cognitive disturbance Diminished libido Impotence	May cause paradoxical hyperactivity
Topiramate (Topamax)	CNS depression Proper hydration to avoid urinary tract calculi	Somnolence, fatigue	Memory dysfunction Weight loss	Urinary tract calculi
Valproate (Depakote)	CNS depression Liver dysfunction Platelet and coagulation tests should be performed periodically	Nausea, vomiting, tremor, thrombo-cytopenia	Weight gain Hair loss Neural tube defect in pregnancy Association with hyperandro-genism	Liver dysfunction

CNS, central nervous system.

compliance. For example, phenytoin may be preferred to other drugs because it can be taken once a day. Of the antiepileptic medications, the highly protein-bound drugs like phenytoin and valproate are affected more by hypoalbuminemia, renal dysfunction, and interactions with other highly protein-bound drugs. The route of elimination may also influence the selection of antiepileptic drug. The liver metabolizes most of these drugs, and many of them induce liver enzymes. Gabapentin is unique in that it is eliminated entirely through the kidney. Two other drugs eliminated mainly through the kidney are felbamate and topiramate. Adjust the dose of the antiepileptic drug if the patient has liver or kidney dysfunction.

Drug interactions, which depend on metabolism, enzyme induction, and protein binding, are also important when selecting an antiepileptic drug. Those that induce liver enzymes, including carbamazepine, phenytoin, phenobarbital, and primidone, can reduce the concentrations and effectiveness of other drugs metabolized by these enzymes, such as oral contraceptives, theophylline, corticosteroids, and warfarin. Gabapentin does not interact with other medications. Some of the drug interactions for carbamazepine, phenytoin, and valproate are listed in Table 9–6.

After a patient starts receiving maintenance therapy with an antiepileptic drug, he or she should be followed up with clinical evaluations and laboratory testing. Clinical evaluation is more useful than laboratory testing. Drug levels should be used only as a guide to therapy. The dosage of an antiepileptic drug should not be changed on the basis of a drug level. The drug level can guide the decision about dosage, based on whether the patient is having seizures or toxic side effects. The level of an antiepileptic drug is not meaningful until the drug has reached steady state (see Table 9–4). Circumstances that may change drug dosage and level include growth in children, aging, weight change, medical illness, or drug interactions. You may need to monitor the free fraction of an antiepileptic drug that has high protein binding (carbamazepine, phenytoin, or valproate) in conditions that affect protein binding, for example, liver and kidney disease, pregnancy, and hypoalbuminemia.

Liver function tests and complete blood counts are often performed to determine whether the serious complications of hepatitis or hematologic suppression have developed. However, it is more important that the patient recognize the early symptoms of these serious complications. Often, minor laboratory abnormalities are not clinically significant. Laboratory values that are significant include a leukocyte count less than 3,000 cells/mm³, a neutrophil count less than 1,500/mm³, platelets less than 100,000/mm³, and liver enzymes greater than 2.5 times normal. Asymptomatic patients with any of these values should be followed closely, and the dose of the antiepileptic drug should be decreased.

EPILEPSY IN WOMEN

When treating women for seizures or epilepsy, several special issues need to be considered. Seizure disorders and antiepileptic drugs affect oral contraceptives, the

TABLE 9–6. ANTIEPILEPTIC DRUG INTERACTIONS

Carbamazepine

Carbamazepine decreases—doxycycline, folic acid, haloperidol, oral contraceptives, theophylline, warfarin
Drugs increasing carbamazepine levels—cimetidine, danazol, diltiazem, erythromycin, fluoxetine, imipramine, isoniazid, propoxyphene, verapamil
Drugs decreasing carbamazepine levels—alcohol (long-term use), folic acid, phenobarbital, phenytoin

Phenytoin

Phenytoin decreases—chloramphenicol, cyclosporine, dexamethasone, doxycycline, folic acid, furosemide, haloperidol, meperidine, methadone, oral contraceptives, quinidine, theophylline, vitamin D
Phenytoin increases—warfarin
Drugs decreasing phenytoin levels—alcohol (long-term use), antacids, carbamazepine, folic acid, rifampin, valproate
Drugs increasing phenytoin levels—alcohol (short-term use), amiodarone, chloramphenicol, chlordiazepoxide, cimetidine, disulfiram, fluconazole, fluoxetine, imipramine, isoniazid, metronidazole, omeprazole, propoxyphene, sulfonamides, trazodone

Valproate

Valproate decreases—carbamazepine, oral contraceptives, phenobarbital, phenytoin
Valproate increases—alcohol, aspirin, benzodiazepines, cimetidine

menstrual cycle, and pregnancy. Tell women who have seizures that the failure rate of oral contraceptives is four times higher than normal when being treated with an enzyme-inducing antiepileptic drug (phenytoin, carbamazepine, or phenobarbital). Valproate, gabapentin, lamotrigine, and the benzodiazepines do not have this effect. Thus, an oral contraceptive with a higher hormone dose or an alternate contraceptive may need to be considered.

Menstrual dysfunction—anovulatory cycles, amenorrhea, oligomenorrhea, and abnormal cycle intervals—is more common in women with epilepsy than in those without epilepsy. Seizures affect the hypothalamic-pituitary-gonadal axis. In addition, antiepileptic drugs affect hormone-binding globulin, which in turn can disrupt estrogen and progesterone binding. Up to 50% of women with epilepsy report that their seizures vary with the menstrual cycle.

There are many important issues related to seizures, antiepileptic drugs, and pregnancy. At the beginning of the therapeutic relationship with a woman of childbearing age, discuss seizures, antiepileptic drugs, and pregnancy. Although more than 90% of women with epilepsy have uneventful pregnancies, they need to know about the teratogenic potential of antiepileptic drugs and the potential harm to the fetus from a seizure. Seizure frequency can increase during pregnancy, and the importance of compliance with medication and close medical follow-up should be emphasized. Recommend a multivitamin with folate (4 mg) for all women of childbearing age. Folate must be present within the first 25 days after conception to protect against neural tube defects.

Discontinuing or switching to another antiepileptic drug should be done before the patient becomes pregnant. If the patient has been seizure-free for a time, consider withdrawal of the drug treatment. Withdrawal of drug treatment is most likely to be successful in patients who have been seizure-free for 2 to 5 years while taking an antiepileptic drug, have a single type of partial or generalized seizure, have normal findings on neurologic examination, have a normal I.Q., and whose EEG results normalized with treatment. Most seizures recur in the first 6

months after withdrawal of an antiepileptic drug; thus, advise the patient that during this period she should not become pregnant or drive a motor vehicle.

If withdrawal of the antiepileptic drug is not a possibility, the patient should receive maintenance therapy with the one drug that, at the lowest dose possible, best controls her seizures. It is best for the patient to receive maintenance therapy with the antiepileptic drug that she already takes. The risk of fetal injury is twice normal and is increased with higher doses and with multiple medications. Antiepileptic drug monotherapy with divided doses is recommended. The free fraction of the drug should be determined before conception and checked every 3 months throughout pregnancy. Major malformations can be detected with ultrasonography, alpha-fetoprotein testing, amniocentesis, and chorionic villus sampling. Enzyme-inducing antiepileptic drugs (carbamazepine, phenytoin, and phenobarbital) have been associated with an increased risk of neonatal bleeding due to low levels of vitamin K. Thus, vitamin K, 10 mg/day, should be taken during the final month of gestation.

Breastfeeding in women taking antiepileptic drugs is usually successful despite the concentration of these drugs in the breast milk. The amount of drug in the breast milk is inversely related to the degree of protein binding. Breastfeeding should be discontinued if sedation, poor feeding, or irritability occurs in the infant.

SLEEP DISORDERS

A 50-year-old woman comes for evaluation after two spells. She reports that on two stressful occasions, while talking to her employer, she suddenly fell to the floor. She did not lose consciousness. She has been having difficulty at work because of her sleepiness. She has always had a problem with falling asleep easily and reports that her dentist was amazed when she fell asleep while having a tooth repaired. At work, she often needs to get up from her desk to avoid falling asleep. She stopped driving to work because of her sleepiness, but she has fallen asleep on the bus and missed her stop, making her late for work. She was explaining this problem to her boss when she had her first spell. She also reports having a frightening episode in which she was dreaming about her work and could not move. Her husband thinks she just does not want to go to work. What are the diagnostic possibilities and how do you manage this patient?

The more than 100 sleep/wake disorders can be divided into four major categories: (1) excessive daytime somnolence, (2) insomnia, (3) disorders of the sleep/wake cycle, and (4) parasomnias. Parasomnias are undesirable motor or experiential phenomena that arise during sleep.

Begin an evaluation of a patient with a sleep disorder with a thorough history and physical examination. Obtain information about the patient's sleep pattern: what time the patient goes to bed, length of time before falling asleep, time in bed, hours of sleep at night, time awake, time needed to feel restored and rested, and the number of daytime naps. You often will need to get information from bed partners, other family members, coworkers, or caregivers. Sleep diaries covering a 2- to 3-week period may be needed to provide an accurate accounting of the patient's sleep pattern.

A formal sleep evaluation can include polysomnography, multiple sleep latency test, maintenance of wakefulness test, pupillography, and actigraphy. Basic polysomnography involves monitoring eye movements, respiratory variables, electrocardiography, electromyography, and EEG. The multiple sleep latency test is a standardized measure of the physiologic tendency to fall asleep during normal waking hours; it measures the same variables that are monitored in polysomnography. The maintenance of wakefulness test is similar to the multiple sleep latency test but measures the ability to remain awake. Pupillography measures pupil size; the interpretation of results is based on the observation that pupils constrict during drowsiness and sleep. Actig-

raphy records movement and nonmovement over time, to supplement the sleep diary.

EXCESSIVE DAYTIME SOMNOLENCE

Most often, excessive daytime somnolence is the result of sleep deprivation. The amount of sleep needed by a person is the amount required to feel rested and restored after awakening. For adults, the range is from 4 to 10 hours, with 8 hours being the average. Make-up sleep is the only way to diminish sleepiness due to sleep deprivation. If excessive daytime sleepiness is not associated with sleep deprivation, evaluate for narcolepsy, idiopathic central nervous system hypersomnia, or sleep apnea.

The woman in the case above describes symptoms compatible with narcolepsy, whose characteristic features are excessive daytime somnolence, cataplexy, sleep paralysis, and hypnagogic hallucinations. Narcolepsy is a sleep disorder in which sleep/wake phenomena are dissociated. The components of rapid eye movement (REM) sleep and nonrapid eye movement (NREM) sleep appear in the wakeful state. The control of the onset and offset of both REM and NREM sleep is impaired, causing nighttime sleep fragmentation and intrusion of REM and NREM sleep components into daytime wakefulness.

The sleepiness of narcolepsy is defined as the tendency to fall asleep easily in a relaxed or sedentary situation. Patients without sleepiness but with complaints of fatigue and tiredness tend not to fall asleep in these situations. The patient's sleep pattern may help distinguish between narcolepsy and sleep deficiency. A person with sleep deprivation tends to have different sleep patterns on weekdays and weekends, whereas a person with narcolepsy tends to have the same sleep pattern (time in bed, hours of sleep, and number of daytime naps) throughout the week.

Cataplexy, which occurs in about two-thirds of patients with narcolepsy, is the sudden loss of muscle tone induced by emotion. The duration of cataplexy is short, and there is no impairment of consciousness or memory. "Hypnagogic hallucinations" are hallucinations that occur during the transition from sleep to waking. They may have vivid features, similar to dreams, but the person can be aware of his or her surroundings. Sleep paralysis is the inability to move during the onset and offset of sleep; it can last from seconds to minutes.

Fewer than half of the patients with narcolepsy have all four symptoms characteristic of the disorder. Furthermore, sleep paralysis and hypnagogic hallucinations can occur in persons who do not have narcolepsy. Cataplexy may be part of somatization disorder or atonic seizures. Myoclonus may be mistaken for cataplexy. The diagnosis of narcolepsy can be confirmed by a formal sleep evaluation. The investigation includes all-night polysomnography, followed by the multiple sleep latency test to determine the quality and quantity of the preceding night's sleep.

The hypersomnolence of narcolepsy is treated with central nervous system stimulants. Modafinil, a new α_1-adrenergic stimulant, has recently been approved in the United States for this use. Cataplexy, sleep paralysis, and hypnagogic hallucinations are treated with tricyclic antidepressants, monoamine oxidase inhibitors, selective serotonin reuptake inhibitors, and anticholinergic medications. The mechanism of tricyclic antidepressants and monoamine oxidase inhibitors is likely suppression of REM sleep.

The term *idiopathic hypersomnia* describes a heterogeneous disorder of the central nervous system characterized by excessive daytime somnolence. Excessive daytime somnolence in the absence of symptoms suggestive of sleep deprivation, narcolepsy, or sleep apnea suggests idiopathic hypersomnia. If this rare disorder is suspected, consult a sleep disorder specialist.

After sleep deprivation, the most common cause of excessive daytime somnolence is sleep apnea, which is defined as repeated episodes of obstructive apnea and hypopnea during sleep. Its clinical features include complaints of fatigue and loud snoring. It is common among adults, especially males, postmenopausal women, and overweight persons. Remember that 25% to 30% of patients with sleep apnea are *not* overweight. A formal sleep study can confirm the diagnosis.

Behavioral interventions for sleep apnea include weight loss, avoidance of alcohol and sedatives, avoidance of sleep deprivation, and nocturnal positioning. First-line medical therapy includes positive pressure through a mask (continuous positive airway pressure [CPAP]). Other medical treatments include the use of an oral appliance, fluoxetine, protriptyline, and nocturnal oxygen. Upper airway bypass with tracheostomy and upper airway reconstruction are surgical options.

INSOMNIA

Insomnia, the most common sleep-related complaint, can be caused by medical, psychiatric, and drug-induced disorders. Neurologists often manage insomnia because of its frequent association with extrapyramidal diseases. Insomnia is also a major complication of restless legs syndrome.

Restless legs syndrome is characterized by an unpleasant sensation in the lower extremities. These leg paresthesias are prominent during periods of inactivity and particularly during the transition from wakefulness to sleep. Movement of the legs provides temporary relief. The discomfort is difficult to describe, and patients describe it as "creeping," "crawling," "itching," "pulling," and "drawing."

Most patients with restless legs syndrome also demonstrate periodic movements of sleep. These are brief (1 or 2 seconds) jerks of one or both legs. Movement may involve only dorsiflexion of the big toe or flexion of the entire leg(s). The movements occur periodically (every 20 to 40 seconds). The patient is often aroused during sleep but is not aware of the arousal. Periodic movements of sleep can be extremely disruptive for the bed partner. Although up to 80% of patients with restless legs syndrome have periodic movements of sleep, not all those with periodic movements of sleep have restless legs syndrome. Periodic leg movements of sleep may have no clinical significance.

The cause of restless legs syndrome is not known. Idiopathic and familial cases have been described. The syndrome is associated with several medical conditions, including pregnancy, iron deficiency anemia, peripheral neuropathies, thyroid disease, rheumatoid arthritis, and uremia. Peripheral neuropathies may mimic restless legs, but movement does not relieve the paresthesias. Patients with fi-bromyalgia may have lower extremity pain that resembles the condition, but the pain does not increase with rest and inactivity. Akathisia, the motor restlessness often caused by dopamine receptor blocking drugs, is included in the differential diagnosis of restless legs syndrome. The restless movements or inner restlessness of akathisia is not worse at night or with lying down.

Treatment of restless legs should include a reduction in caffeine and alcohol consumption. The patient should stop smoking. Effective medications are dopamine agonists, benzodiazepines, and opiates. Some of the medications used for restless legs syndrome are listed in Table 9–7. If the patient does not have a response to one medication, try a different agent, even in the same class. A combination of these drugs may be necessary to control the symptoms. Dopamine agonists are often used before benzodiazepines and opiates. Although there is a potential for abuse and tolerance of benzodiazepines and opiates, the incidence is low. The term "daytime augmentation" describes increasing symptoms earlier in the day, which can be a problem with carbidopa-levodopa preparations; if daytime augmentation occurs, consider switching to another dopamine agonist.

PARASOMNIAS

Parasomnias refers to undesirable behavioral or experiential events that occur during sleep or are exacerbated by sleep. Common examples include nightmares and sleepwalking. The differential diagnosis of paroxysmal nocturnal events or nighttime spells includes seizures and parasomnias.

Parasomnias are often categorized by the stage of sleep in which they occur. The disorders of arousal include confusional arousals, sleepwalking, and sleep terror. The disorders occur during stages 3 and 4 of NREM sleep. Patients often have a positive family history for these events, suggesting a genetic component. These disorders are common in childhood and decrease in frequency with increasing age. Arousal disorders are characterized by confusion and automatic behavior following sudden arousal. Sleep terror is the most

---

TABLE 9–7. MEDICATIONS FOR RESTLESS LEGS SYNDROME

Dopamine Agonists

Carbidopa-levodopa (Sinemet)
Bromocriptine (Parlodel)
Pergolide (Permax)
Pramipexole (Mirapex)
Ropinirole (Requip)

Benzodiazepines

Diazepam (Valium)
Clonazepam (Klonopin)
Triazolam (Halcion)

Opiates

Codeine (Tylenol #3)
Oxycodone (Percocet)
Propoxyphene (Darvocet)
Tramadol (Ultram)

Anticonvulsants

Carbamazepine (Tegretol)
Gabapentin (Neurontin)

Others

Baclofen (Lioresal)
Clonidine (Catapres)
Phenoxybenzamine (Dibenzyline)

---

dramatic type, with the aroused person having a piercing scream or cry with automatic and behavioral manifestations of intense fear. The person cannot be consoled, but he or she is usually amnestic for the event.

These disorders may not need to be evaluated, but polysomnography is recommended if the episodes are frequent or if there is violent behavior, excessive daytime somnolence, or atypical clinical features. Treatment should include removing anything that may precipitate arousal and avoiding caffeine and alcohol. Clonazepam can be effective by increasing the arousal threshold.

REM sleep behavior disorder, a parasomnia that occurs during REM sleep, is often mistaken for psychiatric disease. This sleep disorder is characterized by the loss of the atonia characteristic of REM sleep; thus, the person is able to act out his or her dream. The result may be an elaborate motor behavior that is potentially injurious to the person or bed partner. Unlike the arousal disorders during NREM sleep, the person may recall the dream associated with the motor behavior. REM sleep behavior disorder is often confused with hallucinations or post-traumatic stress disorder.

REM sleep behavior disorder is frequently associated with such neurologic diseases as Parkinson disease, dementia, and stroke. It may be the first symptom in Parkinson disease. Drug withdrawal, fluoxetine, and tricyclic antidepressants can induce the syndrome. Clonazepam is an effective treatment.

SUGGESTED READING

Aldrich, MS: Diagnostic aspects of narcolepsy. Neurology 50(Suppl 1):S2–S7, 1998.

Britton, JW, and So, EL: Selection of antiepileptic drugs: A practical approach. Mayo Clin Proc 71:778–786, 1996.

Chabolla, DR, et al: Psychogenic nonepileptic seizures. Mayo Clin Proc 71:493–500, 1996.

Drislane, FW: Transient events. In Samuels, MA, and Feske, S (eds): Office Practice of Neurology. Churchill Livingstone, New York, 1996, pp 111–121.

Hauser, WA, et al: Seizure recurrence after a 1st unprovoked seizure: An extended follow-up. Neurology 40: 1163–1170, 1990.

Hauser, WA, et al: Risk of recurrent seizures after two unprovoked seizures. N Engl J Med 338:429–434, 1998.

Jack, CR, Jr: Magnetic resonance imaging in epilepsy. Mayo Clin Proc 71:695–711, 1996.

Mahowald, MW, et al: Sleep disorders. Continuum 3: 9–158, 1997.

Mayo Medical Center Drug Formulary 1997–98. Mayo Press, Rochester, Minnesota, 1996.

Morrell, MJ: Guidelines for the care of women with epilepsy. Neurology 51(Suppl 4):S21–S27, 1998.

Mosewich, RK, and So, EL: A clinical approach to the classification of seizures and epileptic syndromes. Mayo Clin Proc 71:405–414, 1996.

Report of the Quality Standards Subcommittee of the American Academy of Neurology: Practice parameter: A guideline for discontinuing antiepileptic drugs in seizure-free patients—summary statement. Neurology 47:600–602, 1996.

Roberts, R: Differential diagnosis of sleep disorders, non-epileptic attacks and epileptic seizures. Curr Opin Neurol 11:135–139, 1998.

Shuster, EA: Epilepsy in women. Mayo Clin Proc 71:991–999, 1996.

Strollo, PJ, Jr, and Rogers, RM: Obstructive sleep apnea. N Engl J Med 334:99–104, 1996.

Trenkwalder, C, Walters, AS, and Hening, W: Periodic limb movements and restless legs syndrome. Neurol Clin 14:629–650, 1996.

Walters, AS: Toward a better definition of the restless legs syndrome. Mov Disord 10:634–642, 1995.

Westmoreland, BF: Epileptiform electroencephalographic patterns. Mayo Clin Proc 71:501–511, 1996.

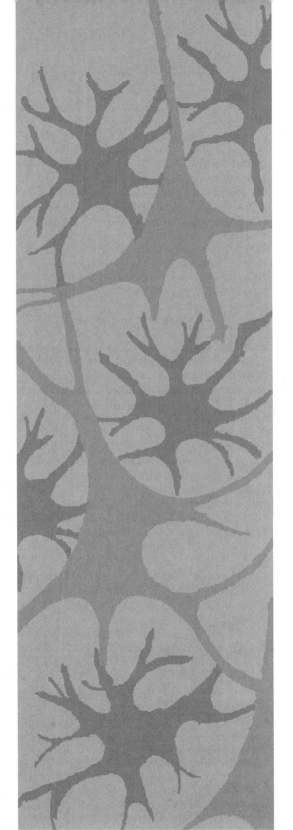

CHAPTER 10

Pain

CHAPTER OUTLINE

General Management Principles
Diagnostic Approach
Treatment
Painful Polyneuropathy
Complex Regional Pain Syndromes
Postherpetic Neuralgia
Central Pain
Neuropathic Cancer Pain
Mental Disorders and Pain

171

A 66-year-old woman had gradual onset of paroxysmal pain in the right lower quadrant of the abdomen. She described the pain as a "zing." Her medical history was significant for breast cancer, which was treated with lumpectomy 6 years before the onset of the abdominal pain. Follow-up evaluations have been negative for recurrence of breast cancer. The "zinging" abdominal pain has been present for 4 years, and extensive diagnostic testing has not revealed any cause of the pain. Testing has included several imaging studies, gastrointestinal procedures, and exploratory laparoscopy. She has received treatment with numerous medications, physical therapy, transcutaneous electrical nerve stimulation (TENS), and acupuncture and has been to two university pain clinics without relief. She expressed interest in trying illicit drugs to get some relief. The paroxysms of pain have become more severe and frequent and have prevented her from enjoying her retirement. How do you manage this patient's pain?

The word *pain* is derived from the Latin word *poena*, meaning fine or penalty. The International Association for the Study of Pain has described pain as an unpleasant sensory and emotional experience primarily associated with tissue damage and/or described in terms of such damage. The sensation of acute pain is familiar to everyone and is one of the earliest and common symptoms of disease. Pain is the number one reason that patients seek medical attention. It is an alarm mechanism warning of tissue damage and potential danger. However, chronic pain is a unique sensory experience. Patients who complain of chronic pain are extremely challenging, and frustration is common on the part of the patient and the clinician.

Pain can be categorized as "neuropathic," "nociceptive," or "idiopathic" (Table 10–1).

This chapter discusses neuropathic pain, which is pain caused by dysfunction of the nervous system in the absence of tissue damage. Nociceptive pain is the result of tissue damage that may or may not include damage to the nervous system. A well-known type of nociceptive pain is arthritis pain. Idiopathic pain encompasses several poorly understood pain disorders that are not associated with tissue damage and includes many pain disorders that have been called psychogenic in origin.

The evaluation of chronic pain has many diagnostic problems. A major problem is the inability to establish a cause for the pain. It is not possible to test for several conditions because of limitations of available technology; for example, electromyography will not reveal small-fiber neuropathies, and bone scan is of no use in early reflex sympathetic dystrophy. Examples of conditions not amenable to diagnostic tests are myofascial pain syndromes and postconcussive headache. Other conditions, such as atypical facial pain and fibromyalgia, have no etiologic specificity. Also, psychiatric issues, including depression, personality disorders, and post-traumatic stress disorder, can complicate the diagnosis. Other

TABLE 10–1. CATEGORIES OF PAIN AND EXAMPLES

Nociceptive

Arthritic
Acute postoperative
Post-traumatic

Neuropathic

Polyneuropathies
Complex regional pain syndrome (causalgia, reflex sympathetic dystrophy)
Central pain syndromes
Postherpetic neuralgia

Idiopathic

Myofascial pain syndrome
Somatoform pain disorder

factors that complicate the evaluation of pain are medical-legal issues, drug abuse, and physical and sexual abuse. Many chronic pain disorders, including fibromyalgia, somatization disorder, factitious disorder, and malingering, need to be understood from a historical perspective. Previous medical records are essential in the evaluation of a patient with chronic pain and often constitute the most important "diagnostic test."

A question that further complicates the evaluation of pain is why some patients have a chronic pain syndrome after an injury to the nervous system and others with the same type of injury do not. The information available about the anatomy and physiology of pain provides only partial answers. Two aspects of pain need to be considered: the sensory-discriminative aspect and the motivational-affective aspect. The sensory-discriminative aspect involves identifying a nociceptive (pain) stimulus (mechanical, thermal, or chemical) and determining its location, intensity, and timing (onset and duration of the stimulus). The motivational-affective aspect involves recognizing the unpleasantness and aversive quality of the stimulus and reacting to it. This is the "suffering" aspect of pain and is unique to the person. In addition to systems involved in the transmission of pain, there is an antinociceptive system that modulates pain.

Pain can result in a change in the nervous system. For example, sensitization is a feature of nociceptors (pain receptors) in which noxious stimuli lower the threshold of the receptors to subsequent stimulation, even to the point that innocuous stimuli can activate the receptors. It also is important to understand that pain is an alarm system that changes the psychologic state of the person and causes a behavioral response. This emphasizes the importance of addressing the psychologic issues that are present in patients experiencing chronic pain.

GENERAL MANAGEMENT PRINCIPLES

Pain, like any other presenting complaint, warrants an appropriate investigation. However, several management principles in the treatment of chronic pain apply to pain in general. First, the pain is real. You must convey to the patient your belief that the symptom is genuine. Believing the patient, caring about the patient's welfare, and showing a willingness to work with the patient to improve the functional aspects of his or her life are keys to successful management of chronic pain. Doubting the authenticity of the complaint has no therapeutic benefit. Instances in which the patient cannot be believed (for example, malingering and factitious disorders) are rare.

Treat any pain aggressively and as early as possible. Treating pain early may avoid the structural-functional changes in the nervous system that lead to chronic pain. The psychologic issues associated with the patient's pain must be incorporated into the management plan. Some of these issues are depression, fear, interpersonal relationships, financial compensation, and disability. The patient needs to understand that these psychologic factors can influence the intensity and tolerance of pain. Ask the patient to imagine how the pain would be if he or she won a million-dollar lottery and to compare this with how the pain would be if his or her spouse died or the house burned down.

It is essential to establish appropriate goals before initiating treatment. A complete "cure" is not a realistic goal, but a reduction in the patient's level of pain with improvement in functional status is a realistic goal. Factors that influence pain, such as depression, physical inactivity or regression, drug addiction, and emotional regression, can be treated.

DIAGNOSTIC APPROACH

Begin your evaluation of a patient with a complaint of chronic pain by obtaining previous medical records. Because these patients tend to have had extensive diagnostic testing, obtaining previous medical records is an important and cost-effective diagnostic tool.

The pain history should include the temporal course of the symptoms, the location and intensity of the pain, and associated symptoms. The patient's description of the pain may provide diagnostic information as well as help in decisions about treatment.

Neuropathic pain is often described as "sharp," "burning," and "shooting" and is associated with skin sensitivity. Patients with peripheral nerve or nerve root pain report an aching sensation "like a toothache." Neuropathic pain is often described as "icky" or as an abnormal noxious sensation (dysesthesia). Features of neuropathic pain include allodynia (a nonnoxious stimulus is perceived as painful) and hyperalgesia (increased pain response to a noxious stimulus).

The pain history also should include an evaluation of the patient's mood, functional status, and sleep pattern and how the patient copes with the pain. It is important to know how the pain has affected the patient's employment, recreational activities, and relationships with family and friends. It also is important to know about the use of alcohol or illicit drugs for the pain or the use of these substances before the onset of pain. Although the medical records provide information about previous treatments, you should get the patient's perspective by asking what treatments have been tried and the response. It also is important to know the medication dose and length of use. If this information is not known, repeat trials of medication can be attempted.

The patient's behavior while the medical history is being taken may be significant in determining reasons for previous treatment failure and may color what is found on examination. Excessive pain behavior, a description of severe disabling pain with little objective evidence of pain, anger, a sense of entitlement, depression, and information that previous treatment was negligent are all meaningful. The history should identify psychosocial stressors and the patient's expectations. It may be useful to ask the patient what his or her plans are if the pain gets better or if it does not. The absence of future plans or goals may indicate that the patient does not plan to get better. Before beginning treatment, it is important to know if the illness is being used to avoid responsibilities or problems. Identify financial and disability issues. If the pain gets better, does it change the patient's financial or legal status?

The physical examination should include systemic, musculoskeletal, dermatologic, and neurologic evaluations. Testing the range of motion of the spine and joints and palpating soft tissues for tightness and tenderness are important in the evaluation of myofascial pain disorders. Complex regional pain disorder or reflex sympathetic dystrophy can be associated with abnormalities in skin color, swelling, and temperature. The neurologic examination should focus on the sensory examination. Central pain, or pain due to damage of the central nervous system, is associated with a deficit in thermal sensation. In addition to evidence of sensory deficit, the presence of allodynia or hyperalgesia suggests a neuropathic pain condition.

TREATMENT

The treatment of chronic pain may involve several types of therapy—medications, physical and occupational therapy, injections of anesthetic agents, and behavioral therapy—and the participation of many healthcare professionals. Referral to a pain specialist should be considered and not necessarily as a last resort.

Many pharmacologic agents are available for treating pain (Table 10–2). Sequential drug trials may be needed to find a drug that provides significant pain relief. The response of a patient to one drug may vary, even among drugs of the same class. It is important to titrate one drug at a time, beginning with the lowest dosage and increasing until significant pain relief is obtained or intolerable side effects develop. Slow increments in dosage can reduce the chances of side effects. Only a few medications (tricyclic antidepressants and mexiletine) have toxic serum levels. The addition of a second drug should be avoided unless the first drug produces only partial pain relief or higher doses cause intolerable side effects.

Whether narcotics should be used to treat chronic pain is a difficult question. Narcotic analgesia is well accepted as a treatment for pain due to malignancy but not for pain due to a nonmalignant cause. Some clinicians advocate early and aggressive use of these agents, whereas others think they should be used only after all reasonable attempts at analgesia have failed. The problem with narcotics is the rapid development of tolerance,

TABLE 10–2. PAIN MEDICATIONS

Drug	Type of Drug or Mechanism	Initial Dosage (Oral Unless Specified)	Adverse Effects
Acetaminophen (Tylenol)	Nonopioid analgesic	650 mg every 4–6 hr	Hepatotoxicity
NSAIDs	Nonsteroidal anti-inflammatory		Gastropathy
Aspirin		650 mg every 4–6 hr	Platelet inhibition
Ibuprofen (Motrin)		400 mg every 4–6 hr	Renal and hepatic dysfunction
Naproxen (Naprosyn)		250 mg every 6–8 hr	
Opioids	Opioid		Constipation, sedation, impaired ventilation
Codeine		15–60 mg, titrate	Toxicity > 1.5 mg/kg
Morphine		15–30 mg, titrate	
Hydromorphone (Dilaudid)		4–8 mg, titrate	
Oxycodone (aspirin and acetaminophen combination) (Percocet/Percodan)		7.5–10 mg, titrate	Hepatotoxicity from acetaminophen, gastropathy from aspirin
Fentanyl (Duragesic)		25 µg/hr, titrate (transdermal)	
Tramadol (Ultram)	Mu-opiate receptor agonist, serotonin and norepinephrine reuptake inhibitor	50 mg every 4–6 hr, titrate	Dizziness, nausea, sweating
Antidepressants			
Tricyclics	Block the reuptake of serotonin and norepinephrine, sodium channel blockade		Drowsiness, dry mouth, constipation, weight gain
Amitriptyline (Elavil)		10–25 mg at bedtime	
Nortriptyline (Pamelor)		10–25 mg at bedtime	
SSRIs	Selective serotonin reuptake inhibitors		
Fluoxetine (Prozac)		20 mg every A.M.	Insomnia, nausea
Paroxetine (Paxil)		10 mg every A.M.	
Mixed Reuptake Inhibitors	Block reuptake of serotonin and norepinephrine, sodium channel blockade		
Venlafaxine (Effexor)		25 mg 2 or 3 times daily	Hypertension
Nefazodone (Serzone)		100 mg twice daily	Headache, insomnia

TABLE 10–2. PAIN MEDICATIONS *(continued)*

Drug	Type of Drug or Mechanism	Initial Dosage (Oral Unless Specified)	Adverse Effects
Anticonvulsants			
Carbamazepine (Tegretol)	Sodium channel blocker	100 mg twice daily	Hepatotoxicity and hematologic
Phenytoin (Dilantin)	Sodium channel blocker	200 mg daily	Rash
Lamotrigine (Lamictal)	Sodium channel blocker	50 mg daily	Rash
Gabapentin (Neurontin)	GABA mimetic?	300 mg daily	Sedation
Clonazepam (Klonopin)		0.5 mg daily	Sedation
Valproic acid (Depakote)		10 mg/kg daily	Weight gain, tremor
Antiarrhythmics			
Mexiletine (Mexitil)	Sodium channel blocker	150 mg daily, titrate	Cardiac (consider cardiology consultation), nausea, anxiety
Sympatholytics			
Clonidine (Catapres)	α_2-Agonist	0.1 mg (transderm)	Hypotension
Topical Agents			
Lidocaine and prilocaine (EMLA)	Sodium channel blocker	See package insert	Caution in liver disease
Capsaicin (Zostrix)	Depletion of substance P	0.075% applied 3 times daily	Burning sensation
NMDA Antagonists	Block NMDA receptors		
Ketamine (Ketalar)		10 mg/mL (intravenous), titrate	
Dextromethorphan (several over-the-counter cough preparations)		15 mg daily, titrate	
Benzodiazepines	GABA-ergic		
Clonazepam (Klonopin)		0.5 mg 1–3 times daily	Drowsiness, physical and psychologic dependence
Antipasmodic	? GABA-ergic		
Baclofen (Lioresal)		5 mg 3 times daily	Drowsiness, hypotension, seizures with abrupt withdrawal

GABA, gamma-aminobutyric acid; NMDA, *N*-methyl-d-aspartate; SSRIs, selective serotonin reuptake inhibitors.

with the patient taking the medicine for withdrawal symptoms instead of pain relief. The risk of opioid narcotic abuse is considered small if the patient has been evaluated for psychologic comorbid conditions, disability, and a history of substance abuse. If the patient is seeing several clinicians, only one practitioner should be designated to prescribe opioid narcotics. Close follow-up is needed, with attention to pain relief, adverse effects, and aberrant drug-related behavior. If these medications are used, specific narcotic guidelines and pain specialists may be very helpful.

Many antidepressant medications are considered adjuvant analgesics and are effective in treating neuropathic pain. The analgesic effect of antidepressant medication is independent of an antidepressant response. Tricyclic antidepressants, such as amitriptyline and nortriptyline, block the reuptake of serotonin and norepinephrine, and the change in serotonin and norepinephrine activity is thought to be the mechanism of the analgesic properties of these antidepressants. There is increasing evidence that tricyclic antidepressants may act like local anesthetics and block sodium channels, decreasing the generation of ectopic discharges. Tricyclic antidepressants also act at cholinergic, histaminergic, and adrenergic receptor sites. The common side effects of the drugs include anticholinergic symptoms of blurred vision, dry mouth, and constipation and antihistaminergic symptoms of sedation and weight gain. The side effects can be minimized if the dose is titrated very slowly. Amitriptyline can be started at 10 to 25 mg at bedtime and increased every week by the same amount. It rarely is necessary to exceed 100 mg, and serum levels can be determined if necessary. Nortriptyline has fewer side effects than amitriptyline. The patient needs to know that it may take up to 6 weeks before a therapeutic effect occurs and that adverse symptoms tend to diminish as the patient becomes used to the medication.

Selective serotonin reuptake inhibitors (SSRIs) have not been as effective as tricyclic antidepressants for treating neuropathic pain. SSRIs are effective antidepressants and should be considered when depression is a prominent symptom. Antidepressants categorized as "mixed reuptake inhibitors" inhibit reuptake of serotonin and norepinephrine and have some local anesthetic properties. They may have fewer adverse effects than tricyclic antidepressants.

Many anticonvulsants can be effective in treating neuropathic pain. Paroxysmal pain or neuralgia-like pain (sharp, lancinating pain) is often responsive to anticonvulsants. Anticonvulsant medications include carbamazepine, phenytoin, and lamotrigine, which act by blocking sodium channels, and valproic acid, clonazepam, and vigabatrin, which interact with GABA-ergic transmission. The mechanism of action for gabapentin, another anticonvulsant, is not known, but it is thought to work through an inhibitory mechanism. These medications have variable effects at different doses and serum levels. Slow titration can reduce the problem of adverse effects.

Gabapentin, approved as an adjunctive medication in the treatment of partial seizures, has been prescribed extensively for neuropathic pain. It has no drug interactions and a low incidence of adverse effects. The initial dose is 300 mg per day, and this can be increased by 300 mg every 3 to 7 days until a therapeutic effect is achieved or intolerable side effects develop. The effective dose varies (usual range, 2,100 to 3,600 mg daily), and 6,000 mg is considered the maximal dose.

Sodium channel antagonists inhibit the spontaneous discharge from nerve sprouts and cell bodies of injured primary afferent neurons. This inhibition is the presumed mechanism of action of mexiletine and lidocaine, two local anesthetic antiarrhythmic agents effective in treating some neuropathic pain problems. Before mexiletine treatment is initiated, be sure the patient has no evidence of cardiac disease. Furthermore, monitor the patient closely for any cardiac adverse effects. Cardiology consultation should be considered if the patient has a history of cardiac abnormality, abnormal electrocardiographic findings, or cardiac symptoms. In pain clinics, an intravenous infusion of lidocaine is often used to predict the response to oral mexiletine.

Several chronic neuropathic pain syndromes, including complex regional pain syndrome and some peripheral neuropathies, may be due partly to abnormal activity in the sympathetic nervous system. Sympatholytic agents used to treat pain include adrenergic receptor blockers such as phentolamine and prazosin and the α_2-agonist clonidine. Intravenously administered phentolamine has been used to identify which patients with sympathetically mediated pain may respond to sympathetic blocks or surgical sympathectomy. Transdermal clonidine has some efficacy in treating painful peripheral neuropathies. Hypotension, impotence, and other autonomic side effects limit the use of sympatholytic agents.

Several topical agents have been useful in treating some neuropathic pain syndromes. Capsaicin cream, an extract of chili peppers, has been used to treat peripheral neuropathies and postherpetic neuralgia. The efficacy of this treatment has been mixed. The mechanism of action is thought to involve the depletion of substance P from small nociceptive fibers, which in turn reduces spontaneous and evoked input from damaged afferent nerves. The cream is applied three times a day. Burning pain is noted after each application and usually resolves after approximately 1 week of use. Some patients have reported that this treatment exacerbated their pain. Care must be taken to avoid contact with the mouth or eyes, but capsaicin has no systemic side effects. Some local anesthetics (lidocaine and a combination of lidocaine and prilocaine) are available as topical agents. These preparations have little systemic effect but are often limited by poor absorption.

Antagonists of the N-methyl-D-aspartate (NMDA) receptor for glutamate are being investigated for the treatment of neuropathic pain. Dextromethorphan, the active ingredient in many over-the-counter cough medicines, has a modest effect on painful neuropathies. The doses that have been used are high (380 mg/day), and sedation and ataxia have been common side effects. NMDA antagonists also may have a role in opioid medication. They potentiate the analgesic effect of opioids and may block or reduce tolerance to opioids.

Baclofen, considered a nonopioid analgesic and skeletal muscle relaxant, has been used to treat spasticity in multiple sclerosis and spinal cord injury. It has some efficacy in painful paroxysms that occur in certain neuropathic pain conditions.

Transcutaneous electrical nerve stimulation is a physical method that can provide pain relief in a few neuropathic pain disorders. The mechanism of action of the TENS unit is to evoke sensation proximal to a nerve injury to inhibit the pain sensation. For this method to be effective, paresthesias need to be induced in the painful area. Local skin irritation is the only adverse effect.

Some clinicians advocate the use of acupuncture to treat several pain conditions. There are several methods of acupuncture, and all of them require inserting needles into various points on the body. Evidence suggests that acupuncture needling causes the release of enkephalin and dynorphin in the spinal cord, activation of the periaqueductal gray matter and release of norepinephrine and serotonin, and the release of adrenocorticotropic hormone and β-endorphin from the pituitary gland. Little information is available on the use of acupuncture in the treatment of neuropathic pain.

PAINFUL POLYNEUROPATHY

Polyneuropathies are discussed in Chapter 6. Painful polyneuropathies include neuropathies due to diabetes mellitus, vasculitis, amyloid deposition, human immunodeficiency virus (HIV), chronic alcoholism, toxic effects of arsenic or thallium, paraneoplastic disease, and Fabry disease. Hereditary sensory neuropathy is also associated with pain.

The most common of these is diabetic neuropathy. Pain can be associated with distal neuropathy as well as with the proximal asymmetric form. The pain is thought to result from axonal injury caused by the metabolic disturbance from diabetes and by diffuse microvascular infarcts of the nerve. Proximal asymmetric neuropathy may involve immune-mediated occlusion of arterioles that supply the nerves. A reasonable treatment for proximal neuropathy is narcotic opioids, because remission usually occurs within 3 to 6 months from onset. Immunosuppressant medication is being investigated for treating diabetic neuropathy.

Tricyclic antidepressants and mixed reuptake inhibitors (venlafaxine or nefazodone) are effective in treating painful polyneuropathies. The effectiveness of SSRIs has been disappointing, and they are not recommended. Gabapentin is efficacious and has few side effects. Treatment with mexiletine is beneficial; however, this drug can be used only if the patient has normal heart function. Transdermal clonidine has been beneficial in some cases of diabetic neuropathy, and this reflects the heterogeneity of painful disorders and the role of the sympathetic nervous system.

COMPLEX REGIONAL PAIN SYNDROMES

Complex regional pain syndrome type I (CRPS I), previously known as "reflex sympathetic dystrophy," is usually caused by minor trauma to an extremity (sprain, fracture) or a medical event such as a myocardial infarction. After the trauma or event, sensory and inflammatory symptoms develop and spread. The symptoms are disproportionate to the injury. CRPS I is characterized by burning pain, swelling, abnormal regulation of skin temperature, motor impairment, osteopenia, severe tenderness, and hyperalgesia.

CRPS II is used to describe causalgia. CRPS II is caused by partial injury of a peripheral nerve. The clinical features of CRPS II are comparable to those of CRPS I and include burning pain, allodynia, edema, and skin changes. The distinction between type I and type II is partial injury of a peripheral nerve in CRPS II.

CRPS I and CRPS II were thought to be due to involvement of the sympathetic nervous system. This concept is being revised. Patients who respond to sympathetic ganglion blockade have "sympathetically maintained pain syndrome" and those who do not respond have "sympathetically independent pain syndrome." The role of the sympathetic nervous system in these pain syndromes is being investigated.

The pain of CRPS is often described as "burning," "throbbing," "shooting," or "aching." It can occur with the patient at rest or be precipitated by movement or other stimulation or it can occur in paroxysms. Painful stimuli can cause delayed pain, pain that outlasts the stimulus and spreads beyond the site of the stimulus (hyperpathia). Autonomic symptoms include sweating abnormalities (hyperhidrosis or hypohidrosis), temperature abnormalities (hot or cold), and swelling. The skin often appears mottled and may turn red, white, or blue.

It is difficult to treat CRPS because specific diagnostic criteria have not been established and the pathophysiologic abnormalities have not been defined. However, the general principles for treating pain apply. The initial management options are analgesics (NSAIDs, opioids, and adjuvants), gentle physical therapy, and psychologic support and therapy. If the response to this treatment is reduced pain and edema at rest, then the therapy is continued with increasing physical activity, active physical therapy, psychologic therapy, and social support. However, if there is no response to treatment, refer the patient for interventional and interdisciplinary pain management.

POSTHERPETIC NEURALGIA

The varicella-zoster virus is omnipresent, and more than 95% of the population of the United States is infected with it. This virus can cause several painful conditions. Preherpetic neuralgia is the radicular pain that precedes the skin eruption, usually by 2 to 4 days. The pain of acute herpes zoster occurs from the time the rash appears to the time of vesicular crusting. Postherpetic neuralgia is the pain that persists for more than 3 months in the region of the cutaneous lesions.

Postherpetic neuralgia occurs in about 10% of patients with herpes zoster. Those at increased risk for postherpetic neuralgia include the elderly and persons with depressed immune function because of malignancy, chemotherapy, surgery, or human immunodeficiency virus (HIV) infection. Also at increased risk are patients who had involvement of the face (especially the ophthalmic branch of the trigeminal nerve), acute herpetic pain intensity, severe skin lesions, or permanent sensory loss in the affected area. Increased psychosocial stress and postherpetic neuralgia appear to be correlated.

The pain of postherpetic neuralgia is described as "constant deep aching" or "burning pain." Intermittent paroxysms of lancinating or jabbing pain with allodynia are also common. Movement and any tactile stimulation of the area, including stimulation produced by clothing, are avoided. Neurologic examination shows a loss of pin and thermal sensation in the affected area.

It is expected that with widespread use of the virus vaccine (only recently available), postherpetic neuralgia will be prevented. Treat with antiviral medication at the time of the infection. Acyclovir decreases herpetic pain in the short term and has a modest effect in reducing the likelihood that postherpetic neuralgias will develop. Newer antiviral agents, famciclovir and valacyclovir, may be more effective than acyclovir in reducing the incidence and severity of postherpetic neuralgia. Corticosteroids may reduce the pain of the acute infection, but they have not been shown to reduce the incidence or severity of postherpetic neuralgia. Nerve blocks early in the course of the disease have not been shown to prevent postherpetic neuralgia.

Tricyclic antidepressants are effective for treating postherpetic neuralgia. As with other painful conditions, these agents are started at a low dose and increased until a therapeutic response is achieved or intolerable side effects develop. Many anticonvulsants have been used to treat postherpetic neuralgia. The initial reports about gabapentin indicate that it may prove to be effective. Topical analgesics are useful because the area involved is well defined and there is an absence of systemic side effects. In addition to the topical agents listed in Table 10–2, aspirin and other NSAID preparations (mixed with chloroform or diethyl ether) can be of benefit. Invasive therapies include dorsal rhizotomy, dorsal root entry zone lesions, cordotomy, cingulotomy, and cortical excision. Currently, none of these is recommended.

CENTRAL PAIN

Central pain is pain caused by a lesion within the central nervous system, such as stroke, spinal cord trauma, or multiple sclerosis. Central pain may be overlooked because of the delay in the onset of painful symptoms. The delay can occur days, months, and (rarely) years after the central nervous system lesion. Further complicating the diagnosis of central pain is the paucity of physical findings. A consistent finding is loss of temperature sensation.

Some of the adjectives patients use to describe central pain are "superficial" and/or "deep pain," "burning," "aching," "pricking," and "lancinating." Temperature changes, emotional stimuli, and movement can trigger the pain. Features of central pain include poor localization, impaired sensory discrimination, prolonged aftersensations, and delayed sensory latency.

Treating central pain can be difficult. Reassure the patient by educating him or her about the cause of the pain, and provide psychosocial support throughout treatment. Antidepressants, anticonvulsants, and opioid analgesics are first-line drug therapy. TENS may be beneficial. Clonidine and mexiletine (if the patient has no cardiac contraindications) are reasonable second-line treatments. Third-line treatments may include spinal cord or deep brain stimulation.

NEUROPATHIC CANCER PAIN

Neuropathic cancer pain can be due to direct involvement of neural structures by tumor or it can be related to cancer therapy. Toxic neuropathies result from treatment with chemotherapeutic agents, including cisplatin, vincristine, and paclitaxel. Postsurgical pain due to thoracotomy, mastectomy, or amputation is an example of a clinical pain syndrome related to cancer. Other examples of neuropathic cancer pain are postradiation pain (myelotomy, plexopathy), paraneoplastic pain (sensory neuronopathy), and postherpetic neuralgia. Many of these pain syndromes are heterogeneous and involve neural, myofascial, bone, and visceral pain symptoms.

The most important aspect in the evaluation of pain in a patient with cancer is to determine whether the cancer causes the symptom. Post-thoracotomy pain and post-mastectomy pain are distinctly different clinical syndromes. In the cancer population, post-thoracotomy pain should be considered to have a neoplastic origin until repeat evaluations over several months are negative. Recurrent neoplasm has been discovered in more than 90% of patients who had increasing pain after the operation and in those with pain after the incisional pain resolved. In contrast, the pain following mastectomy is often caused by surgical injury to the intercostobrachial nerve. This pain occurs in the distribution of the T2 dermatome and can begin several months to years after the operation (see Fig. 1-12). In this characteristic clinical syndrome, the patient can be reassured and extensive evaluation can be avoided.

Treatment of the underlying cancer is the best treatment of pain in patients with cancer. When pain is caused by a tumor compressing a nerve, consider surgical decompression, chemotherapy, or radiation (or a combination). Because most cancer pain syndromes are heterogeneous, pharmacologic treatment often requires multiple medications. A combination of opioids, tricyclic antidepressants, and anticonvulsants is frequently prescribed for neuropathic cancer pain.

The World Health Organization uses three categories of pain to guide analgesic drug therapy. Nonopioid drugs with or without adjuvant therapy are used first for mild pain (e.g., aspirin and other NSAIDs, acetaminophen). For mild to moderate pain, the addition of opioids such as codeine and oxycodone is considered. Morphine or fentanyl is considered for moderate to severe pain. The dose of the drug that is chosen should be increased aggressively to prevent persistent pain. The appropriate dose is the dose that is effective in relieving the patient's pain without causing intolerable side effects. Around-the-clock dosing should be used to prevent pain. Rescue medications—medications used to provide relief for breakthrough pain—should be available. The approximate dose of the rescue medication should be equal to the regular dose of medication given for the interval. For example, 30 mg of immediate-release morphine every 4 hours is the rescue dose for a patient taking 90 mg of sustained-release morphine every 12 hours.

The route of administration of analgesic drugs is important. If the patient cannot take medication orally, consider a rectal, transdermal, spinal, intrathecal, or intraventricular route. Anticipate the common side effects of the medications so they can be managed or prevented. Constipation is a common side effect of opioid analgesics. If one opioid analgesic is not tolerated, change to another. The initial dose of a sequential analgesic drug should be 25% to 50% less than the estimated equivalent dose to allow for incomplete cross-tolerance. All the adjuvant analgesics listed in Table 10–2 are reasonable to try for treating the heterogeneous pain disorders associated with cancer pain.

MENTAL DISORDERS AND PAIN

Chronic pain is frequently a symptom of mental disorders, including somatization disorder, hypochondriasis, and factitious physical disorders. Pain is also associated with psychologic factors and malingering. Other psychiatric disorders (e.g., depression, anxiety, panic, and post-traumatic stress disorder) exert a strong influence on chronic pain. Psychiatric treatment concurrent with medical treatment is recommended for these disorders.

The concept of abnormal illness behavior is useful in understanding mental disorders and pain. How a person behaves when ill is called "illness behavior." Normal illness behavior is behavior that is appropriate to the level of the disease present. Exaggerated or amplified behavior, out of proportion to the level of the disease present, is abnormal and called "illness-affirming behavior." Illness-affirming behavior is seen in conversion disorder, somatization disorder, hypochondriasis, and pain associated with psychologic factors. All four of these conditions have unconscious motivation and sign and symptom production; that is, the patient is unaware of the production of symptoms or the motivation behind the behavior. However, in malingering and factitious disorder, illness-affirming behavior is associated with conscious sign and symptom production. Patients with malingering are aware of the motive behind the behavior, whereas those with factitious disorder are not aware of this motive.

The diagnostic criteria for somatization disorder include multiple physical complaints before the age of 30 years. The physical complaints occur over several years and cause significant impairment or the seeking of medical attention. The presence of four pain complaints, two gastrointestinal symptoms, one sexual symptom, and one pseudoneurologic symptom complete the criteria. Management of somatization disorder requires that one clinician coordinate medical treatment and schedule regular visits. This prevents the unnecessary use of invasive procedures. Also, with this coordinated treatment, the patient does not need to develop new symptoms to maintain the relationship with the clinician.

Patients with hypochondriasis are preoccupied with the belief or fear that they have serious disease. Normal aches and pains may be misinterpreted as signs of significant disease. The preferred method of management is reassurance and follow-up appointments for reassessment.

Pain associated with psychologic factors was previously called "somatoform" or "psychogenic" pain. Pain is the predominant focus of the clinical presentation and causes distress or functional impairment. Psychologic factors have an important role in the onset, severity, exacerbation, and maintenance of the pain. A previous history of physical complaints without organic findings, prominent guilt, or a history of physical or sexual abuse confirms the diagnosis. Individual, group, and marital therapy, psychiatric treatment, physical therapy, biofeedback, and antidepressant medications are all reasonable treatments.

Factitious disorder should be considered if illness-affirming behavior is present and the symptoms appear to be produced on a voluntary or conscious basis. If there is no apparent motivation for the behavior, factitious disorder should be suspected. A patient with factitious disorder has periods of improvement followed by relapses. The patient often can predict relapses. Other clues to this disorder include a willingness of the patient to undergo invasive procedures, difficulty obtaining previous medical records, and the patient's resistance to psychiatric consultation. Malingering differs from factitious disorder by the identification of a motive behind the behavior, for example, avoiding jail, seeking narcotics, and obtaining disability payments. Psychiatric consultation is recommended.

SUGGESTED READING

Allen, RR: Neuropathic pain in the cancer patient. Neurol Clin 16:869–888, 1998.

Aronoff, GM: Approach to the patient with chronic pain. In Samuels, MA, and Feske, S (eds): Office Practice of Neurology. Churchill Livingstone, New York, 1996, pp 1162–1166.

Backonja, MM, and Galer, BS: Pain assessment and evaluation of patients who have neuropathic pain. Neurol Clin 16:775–790, 1998.

Bajwa, ZH, Lehmann, LJ, and Fishman, SM: Anatomy and physiology of pain. In Samuels, MA, and Feske, S (eds): Office Practice of Neurology. Churchill Livingstone, New York, 1996, pp 1157–1162.

Beric, A: Central pain and dysesthesia syndrome. Neurol Clin 16:899–918, 1998.

Casey, KL, et al: Pain. Continuum 2:7–74, 1996.

Ceniceros, S, and Brown, GR: Acupuncture: A review of its history, theories, and indications. South Med J 91:1121–1125, 1998.

Cluff, RS, and Rowbotham, MC: Pain caused by herpes zoster infection. Neurol Clin 16:813–832, 1998.

Dawson, DM, and Sabin, TD: Pain. In Samuels, MA, and Feske, S (eds): Office Practice of Neurology. Churchill Livingstone, New York, 1996, pp 36–40.

Eisendrath, SJ: Psychiatric aspects of chronic pain. Neurology 45(Suppl 9):S26–S34, 1995.

Galer, BS: Painful polyneuropathy. Neurol Clin 16:791–812, 1998.

Gonzales, GR: Central pain: Diagnosis and treatment strategies. Neurology 45(Suppl 9):S11–S16, 1995.

Levy, MH: Pharmacologic treatment of cancer pain. N Engl J Med 335:1124–1132, 1996.

Rowbotham, MC: Chronic pain: From theory to practical management. Neurology 45(Suppl 9):S5–S10, 1995.

Wasner, G, Backonja, MM, and Baron, R: Traumatic neuralgias: Complex regional pain syndromes (reflex sympathetic dystrophy and causalgia): Clinical characteristics, pathophysiological mechanisms and therapy. Neurol Clin 16:851–868, 1998.

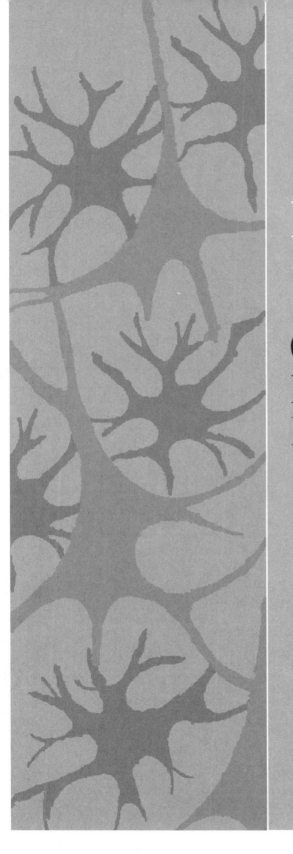

PART III

Common Neurologic Diseases

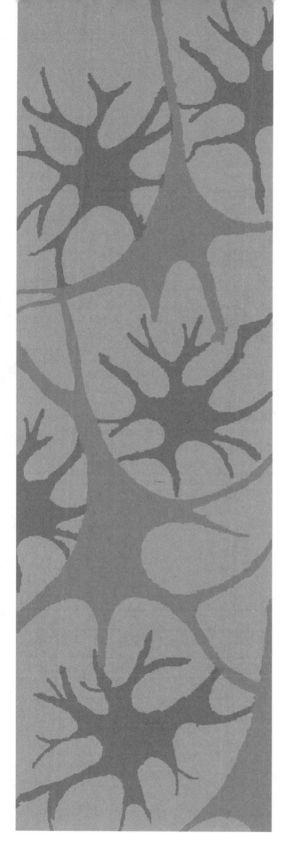

CHAPTER 11

Cerebrovascular Disease

CHAPTER OUTLINE

Diagnostic Approach
  Is It a Vascular Event?
  Is Hospitalization Required?
  Is the Event Hemorrhagic or Ischemic?
  Does the Event Localize to the Anterior
     or Posterior Circulation?
  What Is the Mechanism?
Prevention of a First Stroke
  Strategies
  Modifiable Risk Factors
    Hypertension
    Myocardial Infarction
    Atrial Fibrillation
    Diabetes Mellitus
    Carotid Artery Stenosis
    Cigarette Smoking
    Alcohol Consumption
    Physical Activity
    Dietary Factors
    Other Factors
Symptomatic Carotid Artery Stenosis
Stroke in Young Adults
  Migrainous Stroke
  Arterial Dissection

(continued)

Illicit Drug Use
Hematologic Disorders
Cardiac Causes
Treatment of Acute Stroke:
  Thrombolytic Therapy
Hemorrhagic Stroke

A 67-year-old man with a history of hypertension, coronary artery disease, and hyperlipidemia comes for evaluation of an episode of numbness and speech difficulty that he had the preceding day. While he was playing golf, he suddenly had numbness of the right side of his face and right arm. He turned to his friend to tell him what was going on and "gibberish" came out. The entire episode lasted less than 5 minutes, but the experience was so disconcerting to the patient that he sought immediate evaluation. His neurologic examination findings are normal. What are the diagnostic possibilities? What kind of evaluation and treatment do you recommend? Does the patient need to be hospitalized?

The presentation of this patient is consistent with a transient ischemic attack (TIA). A TIA is an episode of focal neurologic dysfunction caused by ischemia. The length of time for the episode of neurologic dysfunction can be up to 24 hours, but most TIAs last less than 1 hour. The term *reversible ischemic neurologic deficit* (RIND) is used to describe an ischemic episode lasting longer than 24 hours but less than 3 weeks. A *minor stroke* is defined as persistent neurologic deficit that is not disabling. The characteristic temporal profile of a TIA or stroke is sudden onset of neurologic signs or symptoms, with maximal deficit occurring within seconds or a few minutes after onset. Vascular injury to the nervous system presents suddenly, and patients can tell you the exact time of onset unless they awaken with the symptoms or language or if consciousness is involved. TIAs are focal events, and the symptoms and

signs of neurologic deficit should correspond to a known vascular distribution (Figs. 11–1 and 11–2). Patients with TIAs are at risk for developing a disabling stroke. The subsequent risk of stroke is 6% per year for 5 years after the TIA, with the greatest risk within the first year after the TIA. This risk can be even greater, depending on the mechanism of the ischemic event. The risk for subsequent stroke in critical carotid artery stenosis is 13% for 2 years and may be as high as 50% per year if related to a cardiac cause of stroke. Evaluation and intervention need to be initiated immediately.

DIAGNOSTIC APPROACH

Five questions need to be answered in the diagnostic evaluation of a patient with a cerebrovascular event:

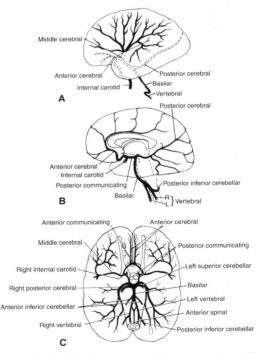

FIG. 11–1. Cerebral vasculature. (A) Lateral surface of brain; **(B)** medial surface of brain; and **(C)** ventral surface of brain.

186

FIG. 11–2. Anatomical distribution of the major cerebral arteries, with common clinical features.

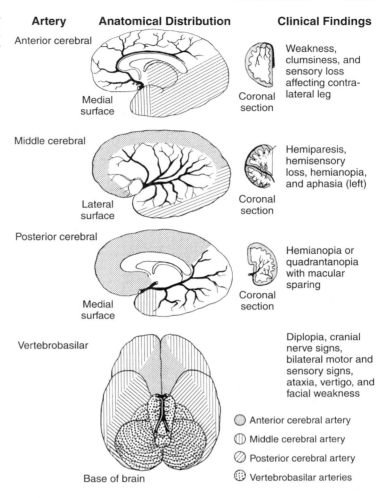

Artery	Anatomical Distribution	Clinical Findings

Anterior cerebral — Medial surface — Coronal section — Weakness, clumsiness, and sensory loss affecting contralateral leg

Middle cerebral — Lateral surface — Coronal section — Hemiparesis, hemisensory loss, hemianopia, and aphasia (left)

Posterior cerebral — Medial surface — Coronal section — Hemianopia or quadrantanopia with macular sparing

Vertebrobasilar — Base of brain — Diplopia, cranial nerve signs, bilateral motor and sensory signs, ataxia, vertigo, and facial weakness

Anterior cerebral artery
Middle cerebral artery
Posterior cerebral artery
Vertebrobasilar arteries

1. Is it a vascular event?
2. Is hospitalization required?
3. Is the event hemorrhagic or ischemic?
4. Does the event localize to the anterior or posterior circulation?
5. What is the mechanism?

IS IT A VASCULAR EVENT?

The first diagnostic consideration is to determine whether the event represents a TIA. TIAs are focal events with focal symptoms, in contrast to the generalized symptoms that can occur in syncope, presyncope, and hypoglycemia. Migraine with neurologic symptoms can often be confused with transient ischemic events because of the abrupt onset of focal symptoms. Migraine symptoms tend to be positive phenomena, for example, scintillating scotomas, fortification spectrum, and tingling paresthesias. Visual or sensory loss is considered a negative phenomenon, and these phenomena more likely occur in ischemic attacks. In the absence of the characteristic headache, a patient with migraine may have a history of previous headaches, a family history positive for headaches, and fewer cardiovascular risk factors than a patient with TIAs.

Partial seizure activity can mimic TIAs. Symptoms of partial seizures, like those of migraine, tend to be positive phenomena. For example, in a partial seizure, focal tonic and clonic movement of an extremity is more likely than motor weakness. The time to maximal deficit is longer in partial seizures, and there is a tendency for the symptoms to "march." For example, motor or sensory symptoms may begin in the hand and, over minutes, spread to the face and then to the leg. Stereotyped spells are characteristic of seizure activity.

An inner ear problem such as labyrinthitis or vestibulopathy may present acutely and is included in the differential diagnosis of TIA. Vertigo without other brainstem or cerebellar symptoms or vertigo associated with auditory symptoms is most often due to an inner ear lesion.

Multiple sclerosis can present with sudden focal neurologic symptoms, but the rapid resolution of symptoms in minutes is uncommon. Neurologic signs and symptoms due to multiple sclerosis are not restricted to a single vascular area. Patients with multiple sclerosis are often younger and have fewer cerebrovascular risk factors than patients with TIAs.

Hemorrhage into a neoplasm can present suddenly, but the signs and symptoms usually are not transient. Focal signs and symptoms from a neoplasm have a stuttering or progressive temporal profile. Neuroimaging will usually resolve any diagnostic questions.

IS HOSPITALIZATION REQUIRED?

After the event has been determined to be vascular, the next step is to determine whether hospitalization is necessary. The patient should be hospitalized if he or she is at high risk for recurrent vascular events or would benefit from intravenous anticoagulant therapy. If a cardiac embolic source is suspected, the patient, like those with atrial fibrillation or recent myocardial infarction, should be hospitalized. The intravenous administration of heparin is recommended for patients with a suspected cardiac source of emboli. Patients who have multiple events and events that are increasing in frequency and duration should also be hospitalized. Conclusive evidence for the use of heparin in other or noncardioembolic mechanisms of stroke has not been established. Temporary treatment with monitoring of anticoagulant activity and platelet counts is reasonable for a patient judged to be at high risk for subsequent stroke. The lack of definite proof of benefit with heparin treatment should be discussed with the patient.

If the patient had only transient monocular blindness (amaurosis fugax) or the event occurred 2 weeks before the assessment, an expedited outpatient work-up in the next 1 or 2 days is reasonable. Immediately start treatment with aspirin, 325 mg per day, while the evaluation is in progress. If the patient has an aspirin allergy, consider hospitalization. The antiplatelet agent ticlopidine does not have the immediate onset of action like aspirin does. Clopidogrel has an initial antiplatelet response in 2 hours, but it takes 3 to 7 days for the peak antiplatelet effect to occur.

IS THE EVENT HEMORRHAGIC OR ISCHEMIC?

The next step in the evaluation of a patient with cerebrovascular symptoms is to determine whether the vascular event is hemorrhagic or ischemic. The majority of vascular events are ischemic. Hemorrhagic stroke is more likely to present with severe headache, fluctuating levels of consciousness, and meningeal signs. Ischemic vascular events are more likely to involve a single vascular territory, and the patient's status may improve early in the course of the event. Often, the distinction between ischemic and hemorrhagic events cannot be made solely on the basis of clinical information. Computed tomography (CT) without contrast is the test of choice for the immediate evaluation of a patient with a cerebrovascular event. CT is able to identify intracerebral hemorrhages, subdural hematomas, and the majority of subarachnoid hemorrhages (see Fig. 2–5). CT findings in a patient with a TIA should be normal and exclude hemorrhage, vascular tumor, and arteriovenous malformation. Early in an ischemic stroke, CT results may be negative or the scan may show only a poorly outlined area of decreased density with subtle gyral flattening. As the interval from the time of the stroke to CT increases, the area of the ischemic stroke becomes better defined and is hypodense to the surrounding tissue. The areas where hypodensity would appear on a CT scan for the major cerebral arteries are illustrated in Figure 11–3. If there is any question about the presence of hemorrhage, repeat imaging may be needed within the next 24 hours.

Magnetic resonance imaging (MRI) is superior to CT for identifying small infarcts, especially those involving the posterior, or vertebrobasilar, circulation. Newer diagnostic methods like diffusion-weighted magnetic resonance, perfusion magnetic resonance, and magnetic spectroscopy are rapidly changing the evaluation of cerebrovascular disorders. These techniques are being developed to identify ischemic changes earlier and are anticipated to improve intervention in acute stroke.

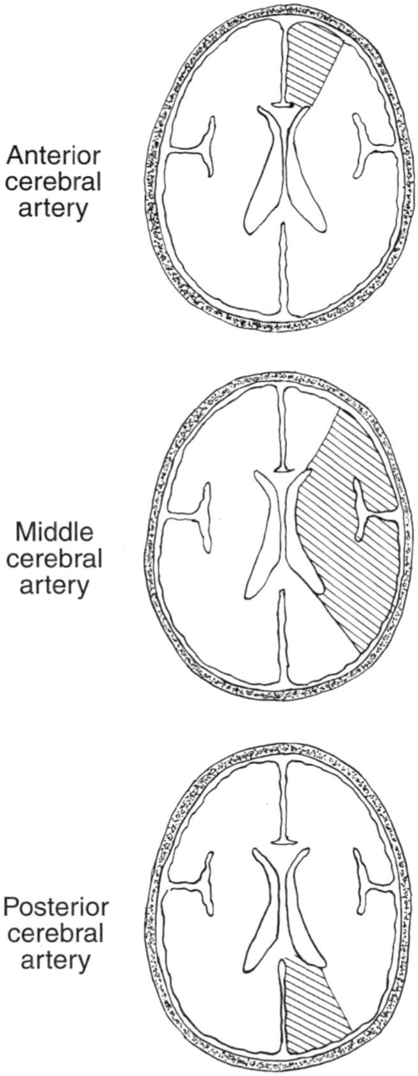

DOES THE EVENT LOCALIZE TO THE ANTERIOR OR POSTERIOR CIRCULATION?

The next diagnostic step is to localize the symptoms to either the anterior or the posterior circulation. The anterior circulation includes the territory supplied by the carotid artery system, which includes the internal carotid, anterior cerebral, and middle cerebral arteries. The posterior circulation includes the vertebral, basilar, and posterior cerebral arteries (Fig. 11–4). Localization is

Anterior cerebral artery

Middle cerebral artery

Posterior cerebral artery

FIG. 11–3. Drawings of cranial computed tomographic (CT) scans showing the areas of hypodensity appearing with infarction of the major cerebral arteries.

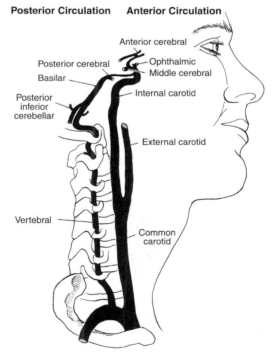

FIG. 11–4. Anterior and posterior cerebral circulations. (Copyright 1983. Novartis. Reprinted with permission from the Netter Collection of Medical Illustrations, Vol 1, Part 1. Illustrated by Frank H. Netter, M.D. All rights reserved.)

particularly important in patients who may have multiple potential mechanisms for stroke. An example is a patient with vertigo and dysarthria, which are posterior circulation symptoms, who has carotid artery stenosis and atrial fibrillation. In this case, the more relevant risk factor for the patient's ischemic symptoms would be the atrial fibrillation. The patient in the case at the beginning of the chapter had symptoms consistent with ischemia of the anterior circulation, specifically within the territory of the left middle cerebral artery, and, if bilateral carotid artery stenosis were found on evaluation, the left carotid artery stenosis would be clinically significant.

WHAT IS THE MECHANISM?

The major portion of the diagnostic evaluation of a patient with a cerebrovascular event is determining the underlying mechanism for the event. Four major groups of diseases are associated with ischemic cerebrovascular disorders: (1) cardiac disorders; (2) large-vessel, or craniocervical, occlusive disease; (3) small-vessel, or intracranial, occlusive disease; and (4) hematologic disorders (Fig. 11–5). Embolus from a proximal artery or from the heart is the most common mechanism of ischemic strokes and TIAs. Atherosclerotic disease of the carotid artery in the region of the carotid bifurcation is a common cause of carotid artery embolus. Cardiac emboli account for 20% of ischemic strokes and TIAs. Another 20% of ischemic strokes and TIAs are related to decreased blood flow or occlusion of small penetrating brain arteries. Poorly controlled hypertension and diabetes mellitus often damage these small blood vessels. Despite extensive investigation, the mechanism of many ischemic events remains unknown or uncertain.

Distinguishing the underlying mechanism by clinical means can be difficult. Suspect cardiac embolism if the patient experienced a recent episode of chest pain, has a pulse irregularity suggestive of atrial fibrillation, has a history or examination findings suggestive of congestive heart failure, has prosthetic heart valves, has the onset of symptoms with a Valsalva maneuver, or has findings of deep vein thrombophlebitis in the lower extremities. Any history, examination, or neuroimaging findings that indicate the stroke involves more than one vascular territory are also suggestive of cardiac embolism.

Carotid artery stenosis is suggested by symptoms consistent with retinal ischemia. Emboli to the first branch of the carotid artery, the ophthalmic artery, cause transient monocular blindness, or amaurosis fugax. Emboli from the carotid artery may lodge in the same branches of the intracranial circulation, causing stereotypic TIAs. The presence of a carotid bruit may indicate carotid artery stenosis.

The occlusion of small penetrating arterioles causes lacunar infarction, or small infarcts, in deep cortical sites and the brainstem (Fig. 11–6). Thus, aphasia, visual field deficits, seizures, or motor and sensory deficits in one limb are uncommon with these ischemic events. Common clinical syndromes associated with lacunar infarctions are pure motor hemiparesis, pure sensory hemianesthesia, and dysarthria–clumsy hand syndrome.

TIA or stroke in a patient younger than 55 years without obvious risk factors for cardiac disease or atherosclerosis should prompt an investigation for atypical causes of stroke. Arteriopathies, such as arteritis and dissection, or coagulation disorders are possible causes that should be investigated.

The initial evaluation of a patient with TIA or ischemic stroke should include CT of the head without contrast medium, to assess for the presence of hemorrhage. Laboratory evaluation should include a complete blood count, platelet count, partial thromboplastin time, prothrombin time, erythrocyte sedimentation rate, serum chemistry panel, and lipid analysis. Lipid analysis should include determining the levels of high-density lipoprotein, low-density lipoprotein, and total cholesterol. The initial cardiac evaluation should include electrocardiography and chest radiography. The clinical presentation of the patient and the results of these initial tests will direct further evaluation. Many of the diagnostic tests used in the evaluation of cerebrovascular disorders and the indications for their use are summarized in Table 11–1.

Cardiac disorders

Valve-related emboli–prosthetic valves, rheumatic heart disease, calcific aortic stenosis, mitral valve prolapse, infective endocarditis, nonbacterial thrombotic endocarditis

Intracardiac thrombus or tumor–atrial fibrillation, sick sinus syndrome, myocardial infarction, cardiac arrhythmias, congestive heart failure, cardiomyopathy, atrial myxoma, cardiac fibroelastoma

Systemic venous thrombi and right-to-left cardiac shunt–atrial or ventricular septal defect, thrombophlebitis, pulmonary arteriovenous malformation

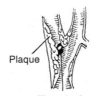

Large-vessel diseases

Atherosclerosis–cervical arteries, aortic arch, and major intracranial arteries

Carotid artery dissection–traumatic, spontaneous, aortic dissection, fibromuscular dysplasia

Other–fibromuscular dysplasia, Takayasu disease, vasospasm, moyamoya disease, homocystinuria, Fabry disease, pseudoxanthoma elasticum

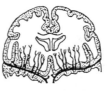

Plaque

Thrombotic blood clot

Small-vessel diseases

Hypertension

Infectious arteritis–from meningitis or any other infective process of the central nervous system

Noninfectious arteritis–systemic lupus erythematosus, polyarteritis nodosa, granulomatous angiitis, temporal arteritis, drug use, irradiation arteritis, Wegener granulomatosis, sarcoidosis, Behçet disease

Hematologic disorders

Polycythemia

Thrombocythemia

Thrombotic thrombocytopenic purpura

Sickle cell disease

Dysproteinemia

Leukemia

Disseminated intravascular coagulation

Antiphospholipid antibody syndromes–lupus anticoagulant anti-cardiolipin antibodies

Protein C and protein S deficiencies
Resistance to activated protein C
Antithrombin III deficiency

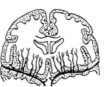

Sickle cell disease

Thrombo-cytopenia

FIG. 11–5. Mechanisms of ischemic stroke.

TIA treatment depends on the mechanism that causes the symptoms. However, all modifiable cerebrovascular risk factors should be treated. Antiplatelet therapy with aspirin is recommended in the absence of a cardiac lesion or high-grade vascular occlusive disease. The dose of aspirin given ranges from 81 mg a day to 650 mg twice a day. Many neurologists start with a dose of 325 mg per day. If the patient cannot tolerate this dose, the lower dose or "baby" aspirin is used. Common adverse reactions to aspirin include gastrointestinal tract irritation, ulceration, and bleeding.

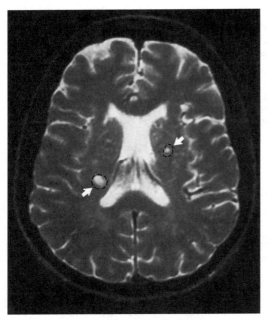

FIG. 11–6. MRI scan showing lacunar infarcts (*arrows*).

For patients who are allergic to or cannot tolerate aspirin, ticlopidine (Ticlid) and clopidogrel (Plavix) are other antiplatelet options. These medications are also options for patients who may have recurrent TIAs while receiving aspirin therapy. The dose of ticlopidine is 250 mg twice a day. The more frequent adverse effects of ticlopidine are diarrhea, abdominal pain, and rash. Neutropenia is rare but requires monitoring with a complete blood count every 2 weeks for the first 3 months of therapy. Clopidogrel is an effective antiplatelet medication that is tolerated much better than ticlopidine and does not require hematologic monitoring. For these reasons, clopidogrel, 75 mg per day, is preferred to ticlopidine.

Anticoagulation with warfarin is recommended if a cardiac source of emboli is identified as the mechanism for the TIA. Warfarin is also prescribed for patients with symptomatic vascular occlusive disease who are not surgical candidates. Anticoagulant therapy may be used for a limited period (3 to 6 months), followed by antiplatelet therapy for patients with low-grade stenosis who have recurrent symptoms while receiving antiplatelet therapy. The therapeutic range of anticoagulation is an International Normalized Ratio (INR) between 2.0 and 3.0. A higher range, 2.5 to 4.5, is used for patients with mechanical heart valves, intracardiac thrombus, or recurrent cardiac embolus. If the patient is receiving anticoagulation with heparin, the treatment is usually continued until the patient reaches the therapeutic range with oral anticoagulation. Bleeding is the major complication of warfarin therapy, and hypertension and increasing age increase the risk for hemorrhagic complications. The usual starting dose is 5 mg per day but is adjusted according to the INR. The INR is monitored daily until the level of anticoagulation has stabilized, and it may be checked every 4 weeks after the maintenance dose of warfarin has been established.

PREVENTION OF A FIRST STROKE

STRATEGIES

Stroke prevention strategies begin with identifying the patients at high risk for stroke and reducing or eliminating modifiable risk factors. Many of the identified cerebrovascular risk factors are listed in Table 11–2. Risk factors that cannot be modified include age, sex, heredity, and race or ethnicity. These nonmodifiable risk factors help identify patients who are at risk and may benefit from more aggressive preventive treatments. Increasing age is a risk factor for stroke, and the risk doubles each decade over the age of 55. Men have a greater risk of stroke than women. Both African-Americans and Hispanic-Americans have an increased incidence of stroke compared with whites. The stroke risk is also greater for persons whose parents had a stroke. The influence of hereditary and environmental factors is an area of ongoing study.

MODIFIABLE RISK FACTORS

Risk factors for which the value of modification has definitely been established in-

TABLE 11-1. DIAGNOSTIC TESTS FOR CEREBROVASCULAR DISORDERS

Diagnostic Test	Indication
Head CT without contrast medium*	Determine hemorrhage from ischemia
Complete blood count with platelet count*	Polycythemia, thrombocytosis, hematologic malignancies
Partial prothrombin time, prothrombin time*	Coagulation disorder
Chemistry screen*	Liver and kidney function, glucose metabolism
Erythrocyte sedimentation rate*	Arteritis, systemic infection, or malignancy
Lipid analysis*	Hyperlipidemia with atheromatous plaques
Electrocardiography*	Cardiac arrhythmia, ischemia
Chest radiography*	Cardiopulmonary status
Additional cardiac evaluation—Holter monitoring, transthoracic echocardiography, transesophageal echocardiography, MRI of heart, cine-CT of heart	Emboli from heart valves, intracardiac thrombi from local stagnation and endocardial alterations, shunting of systemic venous thrombi into the arterial circulation
Arterial evaluation—carotid ultrasonography, transcranial Doppler, MRA, arteriography	Arterial occlusive disease, arteritis, arterial dissection, angiopathy
Homocysteine level, vitamin B_{12}, and folate	Increased homocysteine levels associated with atherosclerotic vascular disease
Hematologic evaluation—anticardiolipin antibodies, lupus anticoagulant, protein C, protein S, antithrombin III, serum fibrinogen, bleeding time, hemoglobin electrophoresis	Hematologic abnormalities, hypercoagulable state
Infectious—treponemal antibody absorption test, blood cultures, CSF analysis	Syphilis, infective endocarditis, central nervous system infections
CSF analysis	Subarachnoid hemorrhage with negative imaging studies, meningitis, neurosyphilis
EEG	Coma, brain death
MRI	Small infarcts, posterior fossa infarcts, tumors, vascular malformations

CSF, cerebrospinal fluid; CT, computed tomography; EEG, electroencephalography; MRA, magnetic resonance angiography; MRI, magnetic resonance imaging.

*Test for initial evaluation.

clude hypertension, atrial fibrillation, cigarette smoking, hypercholesterolemia, heavy alcohol use, asymptomatic carotid artery stenosis, and TIA. Many other medical disorders and lifestyle issues can increase the risk for stroke.

Hypertension

The most prevalent and modifiable risk factor for stroke is hypertension, which is defined as systolic blood pressure of 160 mm Hg or greater and diastolic pressure of 95 mm Hg or greater. Treatment of hypertension reduces the risk of stroke. Meta-analysis has shown that every decrease in diastolic blood pressure of 7.5 mm Hg is associated with a 46% decrease in stroke risk. The National Stroke Association recommends that blood pressure measurement should be part of regular health care visits, blood pressure should be controlled in patients with hypertension who are most likely to develop stroke, and patients with hypertension should monitor their blood pressure at home.

Myocardial Infarction

The risk for ischemic stroke is increased after myocardial infarction, with the greatest risk

TABLE 11–2. CEREBROVASCULAR RISK FACTORS

Nonmodifiable—older age, male gender, race and ethnicity, heredity
Modifiable—hypertension, atrial fibrillation, cigarette smoking, hypercholesterolemia, heavy alcohol use, asymptomatic carotid stenosis, transient ischemic attack, cardiac disease, diabetes mellitus, physical inactivity
Cardiac risk factors
    Established—atrial fibrillation, valvular heart disease, dilated cardiomyopathy, recent myocardial infarction, intracardiac thrombus
    Suspected—sick sinus syndrome, patent foramen ovale, aortic arch atheroma, myocardial infarction within last 2 months, left ventricular dysfunction, atrial septal aneurysm, mitral annular calcification, mitral valve strands, spontaneous echocardiographic contrast (transesophageal echocardiographic finding)
Potential stroke risk factors—antiphospholipid antibodies, increased homocysteine levels, infection (*Chlamydia pneumoniae, Helicobacter pylori,* periodontal infection), systemic inflammation, migraine, oral contraceptive use, sympathomimetic pharmaceuticals, illicit drug use, obesity, stress, snoring

during the first month after infarction. Anticoagulation with warfarin (INR of 2.0 to 3.0) is recommended after myocardial infarction in patients who have atrial fibrillation, decreased left ventricular function (ejection fraction of 28% or less), or left ventricular thrombi. Aspirin is recommended for the prevention of subsequent myocardial infarction. Lipid-lowering agents, particularly 3-hydroxy-3-methylglutaryl coenzyme-A (HMG-CoA) reductase inhibitors (statin agents), reduce the risk for stroke after a myocardial infarction. The United States Food and Drug Administration has approved pravastatin (Pravachol) for patients who have had a myocardial infarction and have average cholesterol levels of less than 240 mg/dL. Simvastatin (Zocor) has been approved for use in preventing stroke and TIA in patients with coronary heart disease and high cholesterol levels.

Atrial Fibrillation

Atrial fibrillation is an important risk factor for stroke. In comparison with patients without atrial fibrillation, the risk is 17 times higher in those with atrial fibrillation associated with valvular heart disease and 5 times higher in those with nonvalvular atrial fibrillation. Recommended guidelines for treating patients with atrial fibrillation depend on age and the associated risk factors of previous stroke or TIA, hypertension, heart failure, and diabetes mellitus. Patients older than 75 years with or without risk factors should be treated with warfarin. Patients 65 to 75 years old who have risk factors should be treated with warfarin, and those without risk factors should be treated with warfarin or aspirin. Patients younger than 65 years with risk factors should be treated with warfarin and those without risk factors should be treated with aspirin.

Diabetes Mellitus

Diabetes mellitus increases the risk of stroke in numerous ways. Large-artery atherosclerosis is accelerated via glycosylation-induced injury, adverse effects on cholesterol level, and promotion of plaque formation through hyperinsulinemia. Diabetes is associated with small-vessel ischemia, or lacunar infarction. Glycemic control has been shown to reduce microvascular complications, but evidence is lacking for macrovascular complications. Glycemic control is recommended to reduce microvascular and other diabetic complications.

Carotid Artery Stenosis

Carotid artery stenosis is another known risk factor for TIA and stroke. The course of action that should be taken for patients with symptomatic carotid artery stenosis is better defined and less controversial than that for patients with asymptomatic carotid artery stenosis. Published guidelines for asymptomatic carotid artery stenosis recommend endarterectomy in patients with stenosis greater than 60%, as defined by angiography, with a perioperative risk less than 3%. Despite this, many neurologists do not recommend endarterectomy because of the low rate of stroke in medically treated patients and several controversial issues concerning the asymptomatic carotid artery studies. The cardiac status and other medical illnesses of a patient need to be factored into the decision about endarterectomy. The status of the other carotid artery and the vertebral arteries is important in the decision about surgery. Patients with bilateral carotid artery occlusive disease or those with rapidly progressive stenosis may be at higher risk for stroke. Neurologic consultation may help identify the patients at high risk for an ipsilateral stroke and also help make a decision about endarterectomy. Medical therapy for asymptomatic carotid artery stenosis includes aspirin, 325 mg per day, or other antiplatelet therapy (e.g., clopidogrel) plus modification of other cerebrovascular risk factors.

Cigarette Smoking

Cigarette smoking is an independent risk factor for ischemic stroke and is dose-related. The mechanisms for this increased risk include progression of atherosclerosis, enhanced platelet aggregation, increased blood pressure, and increased blood viscosity, coagulability, and fibrinogen levels. Smoking cessation leads to a reduction in stroke risk.

Alcohol Consumption

The risk of stroke from alcohol consumption is different for hemorrhagic and ischemic strokes. Alcohol has a direct dose-dependent effect on the risk of hemorrhagic stroke. Moderate alcohol consumption, defined as from one drink per year to two drinks per day, is independently associated with a decreased risk of ischemic stroke. Heavy alcohol consumption, defined as five or more

drinks per day, is associated with an increased risk for ischemic stroke. The mechanisms for the increased risk include induction of hypertension, hypercoagulable state, cardiac arrhythmias, and reduced cerebral blood flow. The mechanisms for the beneficial effect of light to moderate consumption include increasing high-density lipoprotein cholesterol levels and decreasing fibrinogen levels and platelet aggregation.

Physical Activity

Several studies have demonstrated a benefit for stroke risk with physical activity. Regular exercise has well-established benefits for reducing cardiovascular disease and premature death. The protective effect of physical activity may be related to its role in reducing other risk factors, such as hypertension and diabetes. The mechanisms include decreasing fibrinogen levels and platelet activity and increasing high-density lipoprotein concentrations. The Centers for Disease Control and Prevention have recommended at least 30 minutes of moderately intense physical activity daily.

Dietary Factors

Many potential dietary factors may be risk factors for stroke. Increased homocysteine levels have been associated with stroke and atherosclerotic vascular disease. Dietary deficiencies of vitamin B_6, B_{12}, or folic acid can increase homocysteine levels. Increased sodium intake is associated with hypertension. Fruits and vegetables may be protective from an antioxidant effect. A high intake of saturated fat may increase the risk of stroke because of its effect on the patient's lipid profile.

Other Factors

Other potential risk factors for stroke are being investigated (Table 11–2). Antiphospholipid antibodies, acquired autoantibodies directed against various phospholipids, are potential stroke risk factors. These autoantibodies, which include lupus anticoagulant, anticardiolipin, and antiphosphatidylserine antibodies, are often found in patients with autoimmune disease and are a risk factor for arterial and venous thrombosis. Inflammation and infection are also potential stroke risk factors. Improved stroke prevention strategies will occur as cerebrovascular risk factors become better defined.

SYMPTOMATIC CAROTID ARTERY STENOSIS

A 58-year-old man experienced two brief episodes of visual loss in the left eye. He describes the episodes "like a shade being pulled down" over the eye. Each episode lasted only a few minutes. He has been taking one aspirin per day since he had a myocardial infarction 2 years ago and has had no additional cardiac symptoms. On physical examination, a bruit is heard over the left carotid artery. Carotid ultrasonography demonstrates 70% narrowing of the left carotid artery and 40% narrowing of the right carotid artery. How do you proceed to evaluate and manage this patient? Would your management change if he had only 50% narrowing of the left carotid artery?

This patient has transient retinal ischemia or symptomatic carotid artery disease. The symptoms of transient monocular blindness, carotid bruit on examination, and carotid ultrasonographic findings are all consistent with disease of the internal carotid artery. Despite these clinical findings, the patient should be evaluated the same as any other patient who has experienced a TIA, to exclude other lesions and to assess vascular risk factors. The risk for subsequent stroke in a patient with a TIA from high-grade ($\geq$ 70%) carotid stenosis is 13% for 2 years. The risk of stroke is higher for patients with cerebral hemispheric symptoms than for those with retinal symptoms, as in the case of the 58-year-old man.

The internal carotid artery supplies all structures of the frontal, parietal, and temporal lobes and the medial surface of the cerebral hemisphere. Clinical findings of carotid artery disease include transient monocular blindness, contralateral hemiparesis, hemianesthesia, hemianopia, aphasia (left hemisphere), or hemineglect (right hemisphere).

A physical finding that indicates carotid artery disease is the presence of retinal emboli on funduscopic examination. Retinal emboli are seen at the bifurcation of the retinal arterioles. Fibrin-platelet emboli are gray-white, and cholesterol emboli (Hollenhorst plaques) are shiny and orange-yellow. Both types are consistent with carotid embolization from ipsilateral atherosclerotic lesions.

A bruit (the sound of turbulent blood flow in the underlying artery) can be detected with auscultation by gently placing the bell of the stethoscope over the carotid artery. The presence of a localized or diffuse carotid bruit in a patient with cerebrovascular ischemic symptoms is 85% predictive of a moderate or high-grade stenosis. However, bruits are absent in more than one-third of patients with high-grade stenosis. A carotid bruit in an asymptomatic patient is a poor predictor of stenosis.

Clinical features alone are not sufficient for determining which patients would benefit from surgery. Carotid ultrasonography (duplex scanning) can measure blood velocity and arterial morphology with a high degree of accuracy. The study is useful for the initial screening of patients with carotid artery disease. Carotid duplex scanning cannot detect intracranial occlusive disease or provide information about collateral circulation (Fig. 11–7). Currently, cerebral angiography is the best test for assessing arterial status (Fig. 11–8). Angiography is an invasive test, and the complication rate in experienced hands has been estimated to be 1.2%. Magnetic resonance angiography (MRA) is an alternative technique, without the risks associated with conventional angiography. The combination of MRA and duplex ultrasonography has been favored for its low morbidity and mortality and cost-effectiveness ratio. Neurologic and neurosurgical consultation can help you select the appropriate diagnostic tests.

Carotid endarterectomy is a beneficial surgical procedure for preventing strokes in patients with symptomatic carotid artery stenosis. The surgical benefit of this proce-

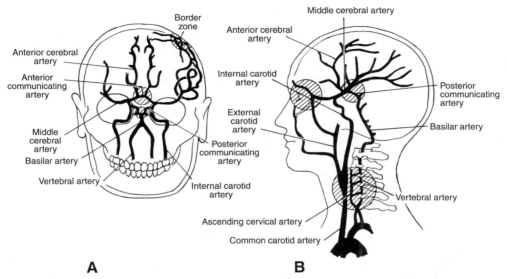

FIG. 11-7. Collateral circulation. (A) Anteroposterior view. Anterior communicating artery connects the right and left carotid circulations. Leptomeningeal anastomoses form collateral pathways among the border zones of major arterial territories. **(B)** Lateral view. Shaded circles indicate important collateral pathways. (From Pessin, MS, and Teal, PA: Cardinal clinical features of ischemic cerebrovascular disease in relation to vascular territories. In Samuels, MA, and Feske, S (eds): Office Practice of Neurology. Churchill Livingstone, New York, 1996, pp 311–329, with permission.)

dure depends on the risk of surgery. Combined morbidity and mortality with carotid endarterectomy is between 2% and 6% at experienced medical centers. Mortality rates are greater for surgeons and hospitals that perform a low volume of carotid endarterectomies.

Clinical trials have demonstrated that carotid endarterectomy is better than medical therapy in patients with stenosis of 70% or greater associated with retinal or cerebral ischemia (TIA) or minor stroke. The benefit of endarterectomy is greatest within the first 2 to 3 years after the operation.

Endarterectomy provides a moderate reduction in the risk of stroke for patients with symptomatic carotid artery stenosis of 50% to 69%. The modest reduction emphasizes the importance of selecting a surgeon with established surgical skill and a patient with low surgical risk. If the risk of stroke or death from surgery exceeds 2%, the benefit of surgery is lost. Carotid endarterectomy should be performed only by surgeons with a low

rate of complications, as determined by independent monitoring.

Many risk factors can influence perioperative risk and should be considered in the decision of whether to pursue carotid endarterectomy. Medical risk factors include hypertension (blood pressure greater than 180/110 mm Hg), recent myocardial infarction, congestive heart failure, angina, chronic obstructive pulmonary disease, severe obesity, and age older than 70 years. Patients who have neurologic deficits from multiple cerebral infarctions, a progressive neurologic deficit, neurologic deficit less than 24 hours in duration, or daily TIAs are at increased risk for perioperative complications. Angiographic evidence of additional vascular disease is also associated with an increased risk. The long-term benefits of carotid endarterectomy in patients with a 50% to 69% stenosis are better for men than for women, for patients with hemispheric symptoms than for those with retinal symptoms, and for patients with minor stroke than for those with a TIA.

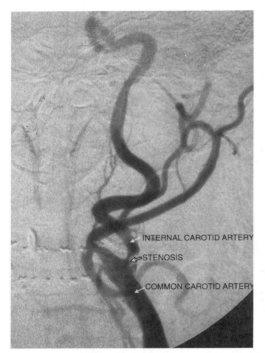

FIG. 11–8. Angiogram showing internal carotid artery stenosis.

The complications associated with carotid endarterectomy, such as wound hematoma and infection, can occur with any surgical procedure. Complications unique to carotid endarterectomy include postoperative carotid occlusion, TIA, and stroke. These complications usually result because of technical errors. Increased cerebral blood flow following the procedure can cause headache, intracerebral hemorrhage, or brain edema. Nerves that are at risk for injury during the procedure include the recurrent laryngeal, superior laryngeal, vagus, spinal accessory, and hypoglossal nerves. The potential complications of endarterectomy emphasize the importance of the skill and experience of the surgical team.

Patients with atherosclerotic carotid artery disease frequently have coronary artery disease. In fact, patients who survive atherosclerotic stroke are more likely to die of a coronary event than a recurrent stroke. Because carotid artery and cardiac disease are coincident, questions arise about the possibility of simultaneous carotid endarterectomy and coronary artery surgery. The few studies that have examined this issue have not demonstrated an advantage of simultaneous surgery. The risk of perioperative stroke during vascular surgery in a patient with asymptomatic carotid artery stenosis is low, and a preoperative or simultaneous prophylactic carotid endarterectomy is not necessary.

The patient described at the beginning of this section, who has had two episodes of transient monocular blindness while taking aspirin and has a 70% carotid artery stenosis, would benefit from carotid endarterectomy. For this patient, current evidence supports surgery over medical management. Management of a patient with a 50% stenosis is more difficult. Surgical and medical management options both are reasonable. Medical management would include treating all modifiable risk factors, changing the antiplatelet medication (increasing the aspirin dose or starting treatment with clopidogrel), and short-term warfarin therapy if the patient continued to have TIAs. The decision ultimately should be based on the perioperative risk factors discussed above and the desire of the patient.

STROKE IN YOUNG ADULTS

A 27-year-old woman with a history of migraine with aura experienced her usual aura of vertigo and facial numbness, followed by a severe throbbing headache. Unlike the previous episodes of migraine, the aura persisted and the patient went to the emergency department. Neurologic examination findings were pertinent for nystagmus, Horner syndrome on the right, and decreased pin and thermal sensation on the right side of the face and on the left side of the body. In the emergency room, CT of the head did not reveal any abnormality. The patient smokes and takes oral contraceptives. One week later, the patient's neurologic deficit persisted and MRI of the head demonstrated a right medullary infarct. What are the diagnostic possibilities for this patient's stroke? How do you manage this patient?

Stroke in persons younger than 45 years is uncommon. In addition to the usual mechanisms for cerebrovascular disease, the investigation of a young person with a stroke should include evaluation of the less common causes of stroke, including angiopathies, unusual cardiac embolic disorders, inflammatory conditions, illicit drug use, and hematologic disorders. There is an association between migraine and stroke, as in the case of the 27-year-old woman, but the mechanism is not entirely understood.

Migrainous Stroke

The criteria for the diagnosis of migrainous stroke have been defined by the International Headache Society Classification of Head Pain. Migrainous stroke occurs in a patient with a previous diagnosis of migraine with aura when the patient has one or more migrainous aura symptoms that are not fully reversible within 7 days, are associated with neuroimaging confirmation of ischemic infarction or both. Migrainous stroke is diagnosed if other causes of infarction have been excluded by appropriate investigation. The four types of migraine-related stroke are the following:

- A stroke that occurs remotely in time from a migraine attack.
- A stroke with migraine symptoms, sometimes called a "migraine mimic" (e.g., arteriovenous malformation that causes the symptoms of a migraine).
- A migraine-induced stroke (preceding symptoms resemble those of a previous migraine attack; other causes of stroke have been excluded).
- Stroke of uncertain cause.

Migraine-induced stroke is a diagnostic possibility for the woman described in the preceding case. This is a diagnosis of exclusion, however, and you need to perform a comprehensive cerebrovascular evaluation to determine whether there are other causes

of stroke and to identify other risk factors. An increase in the risk of stroke has been reported for women with migraine who take oral contraceptives, especially high-dose estrogen preparations. This risk is even higher for patients who smoke. Advise patients to avoid these risk factors. Migraine prophylaxis should be optimized. Also, vasoconstrictive medications should be avoided or their use limited. Taking aspirin daily is reasonable for patients with prolonged or frequent attacks of migraine with aura.

Arterial Dissection

If a young person has a stroke, consider nonatherosclerotic angiopathy. Arterial dissection is a potential cause of stroke by arterial narrowing or the formation of thrombus with secondary embolization. Common sites of dissection are the proximal internal carotid artery beyond the bifurcation and the distal extracranial vertebral artery. Arterial dissection is frequently associated with neck trauma, but it can occur spontaneously or in association with an angiopathy such as fibromuscular dysplasia. Patients with an arterial dissection frequently complain of headache. If the carotid artery is involved, the pain may be referred to the eye, and involvement of the sympathetic fibers coursing along the carotid artery may cause Horner syndrome (see Fig. 1–3). If the vertebral artery is involved, the patient may complain of pain in the neck or back of the head and have lateral medullary syndrome, as in the 27-year-old woman in the case above.

The diagnosis of arterial dissection can be made by angiography or MRA. If more than one vessel is involved, consider diseases of the arterial wall, such as fibromuscular dysplasia, Marfan syndrome, and Ehlers-Danlos syndrome. Treatment options are anticoagulant and antiplatelet therapies.

Illicit Drug Use

Illicit drug use is a potential cause of stroke in young adults. Drugs associated with both ischemic and hemorrhagic strokes include amphetamines, cocaine, heroin, phencyclidine, phenylpropanolamine, and lysergic acid diethylamide (LSD). The mechanisms of stroke include direct vascular effects, inflammatory and noninflammatory arteritis, prothrombotic state, cardiac arrhythmias, and endocarditis.

Hematologic Disorders

Hematologic disorders also can cause both ischemic and hemorrhagic strokes. Sickle cell disease is one of the more common hematologic disorders associated with stroke in young people. Hypercoagulable states due to malignancies and other systemic disorders are potential causes of stroke. Other systemic disorders such as sarcoidosis and connective tissue disease can cause a vasculitis. Syphilis, Lyme disease, tuberculosis, and fungal and bacterial infections can all cause stroke.

Cardiac Causes

In addition to the cardiac causes of stroke seen in older adults, unusual causes of cardiac embolism may be found in young adults, including congenital heart disease, patent foramen ovale, postpartum cardiomyopathy, and cardiac tumors. Transesophageal echocardiography, MRI of the heart, and cardiology evaluation may be needed if you suspect a cardiac source of emboli.

TREATMENT OF ACUTE STROKE: THROMBOLYTIC THERAPY

The treatment of acute stroke has changed remarkably since the publication of the findings of the National Institute of Neurological Disorders and Stroke Study Group on tissue plasminogen activator (t-PA) for acute ischemic stroke. The disability caused by stroke can be effectively reduced by acute early intervention. The effectiveness depends on many factors. Public education is essential so patients recognize a brain attack as a medical emergency. Potential candidates for treatment need to be correctly identified and transported immediately to emergency departments. Emergency departments, hospitals, and medical personnel need acute stroke plans to correctly diagnose and treat patients within the limited therapeutic time.

Patients with an ischemic stroke that is severe or progressive should be considered for thrombolytic therapy. The onset of symptoms needs to be less than 3 hours before treatment is started. For patients who awaken from sleep with a neurologic deficit, the time of symptom onset is the time they went to bed. CT should not show any evidence of intracranial hemorrhage, mass effect, or midline shift.

Exclusion criteria for thrombolytic therapy include patients with:

A rapidly improving deficit
Obtundation or coma
Seizure
Mild deficit
Blood pressure greater than 185/110 mm Hg
Gastrointestinal or urinary tract hemorrhage within the preceding 21 days
Ischemic stroke or serious head trauma within the preceding 3 months
A history of intracranial hemorrhage or bleeding diathesis
Major surgery within the preceding 2 weeks
Arterial puncture at a noncompressible site or lumbar puncture within the preceding week.

Laboratory abnormalities that exclude patients from thrombolytic therapy are (1) heparin treatment within the preceding 48 hours, with an increased activated partial thromboplastin time; (2) anticoagulant treatment, with a prothrombin time greater than 15 seconds, or (3) glucose level less than 50 or greater than 400 mg/dL.

Thrombolytic therapy with t-PA is effective in improving neurologic status if administered within 3 hours after the onset of symptoms. In the treatment trial, a greater proportion (12% greater absolute difference) of patients who received t-PA had minimal or no deficit at 3 months compared with those who received placebo. More importantly, there was no increase in severe deficits or disability.

Intravenous t-PA is given in a 0.9-mg/kg dose (maximum, 90 mg), with 10% given as a bolus and the rest given over 60 minutes. The patient should be monitored in an intensive care unit, and blood pressure should be less than 185/105 mm Hg. Heparin and aspirin should not be taken for 24 hours after t-PA therapy.

The major complication of thrombolytic therapy is intracranial hemorrhage. This complication should be suspected if the neurologic status of the patient deteriorates. If CT confirms hemorrhage, consider replacement therapy with platelets and cryoprecipitate. Hematologic and neurosurgical specialty consultation is very helpful in this situation.

HEMORRHAGIC STROKE

Hemorrhagic stroke, including intracerebral and subarachnoid hemorrhage, accounts for 15% of all strokes. CT can make the diagnosis of hemorrhagic stroke (see Fig. 2–4). The causes of spontaneous intracerebral hemorrhage include hypertension, aneurysms, vascular malformations, bleeding diatheses, drug-related hemorrhage, tumors, and cerebral venous occlusive disease. Hypertensive hemorrhage, the most common cause of intracerebral hemorrhage, is most likely to occur in the putamen, thalamus, cerebellum, pons, and caudate (Fig. 11–9). Lobar hemorrhage, or bleeding into the cerebral cortex and subcortical white matter, can occur in any lobe of the brain and has many causes.

The clinical features of hemorrhagic stroke depend on the location of the hemorrhage. Unlike embolic stroke, which has a maximal deficit at onset, hemorrhagic stroke can progress over minutes to hours. Blood in the form of a hematoma can behave like a mass lesion. Headache, decreased level of consciousness, and seizure are more likely to occur in hemorrhagic stroke than in ischemic stroke.

The diagnostic evaluation of patients with hemorrhagic stroke is the same as for those with ischemic stroke (see Table 11–1). Cerebral angiography is essential to evaluate for aneurysms, vascular malformations, and arteriopathies. Repeat angiography in 2 to 3 months may be necessary if the initial study findings are negative. The hematoma may obscure a vascular abnormality or small tumor. Follow-up CT and MRI may be needed for the same reason.

In hemorrhagic stroke, the management concerns are to identify the cause of the hemorrhage and to control blood pressure and intracranial pressure. Surgical therapy may be necessary for progressively enlarging hematomas. Neurologic and neurosurgical consultation is recommended for management of hemorrhagic strokes.

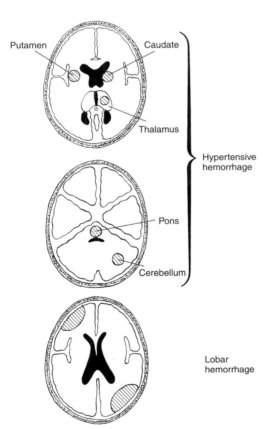

FIG. 11–9. Locations of hypertensive and lobar hemorrhagic strokes.

SUGGESTED READING

Adams, HP, Jr, et al: Guidelines for thrombolytic therapy for acute stroke: A supplement to the guidelines for the management of patients with acute ischemic stroke. A statement for healthcare professionals from a Special Writing Group of the Stroke Council, American Heart Association. Stroke 27:1711–1718, 1996.

Barnett, HJ, et al: Benefit of carotid endarterectomy in patients with symptomatic moderate or severe stenosis. N Engl J Med 339:1415–1425, 1998.

Bendok, BR, et al: Treatment of aneurysmal subarachnoid hemorrhage. Semin Neurol 18:521–531, 1998.

Biller, J, et al: Guidelines for carotid endarterectomy: A statement for healthcare professionals from a Special Writing Group of the Stroke Council, American Heart Association. Circulation 97:501–509, 1998.

Elkind, MS, and Sacco, RL: Stroke risk factors and stroke prevention. Semin Neurol 18:429–440, 1998.

European Carotid Surgery Trialists' Collaborative Group: Randomised trial of endarterectomy for recently symptomatic carotid stenosis: Final results of the MRC European Carotid Surgery Trial (ECST). Lancet 351:1379–1387, 1998.

Executive Committee for the Asymptomatic Carotid Atherosclerosis Study: Endarterectomy for asymptomatic carotid artery stenosis. JAMA 273:1421–1428, 1995.

Gorelick, PB, et al: Prevention of a first stroke: A review of guidelines and a multidisciplinary consensus statement from the National Stroke Association. JAMA 281:1112–1120, 1999.

Kittner, SJ, et al: Cerebral infarction in young adults: The Baltimore-Washington Cooperative Young Stroke Study. Neurology 50:890–894, 1998.

Millikan, CH, McDowell, F, and Easton, JD: Stroke. Lea & Febiger, Philadelphia, 1987, pp 241–245.

The National Institute of Neurological Disorders and Stroke rt-PA Stroke Study Group: Tissue plasminogen activator for acute ischemic stroke. N Engl J Med 333:1581–1587, 1995.

North American Symptomatic Carotid Endarterectomy Trial (NASCET) Steering Committee: North American Symptomatic Carotid Endarterectomy Trial. Methods, patient characteristics, and progress. Stroke 22:711–720, 1991.

Pritz, MB: Carotid endarterectomy. Semin Neurol 18:493–500, 1998.

Sacco, RL: Identifying patient populations at high risk for stroke. Neurology 51(Suppl 3):S27–S30, 1998.

Sacco, RL, et al: The protective effect of moderate alcohol consumption on ischemic stroke. JAMA 281:53–60, 1999.

Samuel, N, et al: Less common vascular causes of stroke. In Samuels, MA, and Feske, S (eds): Office Practice of Neurology. Churchill Livingstone, New York, 1996, pp 294–302.

Shah, MV, and Biller, J: Medical and surgical management of intracerebral hemorrhage. Semin Neurol 18:513–519, 1998.

Wiebers, DO, Feigin, VL, and Brown, RD, Jr: Handbook of Stroke. Lippincott-Raven Publishers, Philadelphia, 1997.

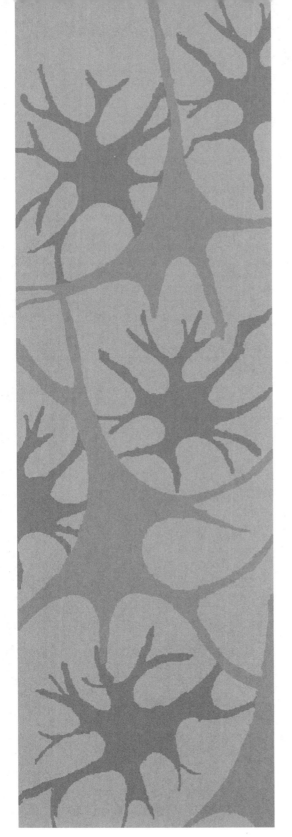

CHAPTER 12

Movement Disorders

CHAPTER OUTLINE

Classifying Movement Disorders
**Diagnostic Approach to Movement
    Disorders**
Parkinsonism
  Features of Parkinsonism
    Tremor
    Bradykinesia
    Rigidity
    Postural Instability
  Other Manifestations
  Differential Diagnosis
  Medical Treatment of Parkinson Disease
  Managing Late Complications of
      Parkinson Disease
    Motor Fluctuations
    Dyskinesias
    Other Late Complications
  Surgical Therapy for Parkinson Disease
Tremor
  Definition
  Types
Dystonia
  Definition and Types
  Treatment

(continued)

Tics and Tourette Syndrome
Definition and Types
Treatment
Tardive Syndromes
Diagnosis
Treatment

CLASSIFYING MOVEMENT DISORDERS

Movement disorders are neurologic syndromes in which movement is either excessive (hyperkinesia) or too little (hypokinesia). *Dyskinesia*, defined as difficulty performing voluntary movement, is a general term used for both hyperkinesia and hypokinesia. The prototypic hypokinetic movement disorder is Parkinson disease. Other terms used to describe this movement disorder are "bradykinesia" (slowness of movement) and "akinesia" (loss of movement). Hyperkinetic movement disorders seen in primary care practice include tremor, tics, and restless legs syndrome (see Chapter 9 for restless legs syndrome). The definitions of many hypokinetic and hyperkinetic movement disorders and common clinical examples are listed in Table 12–1.

Movement is often classified as "automatic," "voluntary," "semivoluntary," and "involuntary." Automatic movements are motor behaviors that are performed without conscious effort, for example, the arm swing associated with walking. Voluntary movements are planned or intentional movements. They can also be induced by external stimuli, as in turning the head in response to a loud noise. Semivoluntary movements include the movements seen with tics, restless legs syndrome, and akathisia. They are induced by an inner sensory stimulus, not unlike the need to scratch an itch. They are also called "involuntary movements," because they are executed to negate an unwanted or unpleasant sensation. Involuntary movements include movements such as tremor and myoclonus. Involuntary movements are often nonsuppressible or only partially suppressible.

Movement disorders frequently are associated with disease or pathologic alterations of the basal ganglia or their connections—the caudate, putamen, globus pallidus, subthalamic nucleus, and substantia nigra (Fig. 12–1). Disorders of the cerebellum are associated with impaired coordination (asynergy, ataxia), impaired judgment of distance (dysmetria), and intention tremor. Myoclonus, or sudden shock-like involuntary movements caused by muscular contractions or inhibitions, can occur from disorders of any part of the central nervous system. Some rare movement disorders such as painful legs and moving toes syndrome are associated with disorders of the peripheral nervous system. Many movement disorders are genetic, and the specific gene has been identified for several of them. Some of the more familiar inherited movement disorders are Huntington disease, Wilson disease, and familial essential tremor.

DIAGNOSTIC APPROACH TO MOVEMENT DISORDERS

If a patient has an abnormal movement, several questions need to be answered to distinguish among the different dyskinesias. (1) Is the movement rhythmical or arrhythmical? Tremor and myoclonus are rhythmical dyskinesias, and athetosis, ballism, chorea, and tics are arrhythmical movements. (2) What is the duration of the movement? Most dyskinesias are brief, nonsustained movements. Focal dystonia like torticollis or writer's cramp is a sustained abnormal movement. (3) What is the continuity of the contractions? Are the movements paroxysmal, as in tics? Are they continual, occurring over and over again, as in chorea? Are they continuous or unbroken, as in tremor? (4) Is there a relationship to sleep? Most dyskinesias are diminished during sleep. However, periodic movements of sleep, hypnogenic dyskinesias, palatal myoclonus, myokymia, and moving toes are dyskinesias that appear or persist during sleep.

TABLE 12–1. DEFINITIONS OF MOVEMENT DISORDERS AND CLINICAL EXAMPLES

Movement Disorder	Definition	Clinical Example
Hypokinetic		
Akinesia/bradykinesia	Absence or slowness of movement	Parkinson disease
Apraxia	Incapacity to execute purposeful movement not due to weakness, sensory loss, or incoordination	Parietal lobe lesion
Blocking tics	Motor phenomenon characterized by a brief interference of social discourse and contact	Tourette syndrome
Catatonia	Syndrome of psychomotor disturbances characterized by periods of physical rigidity, negativism, and bizarre mannerisms	Schizophrenia
Freezing phenomenon	Transient period of several seconds in which the motor act is halted	Parkinson disease
Hesitant gait	Slow cautious gait with wide base and short steps associated with a fear of falling	Hydrocephalus
Rigidity	Increased muscle tone to passive motion	Parkinson disease
Stiff muscles	Continuous muscle contraction without muscle disease, rigidity, or spasticity	Stiff-person syndrome
Hyperkinetic		
Akathisia	Inability to sit still, motor restlessness	Adverse effect of antidopaminergic drugs, e.g., antipsychotic agents
Asynergia or dyssynergia	Decomposition of movement due to breakdown of normal coordinated execution of a voluntary movement	Cerebellar disease
Ataxia	Incoordination	Cerebellar disease
Athetosis	Slow, writhing, continuous involuntary movement	Perinatal injury
Ballism	Large jerking or shaking movements	Infarct of subthalamic nucleus (hemiballism)
Chorea	Involuntary, irregular, purposeless, nonrhythmic, abrupt, rapid, unsustained movements that seem to flow from one body part to another	Huntington disease
Dysmetria	A form of dyssynergia	Cerebellar disease
Dystonia	A state of abnormal tone; twisting movements tend to be sustained at peak of movement and can be repetitive and progress to prolonged abnormal postures	Torticollis (focal dystonia)

(continued)

TABLE 12–1. DEFINITIONS OF MOVEMENT DISORDERS AND CLINICAL EXAMPLES
(continued)

Movement Disorder	Definition	Clinical Example
Hemifacial spasm	Unilateral facial muscle contractions	Compression of facial nerve by aberrant blood vessels
Myoclonus	Sudden, brief, shock-like involuntary movements caused by muscle contractions or inhibitions	Asterixis (brief flapping of of outstretched arms) from metabolic encephalopathy
Myokymia	Fine persistent quivering or rippling of muscles	Pontine lesion from multiple sclerosis
Stereotypy	Coordinated movements that are repeated continually and identically	Obsessive-compulsive disorder
Tics	Stereotyped, voluntary-appearing, purposeless movements	Tourette syndrome
Tremor	Oscillatory movement affecting one or more body parts	Essential tremor

After initially observing the patient, determine whether the abnormal movement occurs at rest or with action. This is the major focus when evaluating a patient with tremor. The tremor of Parkinson disease diminishes with action, whereas essential tremor occurs with action. Akathisic movement and restless legs are also associated with rest. The distribution of movement (focal or generalized), speed (fast or slow), and associated features help distinguish the various movement disorders.

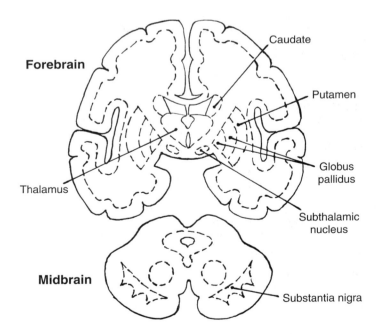

FIG. 12–1. Location of the basal ganglia (caudate, putamen, and globus pallidus), thalamus, subthalamic nucleus, and substantia nigra. Abnormalities of the structure and function of these structures are associated with abnormal movements, including tremor.

PARKINSONISM

A 61-year-old man is evaluated because of his hand tremor. He has been in good health except for right shoulder stiffness, which he attributes to arthritis. His wife first noticed that his right hand would shake when he watched television. Other symptoms elicited from him included generalized slowing of movement, trouble getting out of a deep chair, and stiffness. His wife volunteers that he shuffles his feet while walking and she has a hard time understanding him because of his soft voice. Their children have commented that "Dad looks depressed."

Neurologic examination demonstrates reduced facial expression. The patient rarely blinks. His voice is soft, consistent with a hypokinetic dysarthria. He has reduced arm swing with walking. He has a resting tremor of the right hand while walking and at rest. Muscle tone is increased on the right. When he is pulled backward (the pull test), he can maintain his posture with one step. What are the diagnostic considerations? How do you manage this patient?

The clinical presentation of this patient is typical of parkinsonism. The diagnostic criteria for parkinsonism include bradykinesia, rest tremor (also called "resting tremor"), rigidity, and loss of postural reflexes. Other diagnostic features are flexed posture and freezing or motor blocks. The diagnosis is considered definitive if the patient has at least two of these features, with one of them being rest tremor or bradykinesia. The diagnosis of probable parkinsonism is made if rest tremor or bradykinesia is present alone. Without bradykinesia or rest tremor, at least two of the other features must be present for the diagnosis of possible parkinsonism.

The four major categories of parkinsonism are primary, secondary, heredodegenerative, and multisystem degeneration. Primary parkinsonism is the most common form and is called *Parkinson disease*. Secondary (acquired or symptomatic) parkinsonism can result from anything that damages or interferes with the normal functioning of the motor control circuitry of the brain (for example, stroke, trauma, toxins, drugs, or infections), but the most common cause is exposure to dopamine receptor blocking drugs (for example, antipsychotic or antiemetic agents). Heredodegenerative parkinsonian disorders are rare. The most familiar ones are Huntington disease and Wilson disease. Multisystem degenerative, or "parkinsonism plus," disorders include progressive supranuclear palsy, cortical-basal ganglionic degeneration, and multiple system atrophy disorders (for example, striatonigral degeneration, Shy-Drager syndrome, and sporadic olivopontocerebellar atrophy).

The diagnosis of parkinsonism is relatively straightforward in the man in the above case, but it is more difficult in the early stages of the disease. The primary focus of the evaluation of a patient with a hypokinetic movement disorder is to determine whether the diagnosis is "Parkinson disease" or "parkinsonism." The distinction is important for prognosis and treatment. Patients with parkinsonism have a poorer prognosis and response to treatment than those with Parkinson disease.

The diagnosis of Parkinson disease is made clinically on the basis of the cardinal motor features of bradykinesia, rest tremor, rigidity, and postural instability. However, these clinical features are not specific and are of limited sensitivity for Parkinson disease. Autopsy studies have shown that the diagnosis of Parkinson disease is incorrect in approximately 25% of cases. The neuropathologic findings in the disease are Lewy bodies and loss of neurons in the substantia nigra.

Patients with early Parkinson disease rarely complain of slow movement. Instead, they usually complain of a feeling of weakness or fatigue. The term "weakness" is often used to describe difficulty with getting started or initiating movement. The most frequent complaints are trouble getting out of a car or bathtub, difficulty with turning in bed, difficulty with buttoning clothing, stiffness, and tremor. Handwriting becomes slow and small (micrographia). Patients often describe the rigidity of Parkinson disease as "stiffness" and think it is related to arthritis. Family members and friends are likely to comment on the change in the patient's gait and voice. Patients are often told that they appear depressed because of reduced animation in their face, or "masked facies."

A large part of the physical examination of a patient with a hypokinetic movement disorder can be conducted while the patient is walking to the examination room and during the history. Trouble getting up from a chair, flexed posture with reduced arm swing while walking, hand tremor, and masked facies are readily apparent physical findings. In patients with subtle disease, the reduced rate of eye blinking will become apparent if you blink only when the patient blinks.

FEATURES OF PARKINSONISM

Tremor

The tremor of Parkinson disease is a distal rest tremor, and it was this characteristic feature that led James Parkinson to refer to the disease as "shaking palsy." The tremor can occur in the hands, legs, or lips. It usually begins on one side. Asymmetric onset of the tremor is more characteristic of Parkinson disease than of the other parkinsonian disorders. The usual tremor is "pill-rolling" of the fingers or flexion-extension or pronation-supination of the hands. The tremor stops with active movement of the limb but reappears when the limb remains in a posture against gravity or "resets" to another resting position. In contrast, postural and action tremors (from essential tremor or cerebellar disease) appear only when the limb is being used.

The absence of a rest tremor often raises the possibility of other parkinsonian syndromes. Rest tremor is estimated to occur in only 75% of Parkinson patients. Furthermore, this tremor can occur in other syndromes, including multiple system atrophy, progressive supranuclear palsy, and dementia with Lewy bodies. The presence of an action tremor or both an action tremor and a rest tremor in a patient with Parkinson disease complicates the diagnosis. Be aware that a patient can have both types of tremor.

Patients often hold their hands or an object to minimize the tremor. You can demonstrate the tremor by having patients place their hands on their legs during the interview. The tremor may also become apparent while you are assessing gait. In Parkinson disease, tremor of the head usually involves the lips, chin, or tongue. Although head (neck) tremor can occur in Parkinson disease, it is more common in essential tremor, cerebellar disease, or dystonic tremor.

Bradykinesia

Bradykinesia is best demonstrated when the patient initiates movement, as in getting up from a chair, or makes a turn while walking. Turning often requires several steps, and the patient turns "en bloc." Reduced facial movement, decreased frequency of blinking, impaired upgaze and eye convergence, hypophonic speech with loss of inflection, drooling of saliva from decreased spontaneous swallowing, and micrographia are all examples of bradykinesia. Voluntary movement is slow and shows a reduction in amplitude. You can demonstrate reduction in amplitude by having the patient perform repetitive finger or foot tapping during rapid alternate motion testing. The range of movement is reduced and the rate appears faster. Bradykinesia can be a feature in other parkinsonian syndromes and in Alzheimer disease, depression, and normal aging.

Rigidity

Rigidity is an increase in muscle tone or resistance to motion. Test muscle tone by moving a patient's extremity (or joint) through its range of movement. Rigidity of the proximal joints can be elicited by swinging the patient's shoulders or rotating the hips. Rigidity can be distinguished from spasticity by the resistance that is present equally in all directions of the passive movement in both flexor and extensor muscles. The rigidity in Parkinson disease is often called "cogwheel rigidity" because of the jerky nature of the resistance, which is due to the superimposed tremor. Rigidity can be painful, and it is not uncommon for shoulder pain to be an initial symptom of Parkinson disease, as in the case above. Rigidity is often associated with the change that occurs in the patient's posture, with flexion of the neck, trunk, elbows, and knees becoming more prominent as the disease progresses.

Rigidity is a feature of many movement disorders and lesions of the central nervous system, including neuroleptic malignant syndrome, tetanus, and decorticate and decerebrate posturing. Cogwheel rigidity may also occur in essential tremor.

Postural Instability

Postural instability is a late manifestation of Parkinson disease. The "pull test" is a useful office procedure to test for postural instability. Stand behind the patient and pull the patient by the shoulders toward you. Carefully explain how the test is performed, and tell the patient to try to maintain his or her balance by taking a step backward. Be prepared to catch the patient if he or she cannot maintain balance. If the patient is large, stand next to a wall for support. Normally, a patient maintains his or her balance by taking one step back.

Two features that contribute to the high rate of fall-related injuries in patients with parkinsonism are the loss of postural reflexes and the freezing phenomenon. Postural instability and flexed truncal posture often cause festination, in which patients walk progressively faster to catch up with their center of gravity to avoid falling. The combination of postural instability, bradykinesia, and axial rigidity causes patients to collapse when they attempt to sit down.

Postural instability is not unique to Parkinson disease. If it occurs early in a patient with parkinsonism, you should consider the diagnostic possibility of progressive supranuclear palsy. Postural instability and falls are the common initial symptoms of this disorder. Postural instability is also seen in many neurologic disorders associated with sensory loss or muscle weakness and in nonneurologic disorders like severe arthritis.

OTHER MANIFESTATIONS

Parkinson disease has many manifestations in addition to rest tremor, bradykinesia, rigid-

ity, and postural instability. Dystonia, or sustained muscle contractions, can be either a symptom of Parkinson disease or a complication of drug therapy. It can result in abnormal posture or painful spasms. The most common types of dystonia in Parkinson disease are morning foot inversion dystonia, blepharospasm, and other focal dystonias.

With the freezing phenomenon (another motor manifestation of Parkinson disease), the patient's gait is affected initially by start-hesitation. Before starting, the patient takes small, shuffling steps. As the freezing phenomenon progresses, it seems as though the patient's feet are "glued" to the floor. This may be aggravated in situations such as going through a revolving door or crossing the street. The phenomenon can affect the arms and speech and is usually a late manifestation of the disease. The presence of the freezing phenomenon early in the course of the disease should raise the possibility of a parkinsonian syndrome.

Behavioral signs that may be found in patients with Parkinson disease include bradyphrenia, depression, and dementia. Bradyphrenia is mental slowness that may be reflected by slow thinking and a slow response to answering questions. Depression is estimated to occur in 30% to 50% of patients with Parkinson disease and is considered a biologic association of the disease and not a reaction to it. The prevalence of dementia in Parkinson disease is about 40%, but it increases with age. The dementia can be due to the neuropathologic changes that occur in the disease itself or in a coexisting condition such as Alzheimer disease or cerebrovascular infarcts.

Sleep disturbance is common in Parkinson disease and includes fragmentation of sleep, restless legs, periodic leg movement of sleep, and rapid eye movement (REM) sleep behavior disorder. Dysautonomia, including orthostatic hypotension, sphincter dysfunction, and erectile dysfunction are often late findings in the disease. Constipation and dysphagia are common gastrointestinal symptoms and seborrhea is a common dermatologic feature. Other manifestations of Parkinson disease include paresthesias, akathisia, and oral and genital pain. It is important to recognize these symptoms as part of the disorder to avoid unnecessary diagnostic evaluation.

DIFFERENTIAL DIAGNOSIS

Several diagnostic features are useful in differentiating Parkinson disease from the other parkinsonian disorders. Features of parkinsonian disorders include little or no tremor, early gait trouble, postural instability, upper motor neuron signs, and poor response to levodopa. If dementia occurs before the onset of motor symptoms, the patient probably does not have Parkinson disease but another parkinsonian disorder. Prominent postural instability, freezing phenomenon, and hallucinations unrelated to medications during the first 3 years after the onset of symptoms are clinical features of parkinsonian syndromes. Dysautonomia unrelated to medications should suggest an alternative diagnosis, such as multiple system atrophy. Combinations of parkinsonism, cerebellar dysfunction, autonomic failure, and corticospinal signs characterize multiple system atrophies. Parkinsonian disorders and their clinical features are summarized in Table 12–2.

Secondary parkinsonism should be considered if the patient has a known cause of parkinsonism, for example, exposure to dopamine receptor blocking medications. Medications

that can induce parkinsonism are listed in Table 12–3. The first line of treatment is to discontinue the medication. Infectious causes of parkinsonism include acquired immunodeficiency syndrome (AIDS) and Creutzfeldt-Jakob disease and other prion diseases. Encephalitis can result in parkinsonism, as it did following the influenza pandemic at the end of World War I. Toxins that cause parkinsonism include carbon monoxide, manganese, mercury, cyanide, methanol, and ethanol. MPTP, a byproduct of meperidine synthesis, caused an outbreak of parkinsonism among drug abusers in northern California in the 1980s. Parathyroid abnormalities and hypothyroidism can cause parkinsonism, as can cerebral infarcts, trauma, brain tumors, paraneoplastic syndrome, and normal-pressure hydrocephalus.

MEDICAL TREATMENT OF PARKINSON DISEASE

The goal of treating Parkinson disease is to keep the patient functioning independently as long as possible. Nonpharmacologic treatment includes education, peer and group support, and professional, legal, financial, and oc-

TABLE 12–2. PARKINSONIAN DISORDERS

Disorder	Clinical Features
Parkinson disease	Resting tremor, bradykinesia, rigidity, asymmetric onset, good response to levodopa
Cortical-basal ganglionic degeneration	Marked asymmetry, focal rigidity and dystonia, apraxia, tremor, myoclonus, cortical sensory deficit, alien-limb phenomenon
Dementia with Lewy bodies	Early-onset dementia, gait impairment, rigidity, hallucinations, poor tolerance of neuroleptic agents, fluctuating cognitive status
Olivopontocerebellar atrophy*	Cerebellar ataxia
Progressive supranuclear palsy	Vertical gaze palsy, oculomotor problems, early postural instability, axial rigidity, neck extension
Shy-Drager syndrome*	Dysautonomia, gait disturbance, mild tremor, dysarthria, inspiratory stridor
Striatonigral degeneration*	Early falls, poor response to levodopa, dysarthria, respiratory stridor, upper motor neuron signs
Vascular parkinsonism	Gait disturbance of legs more than arms, "lower-half" parkinsonism, upper motor neuron signs, pseudobulbar palsy, cerebrovascular risk factors

*Multiple system atrophy.

TABLE 12–3. DRUGS CAPABLE OF INDUCING PARKINSONISM

Amiodarone (Cordarone)
Amoxapine (Asendin)
Chlorpromazine (Thorazine)
Cytosine arabinoside (Cytarabine)
Fluphenazine (Prolixin)
Haloperidol (Haldol)
Lovastatin (Mevacor)
Methyldopa (Aldomet)
Metoclopramide (Reglan)
Perphenazine (Trilafon),
    perphenazine/amitriptyline (Triavil,
    Etrafon)
Prochlorperazine (Compazine)
Promethazine (Phenergan)
Reserpine (Serpasil)
Risperidone (Risperdal)
Thioridazine (Mellaril)
Thiothixene (Navane)
Trifluoperazine (Stelazine)
Verapamil (Calan)

cupational counseling. Encourage the patient to remain active and mobile. Exercise is important in slowing the effects of the disease that limit the patient's functional activity. The exercise program should include aerobic, strengthening, and stretching activities. Formal physical therapy can be beneficial.

Therapy should be individualized and based on the patient's social, occupational, and emotional issues. For example, it may be more important to treat a mild tremor in a patient who is still working than in one who is retired. For younger Parkinson patients, who are more likely to develop motor fluctuations and dyskinesias, consider prescribing a dopamine agonist. The medication regimen should be simplified for older patients, who are more likely to experience the adverse effects of confusion, hallucinations, and sleep-wake alterations. Discuss the specific symptoms that bother a patient, the degree of functional impairment, and the risks and benefits of therapy. Medical therapy, physical therapy, speech therapy, and mental health treatment can all be valuable. Several surgical treatments are also available.

The most effective medicine for the symptomatic treatment of Parkinson disease is levodopa (levodopa/carbidopa [Sinemet]). A favorable response to levodopa supports the diagnosis of Parkinson disease. Levodopa is converted to dopamine by dopa decarboxylase and acts on the postsynaptic dopamine receptors. Carbidopa inhibits peripheral dopa decarboxylase and allows more levodopa to enter the central nervous system. The carbidopa/levodopa combination reduces nausea and orthostatism (Sinemet = "without emesis").

Despite the effectiveness of levodopa, it is not free from controversy. Most patients who take levodopa develop serious complications that include motor fluctuations, dyskinesias, toxicity at therapeutic and subtherapeutic dosages, and a loss of efficacy. Dopamine increases oxidative stress and, theoretically, may accelerate disease progression. Some neurologists argue that levodopa therapy should be delayed to avoid the neurotoxic effects of dopamine and to delay the onset of complications.

Dopamine agonists (Table 12–4) do not generate oxidative metabolites and may have potential neuroprotective benefits. Advocates for delaying the use of levodopa favor the early use of dopamine agonists, especially in younger patients. The major disadvantages of dopamine agonists are their limited effectiveness and the frequency of adverse neuropsychiatric effects.

Evidence that supports the use of levodopa early in the course of Parkinson disease includes the failure to show a correlation between the rate of disease progression and the duration and quantity of levodopa used. Additional support for the early use of levodopa is the improved survival among those taking it. When levodopa treatment was introduced, patients with long-standing Parkinson disease developed motor fluctuations despite receiving the medication for only a short time. This supports the idea that motor fluctuations are more the product of disease duration than levodopa use.

Carbidopa/levodopa (Sinemet 25/100) is recommended for the initial treatment of symptomatic Parkinson disease. The starting dose is ½ tablet 1 hour before meals, three times a day. Instruct the patient to take the medicine on an empty stomach. Emphasize this point, because dietary protein can

TABLE 12–4. DOPAMINERGIC DRUGS FOR TREATING PARKINSON DISEASE		
Drug, Initial Dose	**Clinical Advantages**	**Clinical Disadvantages**
Carbidopa/levodopa (Sinemet) 25/100 ½ tablet 1 hr before meals, increase ½ tablet tid weekly to 3½ tablets tid	Most effective symptomatic treatment, may improve mortality rate	Nausea, orthostatic hypotension, dyskinesias, motor fluctuations, confusion
Dopamine agonists Bromocriptine (Parlodel) 1.25 mg bid Pramipexole (Mirapex) 0.125 mg tid Ropinirole (Requip) 0.25 mg tid	Reduced incidence of levodopa-related adverse events, levodopa-sparing effect	Nausea, hypotension, limited antiparkinson effect, neuropsychiatric adverse side effects
MAO B inhibitor Selegiline (Eldepryl) 5 mg bid	Levodopa-sparing effect, levodopa adjunct with increase in "on" time, neuroprotective effect in laboratory models	Minimal antiparkinson effect, question of increase in mortality, neuroprotection not established
COMT inhibitor Tolcapone (Tasmar) 100 mg tid Entacapone 200 mg tid	Increases levodopa availability to brain, decreased "off" time in patients with fluctuations	Liver failure, diarrhea, dyskinesia
Amantadine (Symmetrel) 100 mg bid	Reduces motor fluctuations, mild symptomatic effect	May contribute to confusion and hallucinations

bid, twice daily; COMT, catechol-*O*-methyltransferase; MAO, monoamine oxidase; tid, three times daily.

compete with levodopa for facilitated transport into the bloodstream of the small intestine, and the delay in gastric emptying has the potential for aggravating motor fluctuations. The dose should be increased by ½ tablet three times a day weekly (i.e., ½ tablet three times daily the first week, 1 tablet three times daily the second week, 1½ tablets three times daily the third week, and so forth), as tolerated and needed, to an initial maximal dose of 3½ tablets three times a day. The majority of patients should have significant improvement with this dose. A lack of response to levodopa therapy suggests that the patient has a parkinsonian syndrome instead of Parkinson disease.

Nausea is one of the most common side effects of levodopa therapy and may be avoided if the patient eats a soda cracker 30 minutes after each dose. Additional carbidopa (Lodosyn) taken 1 hour before each dose may also circumvent the problem. Trimethobenzamide (Tigan) may be effective for nausea, and it is not associated with drug-induced parkinsonism, as are metoclopramide (Reglan) and prochlorperazine (Compazine). Another strategy to combat nausea is to prescribe a controlled-release carbidopa/levodopa preparation (Sinemet CR). The controlled-release preparation is limited because it is expensive, the dose cannot be titrated, and the onset of the therapeutic effect is slow.

Orthostatic hypotension is a serious complication of levodopa therapy. Before getting up, patients should sit on the side of the bed for several minutes. They should drink six to eight glasses of water daily, use salt liberally, and drink a caffeinated beverage with each meal. The problem of hypotension can also be minimized by elevating the head of the bed. Support or pressure stockings are useful, but, practically, they are difficult for hypokinetic patients to put on and to wear. Medications that may be helpful include additional carbidopa, nonsteroidal anti-inflammatory drugs, fludrocortisone (Florinef), and midodrine (ProAmatine).

Hallucinations can be a complication of levodopa therapy and are more prominent in demented patients. Clozapine (Clozaril) is an antipsychotic agent that can be used to treat levodopa-induced psychosis without worsening parkinsonism. With clozapine treatment, the patient's leukocyte count has to be monitored weekly. If the number of leukocytes decreases, the agent has to be discontinued to avoid an irreversible agranulocytosis. One-half of a 25-mg tablet can be taken at bedtime and increased to one tablet in 1 week if needed. Risperidone, olanzapine, and quetiapine are atypical antipsychotic agents that do not require hematologic monitoring. Although they can aggravate parkinsonism, they may reduce psychotic symptoms without causing a significant change in Parkinson disease if used at a low dose.

The dopaminergic medications used to treat Parkinson disease are listed in Table 12–4. The use of selegiline, a monoamine oxidase type B inhibitor, has fluctuated over the last several years. Initially, this drug was thought to have some neuroprotective effect in Parkinson disease, and it was recommended as first-line therapy. After further study, it was shown to have a mild symptomatic benefit, but no neuroprotective benefit was established. Subsequently, conflicting results have been published about whether mortality is increased among patients taking selegiline. Serious drug interactions can occur with the concomitant use of selegiline and antidepressants or meperidine. The combination of selegiline and antidepressants can cause a syndrome of hyperthermia, autonomic instability, and mental status changes. The expense, the potential for drug interactions, and the lack of evidence to support the neuroprotective benefit of selegiline have limited its use.

Catechol-O-methyltransferase (COMT) inhibitors (tolcapone and entacapone) can extend the plasma half-life of levodopa without increasing the peak plasma concentration, prolonging the duration of action of each dose of levodopa. Explosive diarrhea is an adverse side effect that can occur 6 weeks after the patient starts taking the medication. Tolcapone has been associated with serious liver damage and, thus, requires monitoring of liver function tests. Because of this serious complication, many neurologists have stopped prescribing tolcapone. Entacapone (newly released) reportedly does not have the same adverse effects.

Amantadine causes the release of dopamine from nerve terminals, blocks dopamine uptake, has antimuscarinic effects, and blocks glutamate receptors. It has a limited anti-parkinson effect but may be useful in reducing levodopa-induced dyskinesias. Its important adverse effects include livedo reticularis (reddish mottling of skin), edema, and hallucinations.

Parkinson disease is treated with several nondopaminergic agents. Because of the relative cholinergic sensitivity that results from dopamine depletion, the symptoms of Parkinson disease have been treated with anticholinergic agents. The anticholinergic agents trihexyphenidyl (Artane) and benztropine (Cogentin) are prescribed primarily for resting tremor in young Parkinson patients who do not have dementia. Anticholinergic agents are limited by their side effects, including memory impairment, hallucinations, confusion, constipation, and urinary retention. Because antioxidants have a potentially neuroprotective effect, some neurologists recommend large doses of vitamins E and C. However, there is no evidence to support the idea that megadoses of vitamins alter the course of Parkinson disease. Preliminary evidence suggests that estrogen replacement therapy for postmenopausal women has a neuroprotective effect. More information is needed, but if there are no contraindications to estrogen replacement therapy, it is a reasonable option to consider in women with Parkinson disease.

MANAGING LATE COMPLICATIONS OF PARKINSON DISEASE

As Parkinson disease progresses, it becomes increasingly more difficult to treat. The pathogenesis for late complications is not fully known, but it involves altered dopaminergic mechanisms of the degenerating nigrostriatal system.

Motor Fluctuations

The most common complications include fluctuations, or "off" states, when parkinsonian symptoms predominate, and "on" states when dyskinesias are prominent. The first complication that usually appears is a mild wearing-off, or end-of-dose failure. During the first few years of treatment, patients experience a long duration of response to levodopa therapy. Wearing-off is what occurs when the dose no longer lasts 4 hours. Initially, the "off" periods are short, but as the disease progresses, both the "off" and "on" periods shorten. In association with these fluctuations, many patients develop dyskinesias (chorea and dystonia).

The various strategies for managing motor fluctuations and dyskinesias are listed in Table 12–5. Small changes in the dose of levodopa may be necessary to treat motor fluctuations; liquefied carbidopa/levodopa can be used for this. To make liquefied carbidopa/levodopa, dissolve ten 25/100 mg tablets in 1 L of an acidified solution (diet soda, carbonated water, or ascorbic acid solution): 1 mL of solution = 1 mg of levodopa. Because the solution oxidizes easily, it should be prepared daily and stored in the refrigerator. Motor fluctuations can be lessened if gastrointestinal

motility is improved. Cisapride (Propulsid) increases gastrointestinal motility and can reduce the motor fluctuations caused by poor gastric emptying.

When motor fluctuations develop, it is essential for you to find out the timing of the problem and the relationship to the dose, dosage schedule, meals, and sleep. One way to do this is to have the patient keep a diary. This will help you to determine whether the complication is related to being parkinsonian ("off") or "on." Wearing-off, or end-of-dose failure, is apparent when an increase in parkinsonian symptoms occurs before the next dose. A reduction in the dose interval will solve the problem. The distinction between "off" and "on" states for other fluctuations may be difficult. Types of fluctuations include sudden "off," random "off," "yo-yoing," episodic failure to respond, delayed "on," weak end-of-day response, response variability in relationship to meals, and sudden transient freezing. In "yo-yoing," the patient responds to levodopa rapidly, with a

TABLE 12–5. STRATEGIES FOR MANAGING MOTOR FLUCTUATIONS AND DYSKINESIAS

Complication	Management Options
Wearing-off	Add selegiline, change to controlled-release form, add COMT inhibitor, decrease dose interval, add dopamine agonist
Sudden "off" or random "off"	Dissolve carbidopa/levodopa in carbonated water before ingestion, change to dopamine agonist
"Yo-yoing"	Liquid carbidopa/levodopa titration, dopamine agonist
Dose failures	Liquid carbidopa/levodopa
Delayed "on"	Increase morning dose, add cisapride
Weak response at end of day	Increase evening dose
Freezing	Increase dose for "off" freezing, decrease dose for "on" freezing
Peak-dose dyskinesia	Decrease dose, decrease dose interval, decrease levodopa, dopamine agonists, controlled-release levodopa, amantadine
Diphasic dyskinesia	Dopamine agonists
Off dystonia	Dopamine agonists, controlled-release levodopa

COMT, Catechol-*O*-methyltransferase.

peak-dose dyskinesia followed by the wearing-off.

Dyskinesias

Dyskinesias are frequently a late complication of Parkinson disease and usually consist of chorea or dystonia (or both). The types of dyskinesia include peak-dose dyskinesias, diphasic dyskinesias, and "off" dystonia. Peak-dose dyskinesias represent an excessive level of levodopa. A patient with diphasic dyskinesia may have dystonia, followed by improvement and then the return of dystonia. This is thought to be the result of increasing and decreasing levels of levodopa. "Off" dystonia occurs when the level of levodopa is low; painful sustained contractions can develop. Neurologic consultation is helpful in managing these late complications of Parkinson disease.

Other Late Complications

Other late complications that are frequently seen include falling, sleep difficulty, autonomic dysfunction, psychiatric problems, and cognitive difficulty. Any complication that develops suddenly should prompt an investigation for a medical illness such as pneumonia or a urinary tract infection. Scrutinize the patient's medications to determine if they are responsible for any complications.

Falling. Falling is a dangerous complication and the cause of significant morbidity and mortality. The twofold increase in the risk of death in parkinsonism is related directly to the presence of a gait disturbance and falling. The risk factors for falling include older age, advanced stage of disease, gait disturbance, freezing, and postural instability. Mental status changes, dyskinesias, orthostatic hypotension, arthritis, visual impairment, vestibular dysfunction, and sensory loss also contribute to the problem of falling. If a patient has a positive pull test or has a gait disturbance with freezing, he or she is at risk for falling. Prescribe preventive measures for these patients, for example, gait training, physical therapy, the use of a cane or walker, and home safety devices. Gait freezing with the initiation of walking is sometimes improved with visual cues such as stepping over an inverted cane or placing lines on the floor.

Sleep Disturbance. Sleep disturbance can be a problem throughout the course of Parkinson disease. Patients who have difficulty initiating sleep can be given diphenhydramine (Benadryl) or sedating tricyclic antidepressants such as amitriptyline (Elavil) or trazodone (Desyrel). Difficulty staying asleep can result from low levels of levodopa; thus, increasing the dose or using controlled-release levodopa may reduce the problem. REM behavior sleep disorder can be treated with clonazepam (Klonopin).

Cognitive Difficulty. Cognitive difficulty becomes more pronounced as the disease progresses, and the prevalence of dementia in Parkinson disease increases with age and severity of disease. No effective treatment is available for this dementia. It is important to exclude any treatable causes of dementia (see Chapter 8).

Psychiatric Complications. The psychiatric complications of Parkinson disease include hallucinations, psychoses, depression, and anxiety. Most psychiatric problems are treated in the same way they would be if Parkinson disease were not present, except for prescribing antipsychotic medications that can aggravate the disease. Psychiatric consultation is useful for managing these complications.

SURGICAL THERAPY FOR PARKINSON DISEASE

Several surgical options can be considered when patients become refractory to medical therapy. These options include thalamotomy, pallidotomy, deep brain stimulation, and cellular transplantation. Surgery for the treatment of movement disorders has been enhanced by improved surgical technique, stereotactic imaging techniques, and microelectrode cell recording. Selecting the neurosurgeon is as important as determining the most appropriate surgical candidate. The neurosurgeon should be experienced and use intraoperative microelectrode cell recording to ensure proper placement of the ablative lesion or stimulating electrode.

The target area for thalamotomy is the ventral intermediate nucleus of the thalamus. This procedure has been used to treat Parkinson disease, essential tremor, dystonia, and hemiballism. It is effective for tremor but less effective than pallidotomy for rigidity, dystonia, and dyskinesias.

Pallidotomy should be considered for patients who have severe dyskinesias or painful "off" dystonia that is refractory to medical treatment. Patients with dementia or multiple medical problems and those with limited life expectancy are not good surgical candidates. The target area for pallidotomy is the internal segment of the globus pallidus. Potential complications of both pallidotomy and thalamotomy are dysarthria, dysphagia, hemiparesis, and visual field defects. Bilateral procedures have produced dysfunction of speech, swallowing, and cognition.

Deep brain stimulation is a promising alternative to neuroablative surgery and may be preferable when bilateral surgical procedures are needed. Deep brain stimulation has been effective in treating tremor, Parkinson disease, and other movement disorders. It is reversible, and the stimulation can be adjusted over time to respond to the progression of the disease. Deep brain stimulation of the thalamus is effective for tremor, and stimulation of the globus pallidus and subthalamic nucleus can improve parkinsonism. Deep brain electrodes are placed through a bur hole, and an implantable pacemaker is inserted in a subcutaneous pocket, similar to a cardiac pacemaker. A magnet is used to turn the stimulator on and off. The mechanism of action of deep brain stimulation is not completely known.

Fetal nigral transplantation is a potential treatment for Parkinson disease. Small pilot studies have shown that fetal nigral tissue can be transplanted into the postcommissural putamen bilaterally with little morbidity. Clinical improvement in parkinsonian symptoms has been related to the survival and function of transplanted fetal tissue; a long-term clinical benefit has been demonstrated. Further study of this therapy is needed.

TREMOR

 A 63-year-old woman is evaluated for hand tremor. She remembers that her hands would shake in college but only when she was taking an examination. Her tremor has gotten worse in the last year and has made her very self-conscious at work. Alcohol reduces the tremor, and she usually has a drink before dinner to minimize the shaking. The patient's mother had a head tremor, and her maternal grandfather had the diagnosis of Parkinson disease. She is worried about Parkinson disease and wants to know what can be done to reduce her tremor. How do you respond to the patient's concerns?

DEFINITION

Tremor, the most common form of involuntary movement disorder, is a rhythmic oscillation of agonist and antagonist muscles. It can be classified as either a "rest tremor" or an "action tremor" (Table 12–6). Rest tremor is the characteristic tremor of parkinsonism. It occurs when the affected body part is supported against gravity and not actively contracting. Rest tremor is absent or diminished during muscle contraction or during movement. Most tremors are action tremors that become more prominent with voluntary movement, such as writing, eating, or drinking. Action tremors include postural, kinetic, task- or position-specific, and isometric tremors.

TYPES

Postural tremors occur when an antigravity posture is maintained, for example, holding the arms in front of the body. Kinetic tremors are seen with voluntary movement. "Initial tremor," "dynamic tremor," and "terminal tremor" describe kinetic tremor, at the beginning of the movement, during the movement, and when the affected body part approaches the target, respectively. A task-specific tremor occurs with a specific activity,

TABLE 12–6. CLASSIFICATION OF TREMOR

Rest Tremor	Action Tremor
Parkinson disease	Postural
Multisystem degenerations	Physiologic tremor
Multiple-system atrophies	Enhanced physiologic tremor—
Progressive supranuclear	stress-induced, endocrine, drugs,
palsy	toxins
Cortical-basal ganglionic	Essential tremor—autosomal
degeneration	dominant, sporadic
Diffuse Lewy body disease	Parkinsonism
Heredodegenerative disorders	Tardive tremor
Huntington disease	Midbrain (rubral) tremor
Wilson disease	Cerebellar
Neuroacanthocytosis	Neuropathic
Ceroid lipofuscinosis	Kinetic (intention, termination)
Secondary parkinsonism	Cerebellar disorders
Drug-induced	Midbrain lesions
Toxic	Task- or position-specific tremors
Vascular	Handwriting
Trauma	Occupational task-specific
Infectious	Isometric
Tardive tremor	Orthostatic
Severe essential tremor	
Midbrain (rubral) tremor	

for example, a voice tremor that occurs with singing and a hand tremor that occurs only with writing. Position-specific tremors occur only when a specific posture is maintained, for example, holding a cup up to the mouth. An isometric tremor occurs during voluntary muscle contraction not accompanied by a change in position of the body part. An example is orthostatic tremor, in which a fine, fast tremor occurs in the legs with standing.

Physiologic tremor is a postural tremor that everyone has. It can be enhanced by several things, including emotion, exercise, fatigue, anxiety, and fever. If a patient presents with an enhanced physiologic tremor, consider such endocrine disorders as thyrotoxicosis, hypoglycemia, and pheochromocytoma. Drugs that enhance physiologic tremor are listed in Table 12–7. Physiologic tremor can be enhanced by any condition that increases peripheral β-adrenergic activity.

Essential tremor is the most common movement disorder and occurs equally in both genders. The age at onset has a bimodal distribution, with peaks in the second and sixth decades. This tremor is most likely to in-

volve the hands, but it can involve, in descending order, the head, voice, leg, jaw, trunk, and tongue. Patients with essential tremor of-

TABLE 12–7. DRUGS ASSOCIATED WITH ENHANCED PHYSIOLOGIC TREMOR

Bromocriptine (Parlodel)
Carbidopa/levodopa (Sinemet)
Caffeine (coffee, tea)
Cyclosporine (Neoral)
Haloperidol (Haldol)
Fluoxetine (Prozac)
Lithium (Lithobid)
Methylphenidate (Ritalin)
Metoclopramide (Reglan)
Pergolide (Permax)
Phenylpropanolamine (nasal decongestant)
Pramipexole (Mirapex)
Pseudoephedrine (Sudafed)
Ropinirole (Requip)
Terbutaline (Brethine)
Theophylline (Theo-Dur)
Valproate (Depakote)

ten have other associated movement disorders. Acccording to one study, a large proportion of patients with essential tremor have dystonia and parkinsonian signs.

Essential tremor occurs sporadically and is inherited. Familial tremor shows an autosomal dominant inheritance pattern with variable penetrance. An association between essential tremor and Parkinson disease has been suggested by several studies, but the exact relationship has not been identified. Complicating the distinction between essential tremor and Parkinson disease is the presence of both conditions in one patient and an incorrect diagnosis, for example, a patient with essential tremor being diagnosed as having Parkinson disease. The 63-year-old woman in the case above is said to have had a grandparent with Parkinson disease, but this may have been essential tremor that was misdiagnosed. Patients with tremor, like the woman in this case, are often worried about having Parkinson disease.

Essential tremor is a postural tremor that becomes more prominent with voluntary movement. Some patients with parkinsonism have a postural tremor (with the arms outstretched in front of them) that develops after a latency of a few seconds. This probably represents a rest tremor that has been "reset" during posture holding. This tremor is sometimes called a "repose tremor." In essential tremor, the tremor does not occur when the hands and arms are relaxed. Hand tremor that occurs with the arms hanging at the sides is more likely a parkinsonian tremor. Alcohol frequently decreases essential tremor, but it has no effect on a parkinsonian tremor. The differences between es-

sential tremor and the tremor of Parkinson disease are summarized in Table 12–8. It is important to keep in mind that these two tremor types overlap.

The treatment of essential tremor depends on the severity of the tremor and the patient's functional impairment. Some patients with extremely mild tremor may require only reassurance about the absence of a serious problem. Many patients drink alcohol to suppress the tremor. Although the information available about alcoholism and essential tremor is contradictory, drinking alcohol is not a recommended treatment.

Before you start drug therapy for the tremor, obtain a sample of the patient's handwriting. The handwriting or the patient's drawing of a spiral (Fig. 12–2) can be monitored to assess the response to treatment. Having patients maintain a daily sample of handwriting helps them visualize their response to treatment.

Propranolol (Inderal), a β-adrenergic blocking drug, is effective for treating essential tremor. Metoprolol (Lopressor) and nadolol (Corgard) are moderately effective, and atenolol (Tenormin) and timolol (Blocadren) have limited efficacy. The effectiveness of β-adrenergic blocking medications for tremor is not related to lipid solubility. The maintenance dose for propranolol ranges from 80 to 240 mg twice a day. These drugs should not be taken by patients who have congestive heart failure, chronic obstructive pulmonary disease, asthma, or insulin-dependent diabetes mellitus. Frequent adverse effects include fatigue, depression, and lightheadedness.

Primidone (Mysoline) is also effective in treating essential tremor. Its tremor-suppres-

TABLE 12–8. COMPARISON OF ESSENTIAL TREMOR AND PARKINSON TREMOR

Characteristic Feature	Essential Tremor	Parkinson Tremor
Tremor type	Action	Rest
Anatomical distribution	Head and voice Not in leg	Ipsilateral limbs
Symmetry	Symmetric	Asymmetric
Effect of alcohol	Decreases	No effect
Other neurologic signs	None	Bradykinesia, rigidity, postural instability

FIG. 12–2. Spirals, as drawn by a person with no movement disorder (A) and a patient with tremor (B).

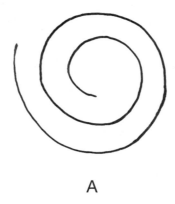
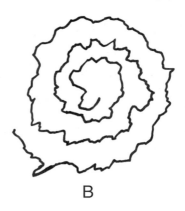

A   B

sant effect is due primarily to the parent compound rather than the metabolites (phenobarbital or phenylethylmalonamide). Treatment should be started at a very low dose (25 mg at bedtime) to prevent the common side effects of sedation, confusion, and ataxia. Doses greater than 250 mg per day are rarely needed.

Gabapentin (Neurontin) has been used to treat many types of tremor. A recent study compared gabapentin (400 mg three times a day) and propranolol (40 mg three times a day) in the treatment of essential tremor and concluded they had a comparable efficacy. The absence of drug interactions and the high tolerability of gabapentin make it a useful alternative for patients who cannot take propranolol or primidone. Other medications used to treat essential tremor are methazolamide (Neptazane), buspirone (BuSpar), and benzodiazepines (e.g., clonazepam [Klonopin]).

Another treatment for tremor is to inject botulinum toxin (Botox) into the muscles that produce the oscillatory movement. When the tremor becomes severe and refractory to medical treatment, consider thalamotomy and deep brain stimulation. The various treatments for tremor are summarized in Table 12–9.

DYSTONIA

A 54-year-old man is evaluated for a painful neck. He was involved in a motor vehicle acci-

dent 5 years ago and sustained a minor flexion and extension injury of the neck. His symptoms improved. About 2 years ago, his neck started to pull toward the right. He has noticed that he can reduce the movement of the neck to the right by placing his hand on his chin. The problem is becoming progressively worse. Except for his neck posture, the findings on neurologic examination are normal. How do you manage this patient? What is the relationship of his condition to the accident?

DEFINITION AND TYPES

This man has a focal cervical dystonia, also called "torticollis" or "wry neck." Dystonia is a syndrome of sustained muscle contractions, frequently causing twisting and repetitive movements or abnormal postures. According to the distribution of the muscles involved, dystonias can be classified as focal, segmental, multifocal, generalized, or hemidystonic. Most patients with dystonia have focal dystonia. Common focal dystonias in addition to torticollis are hand or writer's cramp, voice or spasmodic dysphonia, and blepharospasm.

Primary dystonia includes both familial and sporadic cases. Secondary, or symptomatic, causes of dystonia include stroke, trauma, birth injury, encephalitis, and exposure to dopamine receptor blocking drugs. In the preceding case, the motor vehicle accident is unlikely to have caused the patient's focal dystonia. Although peripheral injury

TABLE 12–9. TREATMENT OF TREMOR

Treatment	Tremor Type
Botulinum toxin (Botox)	Postural, kinetic, rest, task-specific, head, face, voice, tongue
Buspirone (BuSpar)	Kinetic
Carbidopa/levodopa (Sinemet)	Rest, facial, tongue
Clonazepam (Klonopin)	Kinetic, head, orthostatic
Deep brain stimulation	Postural, kinetic, rest
Gabapentin (Neurontin)	Postural, kinetic, task-specific, head, voice, face, tongue, orthostatic
Methazolamide (Neptazane)	Postural, kinetic, head
Pallidotomy	Rest
Propranolol (Inderal)	Postural, kinetic, task-specific, head, voice, face, tongue
Phenobarbital	Orthostatic
Primidone (Mysoline)	Postural, kinetic, task-specific, head, face, tongue, orthostatic
Thalamotomy	Postural, kinetic, rest
Trihexyphenidyl (Artane)	Rest, task-specific

has been reported as a possible etiologic factor for dystonia, most cases of symptomatic dystonia involve pathologic alterations of the basal ganglia, particularly the putamen (see Fig. 12–1). The onset of dystonia from months to years after a cerebral insult has been described in perinatal asphyxia, but other neurologic abnormalities were noted. In the patient described here, the symptomatic improvement after the accident and the normal examination findings are evidence that the accident did not cause the man's dystonia. A unique feature of dystonic movements is a reduction in movement caused by a tactile or sensory stimulus (sensory trick, or *geste antagoniste*). The man touched his chin to reduce the movement. Pain is uncommon in most forms of dystonia, although most patients with cervical dystonia experience neck pain.

TREATMENT

No drug is entirely effective in treating dystonia. Dopamine agonists are prescribed because of the rare dopa-responsive dystonia. Other drugs that have been used include anticholinergic agents, baclofen, carbamazepine, and benzodiazepines. The treatment of choice for focal dystonias is botulinum toxin. Electromyography is useful in selecting the muscles that should be injected with the toxin.

TICS AND TOURETTE SYNDROME

An 11-year-old boy is taken to a doctor by his mother because she is concerned that he has abnormal movements and makes abnormal sounds. About 1 year earlier, he constantly rolled his eyes. She thought he did this to get attention, and after several months, the movement stopped. He then developed frequent sniffing and throat-clearing sounds that were initially attributed to allergies. The boy's teachers commented on his frequent facial grimacing and grunting. He is active in sports and has a "B" average. Except for facial grimacing and grunting sounds, the findings on neurologic examination are normal. The child is able to suppress the movement temporarily. What is your diagnosis, and what do you recommend for treatment?

DEFINITION AND TYPES

The boy has both motor and phonic tics. Tics are brief and intermittent movements (motor) or sounds (phonic) that can be classified as either simple or complex. Simple motor tics involve only one group of muscles and cause a brief jerk-like movement. Phonic, or vocal, tics are essentially motor tics that involve the respiratory, pharyngeal, laryngeal, oral, and nasal musculature. Simple phonic tics consist of grunting, throat-clearing, sniffing, coughing, or blowing sounds. Examples of complex vocal tics include using obscenities and profanities (coprolalia), repeating what is said by others (echolalia), or repeating oneself (palilalia). Complex motor tics consist of coordinated sequenced movements that are inappropriately timed and intense, for example, making obscene gestures (copropraxia) and imitating gestures (echopraxia).

Tics are paroxysmal and occur abruptly for brief moments from a background of normal motor activity. They frequently are diagnosed as habits, allergies, or hyperactivity. Distinguishing a simple motor tic from myoclonus or chorea may be difficult in isolation. Compared with other hyperkinetic movement disorders, tics tend to be repetitive and the patient is more likely to have other complex motor tics. Eye movement abnormalities are often seen in tics but are infrequent in other hyperkinetic movement disorders. Tics are usually induced by an inner sensory stimulus that is relieved by the movement. This premonitory sensation is compared to the urge to scratch an itch. Tics are suppressible and frequently vary in severity over time. Remission and exacerbations are common.

The combination of simple and complex motor and vocal tics is characteristic of Tourette syndrome. This syndrome usually begins in childhood and has been associated with attention deficit disorder, lack of impulse control, and obsessive-compulsive disorder. It is an inherited disorder that is more penetrant in males than females. The genetic relationship among Tourette syndrome, obsessive-compulsive disorder, and attention deficit with hyperactivity has not been defined.

TREATMENT

The treatment of tics and Tourette syndrome begins with educating the patient, family, and those who interact with the patient about the disorder. National and local support groups are an invaluable resource for support and education. Many patients do not require pharmacologic therapy. Medications should be considered when the symptoms interfere with academic or job performance, social interactions, or activities of daily living. Many medications can be used to treat the symptoms of Tourette syndrome, but therapy should be individualized and tailored to the specific needs of the patient. It is important to give the medication an adequate dose and time trial to avoid unnecessary changes in response to the normal variations in symptoms that occur during the natural course of the disease. Fluphenazine (Prolixin), pimozide (Orap), and haloperidol (Haldol), dopamine receptor blocking agents, are prescribed most often for tics.

TARDIVE SYNDROMES

A 72-year-old woman reports a long history of being "nervous." She has been taking perphenazine/amitriptyline (Triavil) for the last 20 years to help her calm down. About 3 months ago, she developed involuntary movements of the mouth. Neurologic examination reveals rapid, repetitive, stereotypic movements involving the oral, buccal, and lingual areas. This movement is making her more "nervous." Her doctor has retired, and she needs the prescription renewed and wants treatment to reduce the movement. How do you manage this patient?

DIAGNOSIS

This woman has a movement disorder called *oral-buccal-lingual dyskinesia*. It is the most common tardive syndrome. Tardive dyskinesia is an iatrogenic syndrome of persistent abnormal involuntary movements that occur as a complication of drugs that block dopamine receptors (Table 12–10). The diagnosis of a tardive syndrome is based on exposure of the patient to a dopamine receptor blocking agent within 6 months before the onset of the movement and the persistence of the movement for 1 month after the patient stops taking the offending drug.

Akathisia can occur as a tardive syndrome. It is described as an inner restlessness of the whole body, but it can involve an uncomfortable sensation in a specific part of the body. Focal akathisias are often described as a burning pain, commonly in the mouth and genital areas. A patient with generalized akathisia has rhythmical, repetitive, stereotypic movements like body rocking, crossing and uncrossing the legs, and moaning. Dystonia can be part of a tardive syndrome. It is not uncommon for patients to have both dystonia and an oral-buccal-lingual dyskinesia. Both akathisia and dystonia can occur acutely after exposure to dopamine receptor blocking drugs. Acute dystonia that affects the ocular muscles is called an *oculogyric crisis*. The acute reactions can be treated with parenteral anticholinergic and antihistamine agents such as diphenhydramine and benztropine.

Unlike drug-induced parkinsonism, in which the symptoms disappear when the drug is withdrawn, tardive dyskinesias can persist and be permanent. This emphasizes the importance of avoiding dopamine receptor blocking drugs unless absolutely necessary. The patient should be informed about the potential complication of these agents, and this should be documented in the medical record. Patients at risk for tardive dyskinesia are older, female, and persons exposed to higher daily doses and greater cumulative amounts of dopamine receptor blocking drugs.

TREATMENT

The first step in treating tardive syndromes is to remove the offending drug. Gradual withdrawal is recommended to avoid an exaggeration of the movement (withdrawal emergent syndrome). If the drug can be avoided, the tardive symptoms may resolve. If it is necessary to treat the symptoms, dopamine receptor depleting drugs (reserpine and tetrabenazine [available in Europe]) can be prescribed. Other useful drugs are clonazepam, alprazolam, baclofen, and anticholinergic agents (for dystonia). If continued treatment with an antipsychotic medication is needed, then clozapine, olanzapine, or quetiapine may be preferred. Neurologic and psychiatric consultation may be required to manage severe tardive syndromes.

TABLE 12–10. DRUGS THAT CAN CAUSE TARDIVE SYNDROMES

Amoxapine (Asendin)
Chlorpromazine (Thorazine)
Clozapine (Clozaril)
Fluphenazine (Prolixin)
Haloperidol (Haldol)
Loxapine (Loxitane)
Mesoridazine (Serentil)
Metoclopramide (Reglan)
Molindone (Moban)
Olanzapine (Zyprexa)
Perphenazine (Trilafon), perphenazine/amitriptyline (Triavil or Etrafon)
Pimozide (Orap)
Prochlorperazine (Compazine)
Promethazine (Phenergan)
Quetiapine (Seroquel)
Risperidone (Risperdal)
Thioridazine (Mellaril)
Thiothixene (Navane)
Trifluoperazine (Stelazine)

SUGGESTED READING

Adler, CH: Differential diagnosis of Parkinson's disease. Med Clin North Am 83:349–367, 1999.
Bennett, DA, et al: Prevalence of parkinsonian signs and associated mortality in a community population of older people. N Engl J Med 334:71–76, 1996.
Charles, PD, et al: Classification of tremor and update on treatment. Am Fam Physician 59:1565–1572, 1999.
Colcher, A, and Simuni, T: Clinical manifestations of Parkinson's disease. Med Clin North Am 83:327–347, 1999.
Gelb, DJ, Oliver, E, and Gilman, S: Diagnostic criteria for Parkinson disease. Arch Neurol 56:33–39, 1999.

Gironell, A, et al: A randomized placebo-controlled comparative trial of gabapentin and propranolol in essential tremor. Arch Neurol 56:475–480, 1999.

Hauser, RA, et al: Long-term evaluation of bilateral fetal nigral transplantation in Parkinson disease. Arch Neurol 56:179–187, 1999.

Lang, AE, and Lozano, AM: Parkinson's disease. N Engl J Med 339:1044–1053; 1130–1143, 1998.

Lou, JS, and Jankovic, J: Essential tremor: Clinical correlates in 350 patients. Neurology 41:234–238, 1991.

Muenter, MD, et al: Treatment of essential tremor with methazolamide. Mayo Clin Proc 66:991–997, 1991.

Olanow, CW, and Koller, WC: An algorithm (decision tree) for the management of Parkinson's disease: Treatment guidelines. Neurology 50(Suppl 3):S1–S57, 1998.

The Parkinson Study Group: Low-dose clozapine for the treatment of drug-induced psychosis in Parkinson's disease. N Engl J Med 340:757–763, 1999.

Stacy, M: Managing late complications of Parkinson's disease. Med Clin North Am 83:469–481, 1999

Uitti, RJ: Tremor: How to determine if the patient has Parkinson's disease. Geriatrics 53:30–36, 1998.

Uitti, RJ: Medical treatment of essential tremor and Parkinson's disease. Geriatrics 53:46–48; 53–57, 1998.

Winikates, J, and Jankovic, J: Clinical correlates of vascular parkinsonism. Arch Neurol 56:98–102, 1999.

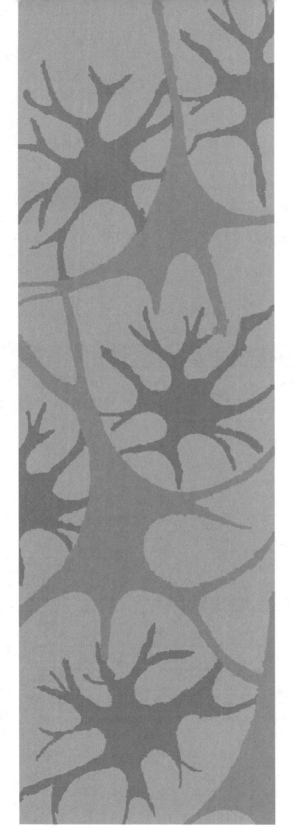

CHAPTER 13

Immune and Infectious Diseases

CHAPTER OUTLINE

Multiple Sclerosis
 Features and Types
 Diagnostic Approach
 Diagnostic Laboratory Support
 Differential Diagnosis
 Epidemiology
 Prognosis
 Pregnancy
 Disease-Modifying Therapy
 Symptomatic Therapy
Optic Neuritis
**Connective Tissue Diseases and the
 Vasculitides**
**Infectious Diseases of the Nervous
 System**
 HIV Infection
 Lyme Disease

Many immune-mediated diseases and infections affect the central and peripheral nervous systems. The common feature that characterizes both immune-mediated diseases and infections is a subacute temporal profile. Immune-mediated diseases can affect only the nervous system or involve the nervous system as part of a systemic illness, as in the vasculitides and connective tissue diseases (Table 13–1). Multiple sclerosis, the most common disabling neurologic illness of young people, is the prototypical immune-mediated disease of the central nervous system. The recent availability of disease-modifying treatments for multiple sclerosis emphasizes the importance of an accurate diagnosis and therapeutic intervention.

MULTIPLE SCLEROSIS

 A 26-year-old woman is evaluated because of right arm numbness and tingling. Two years ago,

---

TABLE 13–1. IMMUNE-MEDIATED DISORDERS OF THE NEUROMUSCULAR SYSTEM

Muscle

Polymyositis
Dermatomyositis
Inclusion body myositis

Neuromuscular Junction

Myasthenia gravis
Lambert-Eaton myasthenic syndrome

Peripheral Nerve

Acute inflammatory demyelinating polyneuropathy (AIDP, or Guillain-Barré syndrome)
Chronic inflammatory demyelinating polyneuropathy (CIDP)
Monoclonal gammopathy of undetermined significance (MGUS)

Central Nervous System

Acute disseminated encephalomyelitis (postviral demyelination)
Multiple sclerosis: prototypical immune-mediated disease of the central nervous system
Optic neuritis
Transverse myelitis
Central nervous system vasculitis

Systemic

Vasculitis: polyarteritis nodosa, Wegener granulomatosis, Churg-Strauss syndrome, Kawasaki
    disease, hypersensitivity vasculitis, giant cell arteritis (temporal arteritis)
Connective tissue disease: systemic lupus erythematosus, rheumatoid arthritis, Sjögren
    syndrome, mixed connective tissue disease, scleroderma
Sarcoidosis
Behçet disease
Cogan syndrome
Hypersensitivity angiitis: drug-induced, serum sickness, cryoglobulinemia
Infection-related vasculitis
Malignancy-related: paraneoplastic, lymphoma, leukemia
Vasculitis in substance abuse: amphetamines, cocaine, heroin

---

she had a 4-week episode of loss of vision in the left eye that was diagnosed as optic neuritis. She was told that this was a symptom of multiple sclerosis. At that time, magnetic resonance imaging (MRI) of her head demonstrated several "white dots." She is concerned about the new sensory symptoms, especially because she and her husband are planning to start a family. Neurologic examination demonstrates an afferent pupillary light defect on the left, diffuse hyperactive reflexes with flexor plantar reflexes, absence of abdominal reflexes, and reduced vibratory sensation in the right upper extremity. She wants to know if she has multiple sclerosis and what will happen to her, whether she should put on hold her plans to have a family, and if she should be treated with any medication. How do you manage this patient?

FEATURES AND TYPES

Multiple sclerosis is a relapsing or progressive immune-mediated disorder of the central nervous system. It is characterized by recurrent patches of inflammation, with damage to the myelin (demyelination) and axons of the brain, spinal cord, and optic nerves. Multiple sclerosis is not a single disease but is several idiopathic inflammatory demyelinating syndromes (Table 13–2). The demyelinating syndromes are defined by their course (monophasic, relapsing-remitting, progressive) and the site of nervous system involvement.

The most common clinical category of multiple sclerosis is "relapsing-remitting." Approximately 80% of patients present with this type of multiple sclerosis. Episodes (relapses, attacks, or exacerbations) of neurologic dysfunction are followed by recovery and a stable phase between relapses

TABLE 13–2. IDIOPATHIC INFLAMMATORY DEMYELINATING DISEASES OF THE CENTRAL NERVOUS SYSTEM

Clinical Category	Description
Relapsing-remitting multiple sclerosis	Episodic neurologic deficits with stable phase between attacks
Secondary progressive multiple sclerosis	Gradual neurologic deterioration from relapsing-remitting course, with or without superimposed acute attacks
Primary progressive multiple sclerosis	Gradual, continuous neurologic deterioration from onset of symptoms
Monosymptomatic demyelinating disease	Single episode of neurologic deficit
Optic neuritis	Visual loss
Transverse myelitis	Bilateral lower extremity motor and sensory deficit, bladder difficulty
Isolated brainstem syndrome	Cranial nerve, motor, and sensory deficits
Fulminant demyelinating disease	
Acute disseminated encephalomyelitis	Postinfectious, monophasic, diffuse white matter encephalopathy
Marburg variant	Fatal multifocal cerebral involvement
Baló concentric sclerosis	Rapidly progressive demyelination presenting as solitary mass lesion
Restricted distribution demyelinating disease	
Devic syndrome	Relapsing bilateral optic neuritis and transverse myelitis
Benign multiple sclerosis	Minimal neurologic disability at 10 years after onset of symptoms

(remission). The length of time for most relapses, or attacks of neurologic deficit, is 4 to 16 weeks.

More than 50% of patients with relapsing-remitting multiple sclerosis go on to develop the secondary progressive stage of the disease. Patients with secondary progressive multiple sclerosis have progressive neurologic deterioration, with or without superimposed acute relapses. "Primary progressive multiple sclerosis" describes patients who have continuous deterioration from the onset of symptoms.

Multiple sclerosis can present as a monosymptomatic illness. Optic neuritis is a common monosymptomatic demyelinating syndrome. The patient presents with unilateral loss of vision, and ophthalmoscopic examination (Fig. 13–1) may reveal a swollen optic nerve head (papillitis) or no abnormality (retrobulbar neuritis). Isolated brainstem and spinal cord (transverse myelitis) syndromes are included in this category.

Fulminant, or severe, demyelinating syndromes include acute disseminated encephalomyelitis, Baló concentric sclerosis, and the Marburg variant. These disorders are associated with high morbidity and mortality. Devic syndrome, or neuromyelitis optica, is a demyelinating syndrome of restricted distribution, affecting only the optic nerves and spinal cord.

DIAGNOSTIC APPROACH

The diagnosis of multiple sclerosis is a clinical diagnosis that can be supported by find-

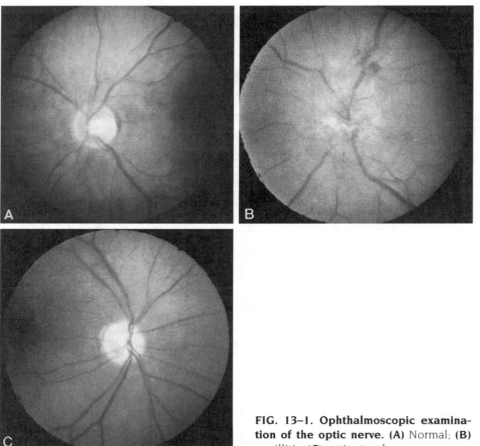

FIG. 13–1. Ophthalmoscopic examination of the optic nerve. (A) Normal; **(B)** papillitis; **(C)** optic atrophy.

ings obtained with MRI, cerebrospinal fluid (CSF) analysis, and evoked potentials. The essential criterion for the diagnosis of multiple sclerosis is the presence of central nervous system lesions disseminated in time and space. Multiple sclerosis is a disorder of young people (between the ages of 10 and 50 years). Diagnostic criteria have been established that can be used in clinical practice to help with therapeutic decision making (Table 13–3). A patient is considered to have clinically definite multiple sclerosis if he or she has two attacks (symptom[s] of neurologic dysfunction persisting longer than 24 hours) and clinical evidence (signs of neurologic dysfunction on examination) of two separate lesions. The young woman in the case above meets the criteria for clinically definite multiple sclerosis. The two attacks must involve different parts of the nervous system and be separated in time by at least 1 month. If the symptoms and signs show progression, then the duration of time needs to be at least 6 months. There can be no alternative clinical explanation for the patient's signs and symptoms.

Although any neurologic symptom can occur in multiple sclerosis, the most frequent initial symptoms are sensory disturbances, motor dysfunction, and monocular visual impairment. Initial somatosensory disturbances may include complaints of tingling, burning, tightness, or numbness. Often, the sensory symptoms do not correlate with a recognizable anatomical pattern. Balance and gait difficulties are common complaints. Bladder disturbance is one of the most disabling symptoms of multiple sclerosis and is seen most often in advanced disease; however, symptoms of urgency and frequency and frequent urinary tract infections may be present early in the disease. Demyelinating disease is one of the first diagnostic considerations in a young man who presents with acute urinary retention. Other signs and symptoms that should raise suspicion of multiple sclerosis include double vision, a "useless hand," trigeminal neuralgia in a person under age 50, and symptoms induced by heat or exercise (Uhthoff sign). Postpartum onset of symptoms and a diurnal fatigue pattern are also significant findings. An electric-like sensation that radiates down the spine with flexion of the neck (Lhermitte sign) is also a characteristic symptom in multiple sclerosis.

TABLE 13–3. DIAGNOSTIC CRITERIA FOR MULTIPLE SCLEROSIS

Clinically definite multiple sclerosis
  1. Two attacks and clinical evidence of two separate lesions
  2. Two attacks, clinical evidence of one lesion and paraclinical evidence of another lesion

Laboratory-supported definite multiple sclerosis
  1. Two attacks, either clinical or paraclinical evidence of one lesion, and CSF OB/IgG
  2. One attack, clinical evidence of two separate lesions, and CSF OB/IgG
  3. One attack, clinical evidence of one lesion and paraclinical evidence of another lesion, and CSF OB/IgG

Clinically probable multiple sclerosis
  1. Two attacks and clinical evidence of one lesion
  2. One attack and clinical evidence of two separate lesions
  3. One attack, clinical evidence of one lesion and paraclinical evidence of another lesion

Laboratory-supported probable multiple sclerosis
  Two attacks and CSF OB/IgG

CSF, cerebrospinal fluid; OB, oligoclonal bands.

Definitions: Attack, symptom(s) of neurologic dysfunction lasting longer than 24 hours; clinical evidence, sign(s) of neurologic dysfunction demonstrated by neurologic examination; and paraclinical evidence, evidence of central nervous system lesions by imaging studies, CSF analysis, evoked potentials.

When performing a neurologic examination on a patient with suspected multiple sclerosis, it is important to check the uninvolved, or "good," side and to attend to subtle asymmetries. The most frequent neurologic deficits found on examination involve the optic nerves, ocular motility, corticospinal pathway, and somatosensory pathways. Cerebellar findings of ataxia, dysmetria, and intention tremor usually occur later in the course of the disease. Cortical (or gray matter) signs such as early cognitive dysfunction, language disturbance, and extrapyramidal features do not suggest multiple sclerosis.

Findings of optic nerve dysfunction include diminished visual acuity, central scotoma, and, on ophthalmoscopic examination, optic nerve pallor (optic atrophy) (Fig. 13–1). Impaired color vision can be detected with the use of Ishihara plates. An afferent pupillary defect (also called a "Marcus Gunn pupil") can be demonstrated by the swinging-flashlight test. When a light source is moved back and forth between the eyes, the eye with the afferent defect appears to dilate when stimulated by the light. Because of the lesion, the direct response is slow in the affected eye and the dilatation that is seen with the swinging-flashlight test is from the consensual response.

Ocular motility problems such as nystagmus and ophthalmoparesis are frequently found on examination and indicate brainstem and cerebellar involvement. Internuclear ophthalmoplegia can be an early manifestation of multiple sclerosis. It is the result of a lesion of the medial longitudinal fasciculus, the nerve tract that connects the nucleus abducens (origin of CN VI) and the oculomotor nucleus (origin of CN III), which produce conjugate lateral eye movements. The eye ipsilateral to the lesion cannot adduct but the contralateral eye can abduct and has horizontal nystagmus. However, the eye ipsilateral to the lesion is able to adduct on accommodation because convergence of the eyes does not require the medial longitudinal fasciculus.

Corticospinal tract abnormalities are frequently elicited on examination. These include hyperactive reflexes, spasticity, extensor plantar reflexes, clonus, and loss of superficial reflexes. The absence or asymmetry of abdominal or cremasteric reflexes is useful when evaluating a person suspected of having demyelinating disease, because the loss or asymmetry of these reflexes indicates upper motor neuron involvement. The sensory examination often reveals reduced vibratory sensation, which precedes any detectable loss in joint position sense.

DIAGNOSTIC LABORATORY SUPPORT

The diagnosis of multiple sclerosis is a clinical diagnosis made on the basis of the history and examination findings of neurologic lesions disseminated in space and time. Although MRI has greatly improved our diagnostic ability, its results can only support the diagnosis of multiple sclerosis. The lesions of multiple sclerosis are of isointensity to low intensity on T_1-weighted images and high intensity on proton density–weighted images and T_2-weighted images. Gadolinium-enhanced lesions represent active inflammation. It is important to remember that white matter abnormalities are nonspecific and can be seen in ischemic and degenerative disorders (Fig. 13–2). MRI results need to be correlated with the clinical evaluation of the patient.

After the history and neurologic examination, the next diagnostic test should be cranial MRI. MRI is the most sensitive test for detecting multiple sclerosis lesions. When the woman in the case above presented with optic neuritis, the MRI findings supported the diagnosis of clinically probable multiple sclerosis. Cranial MRI is recommended for patients who, on clinical grounds alone, meet the diagnosis of multiple sclerosis to exclude other diagnoses (Table 13–4). MRI is an objective test that can indicate disease activity. It also can be used to monitor the effect of treatment.

Guidelines for the use of MRI in the diagnosis of multiple sclerosis are based on the number, size, and distribution of white matter lesions. Four foci larger than 3 mm or three foci with one of them adjacent to the lateral ventricle strongly support the diagnosis of multiple sclerosis. The presence of one lesion larger than 5 mm, the location of the lesion(s)

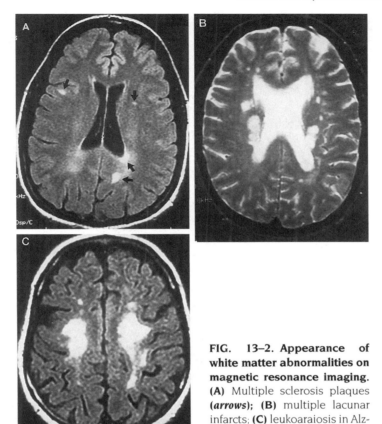

FIG. 13–2. Appearance of white matter abnormalities on magnetic resonance imaging. **(A)** Multiple sclerosis plaques **(*arrows*)**; **(B)** multiple lacunar infarcts; **(C)** leukoaraiosis in Alzheimer disease.

adjacent to the lateral ventricles, or an infratentorial location of at least one lesion supports the diagnosis of multiple sclerosis (Fig. 13–3). Lesions in the corpus callosum (white matter) are consistent with demyelinating disease rather than cerebrovascular disease. To exclude other lesions, MRI of the spine should be performed if the patient presents with myelopathy (Fig. 13–4).

Visual, somatosensory, and brainstem auditory evoked potentials can provide paraclinical evidence of central nervous system lesions and may help to detect a second lesion that is clinically silent. Usually, evoked potentials are performed only when the clinical evaluation and MRI findings do not provide the evidence needed for diagnosis. Evoked potentials may be most useful in patients who do not have multiple sclerosis, when objective evidence is needed to evalu-

ate the optic, somatosensory, and brainstem pathways. (Evoked potentials are discussed in Chapter 2.)

CSF analysis can be useful in supporting the diagnosis of multiple sclerosis. As with evoked potentials, this test may not be necessary if the clinical examination and MRI findings support the diagnosis. CSF immunoglobulins, especially immunoglobulin G (IgG), are increased in most patients with multiple sclerosis, presumably because of immune activation. On electrophoresis, immunoglobulins appear as distinct oligoclonal bands. CSF findings that support the diagnosis of multiple sclerosis include an increased IgG rate of synthesis and oligoclonal bands (not present in the serum). Oligoclonal bands are not specific for multiple sclerosis and can occur with several infectious and inflammatory diseases, including Lyme disease,

TABLE 13–4. DIFFERENTIAL DIAGNOSIS OF MULTIPLE SCLEROSIS

Disease	Distinguishing Clinical or Paraclinical Features
Infectious	
Lyme disease	Rash, arthralgias, arthritis serology
Syphilis	Positive results: RPR, VDRL, FTA-ABS
HTLV-I (myelopathy)	HTLV-I detected
HIV infection	HIV detected
Inflammatory	
Sarcoidosis	ACE increased, meningeal enhancement at base of brain on MRI
Systemic lupus erythematosus	Other organ involvement, MRI abnormalities more subcortical than periventricular, autoantibodies
Sjögren syndrome	Sicca complex, antibodies SS-A and SS-B, MRI lesion may involve gray matter
Behçet syndrome	Mucocutaneous lesions
Degenerative	
Cervical spondylosis (myelopathy)	Cervical spine MRI
Spinocerebellar or olivopontocerebellar degeneration	Family history, normal CSF, pes cavus
Leukodystrophies	Peripheral nerve involvement, increased levels of long-chain fatty acids
Hereditary spastic paraplegia (myelopathy)	Family history
Nutritional	
Vitamin B_{12} deficiency (myelopathy)	Serum vitamin B_{12} level
Neoplastic	
Sphenoid wing meningioma (optic neuritis)	Abnormal MRI findings
Optic nerve tumors (optic neuritis)	Abnormal MRI findings
Primary CNS lymphoma	Abnormal MRI findings
Paraneoplastic syndromes	Paraneoplastic antibodies, other evidence of malignancy
Psychogenic	Absence of objective neurologic signs; inconsistent weakness or sensory loss; normal MRI, CSF, evoked potentials; disability out of proportion to neurologic examination

ACE, angiotensin-converting enzyme; CNS, central nervous system; FTA-ABS, fluorescent treponemal antibody absorption test; HIV, human immunodeficiency virus; HTLV-I, human T-cell lymphotropic virus type I; MRI, magnetic resonance imaging; RPR, rapid plasma reagin test; SS, Sjögren syndrome; VDRL, Venereal Disease Research Laboratory test.

syphilis, human T-cell lymphotropic virus (HTLV-I) myelopathy, sarcoidosis, vasculitis, and chronic meningitis. Rarely, oligoclonal bands have been reported in healthy persons. The CSF of patients with multiple sclerosis may demonstrate a mild leukocytic pleocytosis and increased concentration of protein. Infection or malignancy should be investigated if these values are high. CSF analysis is valuable in excluding other infectious diseases (e.g., neuroborreliosis [Lyme disease] and neurosyphilis) and malignancy.

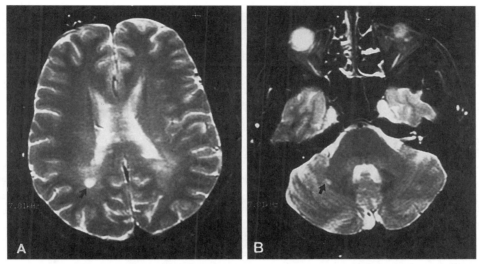

FIG. 13–3. Appearance of white matter abnormalities seen on magnetic resonance imaging in multiple sclerosis. *Arrows* indicate **(A)** periventricular plaque and **(B)** infratentorial plaque (in cerebellum).

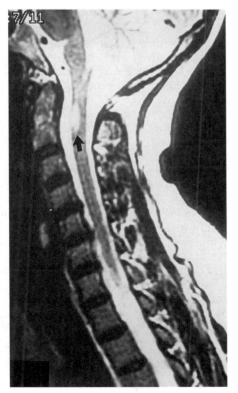

FIG. 13–4. Magnetic resonance imaging of cervical spinal cord, showing a demyelinating lesion *(arrow)* in a patient with multiple sclerosis.

DIFFERENTIAL DIAGNOSIS

You need to consider many infectious, inflammatory, degenerative, and neoplastic diseases of the nervous system in the differential diagnosis of multiple sclerosis (Table 13–4). If the clinical presentation or MRI findings are atypical for multiple sclerosis, further laboratory evaluation is needed to investigate another possible diagnosis. It is important to consider these other diagnoses when patients have progressive deterioration from the onset of symptoms. Evaluation for systemic disease, MRI of the spine, CSF analysis, evoked potentials, and infectious and inflammatory serologic testing may be needed to make an accurate diagnosis.

EPIDEMIOLOGY

Patients often ask what causes multiple sclerosis and if it can be passed on to their children. Currently, multiple sclerosis is considered an autoimmune disease of the central nervous system that is initiated by an undefined environmental trigger in a genetically susceptible person. Environmental factors are suggested by the geographic distribution of multiple sclerosis. Its prevalence increases the greater the distance from the equator. High-risk areas are within the temperate zones in the northern and southern hemispheres. This risk can be affected by migration if the person migrates before puberty. If the person moves during childhood, the prevalence rate will be that of the new residence; however, if he or she moves after puberty, the prevalence rate will be that of the previous location. Epidemics of multiple sclerosis have been reported and support an environmental etiology for the disease. Viruses have been thought to trigger autoimmune demyelination in susceptible persons. Human herpesvirus 6 and many other pathogens (e.g., *Chlamydia*) have been suggested as a cause, but currently, no evidence shows a direct viral involvement as a cause of multiple sclerosis.

Ample evidence supports a genetic component to disease susceptibility. Fifteen percent of patients with multiple sclerosis have a first-degree relative with the disease. The incidence of the disease in studies of twins supports both environmental and genetic factors. The concordance rates in monozygotic twins is 6 to 10 times that of dizygotic twins, but not the 100% that would be expected for a purely genetic disease. Although the lifetime risk that a child of an affected parent will develop multiple sclerosis is low (3% to 5%), it is still 20 to 50 times that of the general population. The risk is increased for children, particularly daughters, of mothers with multiple sclerosis. Multiple sclerosis has also been associated with certain human leukocyte antigen genotypes, and a consistent relationship has been reported with the class II region of the major histocompatibility complex on chromosome 6. Genetic susceptibility to multiple sclerosis is complex, and additional investigation is needed to define the relationship between genetic and environmental factors.

PROGNOSIS

Multiple sclerosis is a disorder that evolves over decades. The clinical course is often unpredictable and the individual variation is considerable, making a discussion about prognosis difficult. Most patients have relapsing-remitting multiple sclerosis, and approximately 50% of these will develop secondary progressive multiple sclerosis. This transition occurs gradually over 10 to 20 years, when clinical relapses become less distinct and recovery is less vigorous. Patients with primary progressive multiple sclerosis (10% to 15% of those with multiple sclerosis) have continuous clinical deterioration from the onset of symptoms.

Multiple sclerosis is seldom fatal, so survival is an insensitive measure of disease outcome. More than one-half of the deaths of patients with multiple sclerosis are not related to the disease. Expected survival is approximately 80% that of an age- and gender-matched population. Prognosis is better discussed in terms of disability and quality-of-life issues. Most patients will be ambulatory 15 years after the onset of disease, but 15% will require a wheelchair.

Several clinical features provide prognostic information. Indicators for a favorable prognosis include sensory symptoms or optic neuritis at the onset, infrequent attacks during the first few years, and good recovery from the attacks. Poor prognostic indicators include age at onset older than 40 years, male gender, progressive disease from onset, early cerebellar signs, more than four attacks in the first 2 years, short intervals between attacks, and permanent disability within 3 years from the onset of symptoms.

MRI is being used as a predictor of clinical outcome. The absence of gadolinium-enhancing lesions on MRI is prognostically favorable in a patient with relapsing-remitting multiple sclerosis. Early studies have shown that the number of gadolinium-enhancing lesions on initial MRI is a predictor of relapses but not of the development of disability. Evidence of inflammatory lesions on MRI in a patient with early disease, such as the woman in the case above, supports the use of disease-modifying therapy.

PREGNANCY

Family planning is an important issue in multiple sclerosis. Many patients are concerned about the effect of pregnancy on multiple sclerosis and about the effect of the disease on pregnancy. An increased risk of relapse has been shown in patients with relapsing-remitting multiple sclerosis during the 6-month postpartum period. However, this increased risk does not appear to have a detrimental effect on the rate of developing sustained disability. The patient's current level of disability may be the most significant factor to consider in family planning. Therapies using disease-modifying medications and many symptom-relieving drugs need to be considered in women anticipating pregnancy.

DISEASE-MODIFYING THERAPY

The medical treatment of multiple sclerosis has changed remarkably with the approval of three drugs: interferon beta-1b (Betaseron), interferon beta-1a (Avonex), and glatiramer acetate (Copaxone). Interferon beta-1b and beta-1a are recombinant interferon beta preparations that have multiple immunomodulatory actions and inhibit cell-mediated inflammation. Glatiramer acetate is a random polymer of basic amino acids that inhibits T-cell recognition of myelin antigens. All three drugs reduce the relapse rate by one-third in patients with relapsing-remitting multiple sclerosis. There is evidence that these drugs are beneficial also in treating secondary progressive disease.

When therapy should be initiated and how long it should be maintained are not known. Generally, therapy is recommended early in the disease, with the idea that patients who have fewer relapses will have less long-term disability. On the basis of studies that showed

reactivation of disease activity after discontinuation of the drug, therapy should be continued indefinitely. MRI and the patient's clinical status are followed to determine disease activity and the effectiveness of treatment.

Neutralizing antibodies can develop with both interferon beta-1a and interferon beta-1b (more with beta-1b than with beta-1a). The clinical efficacy of the interferon drugs was less in patients who had these neutralizing antibodies. Testing for the presence of neutralizing antibodies has been used to monitor treatment with interferon, and another drug is often selected if antibodies are found. However, because patients with neutralizing antibodies also have had higher levels of serum immunoglobulins, the poor response may be independent of the presence of antibodies. Currently, routine testing for neutralizing antibodies is not practical.

The decision about which of the three drugs to use may be based on clinician preference, dosage schedule, and adverse side effects. No study has directly compared the three medications (Table 13–5). During the first few months of treatment with interferon beta-1a or beta-1b, flu-like symptoms are common, and they may be more prominent with beta-1b. The incidence of depression is also higher among patients taking beta-1b, and this medication should not be prescribed if the patient is severely depressed. Interferon therapy should not be given to women who are pregnant or anticipate becoming pregnant. Glatiramer is not recommended for pregnant women (class B pregnancy drug), but the risk may be less than it is with interferon treatment. Periodic neurologic evaluation is recommended for patients

TABLE 13–5. DISEASE-MODIFYING DRUGS FOR MULTIPLE SCLEROSIS

Drug	Dosage	Adverse Effects
Interferon beta-1b (Betaseron)	250 μg subcutaneously every other day	Myalgias, fever, malaise, depression, local rejection reactions
Interferon beta-1a (Avonex)	30 μg intramuscularly weekly	Myalgias, fever, malaise
Glatiramer acetate (Copaxone)	20 mg subcutaneously daily	Transient flushing, chest tightness, palpitations, anxiety

with multiple sclerosis who are receiving disease-modifying therapy.

SYMPTOMATIC THERAPY

Despite the advances in disease-modifying therapy, symptomatic treatment of multiple sclerosis is essential to help maintain function and to improve quality of life. Before you initiate a specific medical therapy, evaluate the patient for factors that may contribute to the symptoms, such as infections or medication side effects. Patients should maintain a well-balanced diet, not smoke, and avoid excessive alcohol consumption. Currently, there is little evidence to recommend a specific diet rather than a well-balanced one. Patient education, rehabilitation (e.g., supervised fitness program for fatigue), and counseling (e.g., for depression) are important nonpharmacologic management measures that may be preferable to drug therapy in some patients (Table 13–6). Many symptoms in patients with multiple sclerosis, for example, pain and depression, are treated just as they are in patients who do not have multiple sclerosis.

Acute attacks or relapses of the disease in patients with significant disability (e.g., visual loss or paraplegia) are frequently treated with corticosteroids. Methylprednisolone given intravenously has a rapid onset of action, produces consistent results, has few adverse effects, and can be administered on an outpatient basis. The recommended therapy is 3 to 5 days of 500 to 1,000 mg given intravenously over 2 to 3 hours. An oral prednisone taper (60 mg/day, decreasing by 10 mg every 2 to 3 days) is optional following intravenous therapy. Corticosteroid treatment accelerates recovery and shortens the duration of the disability. However, no evidence suggests that the outcome is altered.

Occasional adverse effects of intravenous methylprednisolone include flushing, fluid retention, hyperglycemia, depression, and insomnia. The fasting serum glucose level and electrolyte levels may need to be monitored. One study of high-dose oral methylprednisolone treatment demonstrated that it was effective in managing attacks of multiple sclerosis. However, the formulation (4-mg tablets) is a practical limitation to oral therapy.

Depression is relatively common in patients with multiple sclerosis and needs to

TABLE 13–6. SYMPTOMATIC THERAPY FOR MULTIPLE SCLEROSIS

Symptom	Treatment Options
Acute attack	Methylprednisolone (Solu-Medrol), 1,000 mg intravenously every 3–5 days
Bladder problems	Oxybutynin (Ditropan), 2.5–5 mg 3–4 times daily
Depression	All antidepressants
Emotional lability	Amitriptyline (Elavil), 10–25 mg before bedtime
Fatigue	Amantadine (Symmetrel), 100 mg twice daily (early morning and early afternoon)
	Pemoline (Cylert), 18.75–75 mg every morning
	Fluoxetine (Prozac), 20 mg every morning
Muscle spasms	Carbamazepine (Tegretol), titrate dose
	Phenytoin (Dilantin), titrate dose
	Gabapentin (Neurontin), titrate dose
Spasticity	Baclofen (Lioresal), 5 mg 3 times daily (maximum, 80 mg/d)
	Tizanidine (Zanaflex), 2 mg daily–12 mg 3 times daily
	Dantrolene (Dantrium), 25–100 mg 3–4 times daily
	Diazepam (Valium), titrate dose
	Clonazepam (Klonopin), titrate dose
	Cyproheptadine (Periactin), 4 mg twice daily–8 mg twice daily

be taken seriously. Suicide is a leading cause of death among those who are mildly to moderately disabled. Many medications prescribed for multiple sclerosis (interferon beta-1b, baclofen, and benzodiazepines) can aggravate depression. Psychiatric consultation can be useful. Depression in multiple sclerosis is treated with the same medications as those prescribed for treating depression in the general population. Emotional lability or incontinence (pathologic crying and laughing) can be socially disabling. Low-dose amitriptyline is effective in reducing this problem.

Fatigue is the most common symptom in multiple sclerosis and can be extremely disabling. Nonpharmacologic measures that may reduce fatigue include a supervised fitness program, regular rest and sleep routine, the use of air conditioners or fans for cooling, and improved nutrition. Other diagnoses like sleep disorders or depression should be considered. Medication options include amantadine, pemoline, and fluoxetine.

Spasticity is also a common symptom in multiple sclerosis and can be worsened by bladder or bowel distention or by any infection. Regular stretching and exercise can reduce the discomfort and improve function. Many medications are available for treating spasticity (Table 13–6). For all of them, treatment should be started at the lowest dose and increased gradually. The most common adverse effects are increasing weakness, sedation, and hypotension. Dantrolene (Dantrium) is given primarily to nonambulatory patients. The muscle spasms that frequently accompany spasticity can be treated with many of the anticonvulsant medications. These, too, should be started at a low dose and increased until the desired therapeutic effect is achieved or toxicity occurs. If an oral medication is not effective in treating spasticity, consider intrathecal baclofen.

Bladder dysfunction, like fatigue, is an extremely disabling symptom. Urgency, frequency, and incontinence are the most frequent symptoms. Many patients attribute bladder difficulty to the effects of aging. Estrogen deficiency and prostatic hypertrophy can be contributing factors, but you should check for other causes of neurogenic bladder. If the urinary residual volume is less than 100 mL, suspect a spastic bladder. Rec-

ommend that the patient avoid alcohol and caffeine, which stimulate the bladder, drink plenty of fluid to prevent concentrated urine, perform pelvic floor strengthening exercises, and have frequent scheduled voiding times throughout the day. Anticholinergic agents help. Patients with a large postvoid residual volume may need intermittent catheterization. Whenever patients have symptoms of bladder dysfunction, evaluate them for a urinary tract infection. Urologic consultation may be necessary.

OPTIC NEURITIS

Optic neuritis, a syndrome caused by inflammation of the optic nerve, is characterized by painful loss of vision in one eye. As mentioned earlier, multiple sclerosis is a frequent cause of optic neuritis. It is the first symptom in 20% of multiple sclerosis patients and occurs in 70% of patients sometime during the course of the illness. Optic neuritis can also be caused by viral, bacterial (syphilis, Lyme disease, tuberculosis), and fungal (cryptococcosis, histoplasmosis) infections and by such inflammatory disorders as sarcoidosis and systemic lupus erythematosus.

MRI is usually part of the diagnostic evaluation of a patient with optic neuritis. Evidence of other inflammatory lesions provides prognostic information about demyelinating disease and may lead to more aggressive treatment. Other tests you might consider are antinuclear antibodies for connective tissue diseases, fluorescent treponemal antibody absorption (FTA-ABS) for syphilis, and chest radiography for sarcoidosis.

Intravenous methylprednisolone followed by oral prednisone speeds the recovery of visual loss from optic neuritis. Oral prednisone alone is ineffective and increases the risk of new episodes. Also, intravenous methylprednisolone was shown over a 2-year period to reduce the rate of development of multiple sclerosis.

CONNECTIVE TISSUE DISEASES AND THE VASCULITIDES

The systemic inflammatory diseases that affect the neuromuscular system are listed in

Table 13–1. Several potential pathogenic mechanisms can explain how connective tissue diseases and vasculitides affect the nervous system, including direct immune-mediated effects (immune complex, autoantibodies, or cytokine-mediated effects) and indirect effects (vasculopathy, coagulopathy, cardiac emboli). Injury to the nervous system may be due to infections and to metabolic and toxic effects, including the effects of medications. It is important to know how these disorders affect the nervous system because the patient may present initially with a neurologic problem. The neurologic, systemic, and diagnostic features of several of these disorders are highlighted in Table 13–7.

INFECTIOUS DISEASES OF THE NERVOUS SYSTEM

HIV INFECTION

A 33-year-old man with acquired immunodeficiency syndrome (AIDS) is evaluated because of headache. Several years earlier, he tested positive for antibodies against human immunodeficiency virus type 1 (HIV-1). The significant examination findings are fever and a stiff neck. Mild hyperreflexia is noted on the right. How do you proceed to evaluate this patient? What are the diagnostic considerations?

Infectious diseases of the nervous system are well illustrated by considering a patient with HIV infection. The neurologic complications of this infection involve every level of the central and peripheral nervous systems (Table 13–8). Because of the compromised immune status of these patients, every infectious agent needs to be considered in the diagnostic evaluation.

CSF analysis is essential in the diagnostic evaluation of a patient with an infection of the nervous system (see Table 2–1). Infections of the nervous system cause an increase in the leukocyte count ("pleocytosis") and protein level and a decrease in the glucose level, de-

pending on the infectious organism. The CSF leukocyte count and differential need to be interpreted carefully. In general, bacterial infections demonstrate a neutrophilic pleocytosis, but this may be altered if the infection has been partially treated. Some viral infections such as mumps can cause a neutrophilic pleocytosis during the first few days of infection. Eosinophils are seen in allergic and parasitic diseases but can also be present in fungal infections, tuberculosis, and lymphoma. Diagnostic possibilities for the presence of erythrocytes in the CSF include traumatic tap, subarachnoid hemorrhage, and herpes encephalitis. An increased concentration of protein in the CSF occurs in most infections and tends to be greater in bacterial than in viral infections. Neoplasm should be considered if the protein concentration is greater than 400 mg/dL. The CSF level of glucose generally is low in bacterial infections and normal in viral infections, but there are exceptions.

Computed tomography (CT) or MRI should be performed before lumbar puncture. If imaging or examination findings give any evidence of a space-occupying lesion, initiate empirical therapy without delay (Table 13–9). Although treatment may impair CSF culture results, the etiologic agent often can be found with blood cultures or by a positive result on the CSF antigen test. Other diagnostic measures to detect the cause of an infection include culture, serology, antigen detection, and brain biopsy.

In the case above, the man's headache and stiff neck are compatible with meningitis. Meningitis can also present with altered level of consciousness. The stiff neck ("nuchal rigidity") indicates irritation of the meninges. The diagnosis of meningitis is confirmed by an infectious CSF profile (i.e., leukocytosis, increased protein, and decreased glucose). Acute meningitis can present over hours to days and is usually caused by a virus or bacteria in a patient with normal immune status. Chronic meningitis, usually caused by granulomatous diseases, tumor, or syphilis, can be associated with encephalitis. Cortical dysfunction and cranial nerve palsies may occur in chronic meningitis. *Cryptococcus neoformans* is the most common opportunistic organism that causes meningitis in a patient with HIV infection. The CSF findings may be only

TABLE 13–7. NEUROLOGIC, SYSTEMIC, AND DIAGNOSTIC FEATURES OF CONNECTIVE TISSUE DISEASES AND VASCULITIS

Disease	Neurologic Feature	Systemic Feature	Diagnostic Feature
Systemic lupus erythematosus	Encephalopathy, seizure, behavioral changes	Butterfly rash, pleuritic pain, proteinuria	Anti-Sm, anti-DNA antibodies
Sjögren syndrome	Trigeminal sensory neuropathy, autonomic neuropathy	Sicca complex	Anti-SSA
Wegener granulomatosis	Cranial mononeuropathy	Hemoptysis	cANCA, pANCA
Rheumatoid arthritis	Cervical myelopathy, compression neuropathies, peripheral neuropathies	Erosive inflammation of joints	Rheumatoid factor
Polyarteritis nodosa	Mononeuropathy multiplex, polyneuropathy, brachial plexopathy	Renal disease	Angiography, sural nerve biopsy, ANA
Temporal arteritis	Headache, visual impairment, cranial neuropathies	Anemia, weight loss, jaw claudication	Increased ESR, temporal artery biopsy

ANA, antinuclear antibody; ANCA, antineutrophilic cytoplasmic antibody (c, classic; p, peripheral); ESR, erythrocyte sedimentation rate; SSA, soluble substance A antigen.

TABLE 13–8. NEUROLOGIC COMPLICATIONS OF HUMAN IMMUNODEFICIENCY VIRUS (HIV) INFECTION

Muscle—inflammatory myopathy, noninflammatory myopathy, zidovudine myopathy

Peripheral nerve—focal neuropathy, mononeuritis multiplex, polyneuropathy, acute and chronic demyelinating polyneuropathy, distal sensory polyneuropathy, CMV polyneuropathy, nucleoside polyneuropathy, brachial plexitis, autonomic neuropathy

Spinal cord—vacuolar myelopathy

Meninges—aseptic meningitis, cryptococcal meningitis, tuberculous meningitis

Brain—post-infectious encephalomyelitis, CMV encephalitis, AIDS dementia complex, cerebral toxoplasmosis, progressive multifocal leukoencephalopathy, primary CNS lymphoma

AIDS, acquired immunodeficiency syndrome; CMV, cytomegalovirus; CNS, central nervous system.

TABLE 13–9. TREATMENT OF CNS INFECTIONS AND FOCAL CNS DISORDERS IN HIV INFECTION

Infection	Likely Infectious Agent/Disorder	Treatment
Bacterial Meningitis		
Neonate younger than 4 wks	Enteric gram-negative bacteria, group B streptococci, *Escherichia coli, Listeria monocytogenes*	Ampicillin plus cefotaxime or aminoglycoside
Infants and children	*Streptococcus pneumoniae, Neisseria meningitidis, Haemophilus influenzae* type b	Ceftriaxone or cefotaxime plus vancomycin
Adult: community acquired	*Streptococcus pneumoniae, Neisseria meningitidis*	Penicillin G (plus vancomycin) or ampicillin or third-generation cephalosporin
Adult: postneurosurgical	Enteric gram-negative bacteria, *Pseudomonas aeruginosa, Staphylococcus aureus*	Ceftazidime plus oxacillin or vancomycin plus aminoglycoside
Adult: impaired immune status	*Listeria monocytogenes*, staphylococci, enteric gram-negative bacteria, *Haemophilus influenzae* type b, *Streptococcus pneumoniae, Neisseria meningitidis*	Ceftazidime plus ampicillin
Focal CNS Disorders in HIV		
	Cryptococci	Amphotericin B, fluconazole
	Toxoplasma gondii	Pyrimethamine, sulfadiazine (or clindamycin), leucovorin
	Primary CNS lymphoma	Radiation therapy, dexamethasone (not empiric therapy)
	Progressive multifocal leukoencephalopathy	No therapy

CNS, central nervous system; HIV, human immunodeficiency virus.

mildly abnormal (mild pleocytosis, increased protein), so it is important to test for *Cryptococcus* using the India ink preparation, the antigen assay, and fungal culture. Because *Cryptococcus* and other fungal pathogens may be present in low concentrations, it is important to provide the laboratory with several milliliters of CSF for these studies. In a patient with HIV infection, tuberculous meningitis or aseptic meningitis (thought to be secondary to the virus itself) can occur.

In the case of the 33-year-old man, the focal findings (hyperreflexia on the right) suggest the possibility of a mass lesion. The three major diagnostic considerations include cerebral toxoplasmosis, progressive multifocal leukoencephalopathy, and primary central nervous system lymphoma

(Table 13–10). Tuberculous and other fungal brain abscesses can occur. In persons who are not immunosuppressed, brain abscesses can result from such underlying infections as otitis, mastoiditis, sinusitis, head wounds, endocarditis, and pulmonary infections. Brain abscesses cause focal syndromes such as hemiparesis, aphasia, or focal seizures. Infectious disease and neurologic and neurosurgical consultation can be helpful in the diagnosis and treatment of these patients.

Headache in a patient with HIV infection should always prompt an evaluation for an underlying mass lesion of central nervous system infection. When no other cause for the headache can be identified, the diagnosis is "HIV headache." Its cause is not known, but it may be related to the release of vasoactive cytokines.

The most common neurologic complication of HIV-1 is AIDS dementia complex. Other terms used to describe this disorder are "HIV encephalopathy" and "HIV-1-associated cognitive/motor complex." The clinical features include cognitive, motor, and behavioral abnormalities. Early in the course of the disorder, the patient may complain of impaired memory and concentration. Apathy and withdrawal are the usual early behavioral disturbances. Motor features can include ataxia, leg weakness, tremor, and loss of fine motor coordination. The disorder is progressive and, when advanced, can include severe dementia, mutism, paraplegia, and incontinence.

AIDS dementia complex is a late manifestation of the infection and occurs in patients with severe immunosuppression. Evidence suggests that it is the result of HIV infection of the brain. Recommended treatment, for both therapeutic and prophylactic value, is the antiretroviral agent zidovudine.

HIV infection has many neuromuscular complications (see Table 13–8). The pathogenesis of many of these disorders is autoimmune, as in chronic inflammatory demyelinating neuropathy. Treatment includes corticosteroids, plasma exchange, and intravenous immunoglobulin. An important opportunistic infection of the peripheral nervous system can occur with cytomegalovirus (CMV), which can cause a subacute progressive polyradiculoneuropathy. CSF analysis shows pleocytosis with neutrophil pre-

TABLE 13–10. MAJOR FOCAL CNS DISORDERS IN HIV INFECTION

Focal CNS Disorder	Time Course (Onset to Presentation)	Associated Symptoms	MRI Focal Lesion
Cerebral toxoplasmosis	Few days	Altered consciousness, fever, headache, constitutional symptoms	Mass effect with surrounding edema; distinct, ring-like contrast enhancement; located in gray matter of diencephalon and cerebral cortex
Progressive multifocal leukoencephalopathy	Weeks	Progressive focal syndrome, cognitive dysfunction	No mass effect or edema; lesions confined to white matter
Primary CNS lymphoma	1–2 wks	Focal syndrome, headache, confusion, seizures, cranial nerve deficits	Mass effect with surrounding edema; diffuse contrast enhancement, involvement of white matter adjacent to ventricles

CNS, central nervous system; HIV, human immunodeficiency virus; MRI, magnetic resonance imaging.

dominance. Ganciclovir is used to treat this disorder.

The most frequent neuropathy in patients with HIV infection is a distal sensory polyneuropathy. Management of the painful dysesthesias includes many of the medications used to treat other painful disorders, such as painful diabetic neuropathy (see Table 10–2). Several antiviral nucleosides (didanosine, zalcitabine, stavudine) can cause a dose-related painful neuropathy, and zidovudine can cause myopathy.

LYME DISEASE

Lyme disease is a bacterial infection caused by *Borrelia burgdorferi*, a tick-transmitted spirochete that occurs along the U.S. Atlantic coast and in parts of the West and Midwest and in Western Europe. Peripheral nervous system manifestations of the infection include multifocal axonal neuropathy, painful radiculitis, mononeuritis multiplex, sensorimotor neuropathy, facial nerve palsy, and myositis. Central nervous system manifestations include lymphocytic meningitis, focal and diffuse encephalitis, encephalomyelitis, and encephalopathy.

The illness begins (stage 1) with flu-like symptoms and may be associated with an expanding ring-like skin rash that has a clear center (erythema migrans). After several weeks or months (stage 2), the patient may experience meningeal and radicular symptoms, with headache, stiff neck, or cranial nerve (facial nerve) or spinal root involvement. Arthritis is typical at this stage. Late central nervous system complications (stage 3) can include encephalopathy, seizures, and dementia. The late syndrome may resemble multiple sclerosis.

Laboratory tests to detect Lyme disease can be difficult to interpret, and it is important to interpret the results in relation to the clinical findings. Currently, serologic tests are the best measure of infection. Most laboratories use enzyme-linked immunosorbent assays (ELISAs) to measure specific antibodies. The most helpful method of confirming central nervous system infection is to demonstrate the specific antibody in the CSF.

Parenteral ceftriaxone (2 g intravenously every 24 hours for 10 to 30 days) is recommended for meningitis, radiculoneuritis, encephalomyelitis, peripheral neuropathy, and encephalopathy. Oral doxycycline (100 mg orally twice daily for 10 to 30 days) is used to treat cranial neuritis or facial palsy if the results of CSF analysis are normal.

SUGGESTED READING

Andrews, KL, and Husmann, DA: Bladder dysfunction and management in multiple sclerosis. Mayo Clin Proc 72:1176–1183, 1997.

Beck, RW, et al: A randomized, controlled trial of corticosteroids in the treatment of acute optic neuritis. N Engl J Med 326:581–588, 1992.

Beck, RW, et al: The effect of corticosteroids for acute optic neuritis on the subsequent development of multiple sclerosis. N Engl J Med 329:1764–1769, 1993.

The choice of antibacterial drugs. Med Lett Drugs Ther 40:33–42, 1998.

Damek, DM, and Shuster, EA: Pregnancy and multiple sclerosis. Mayo Clin Proc 72:977–989, 1997.

Ebers, GC, and Dyment, DA: Genetics of multiple sclerosis. Semin Neurol 18:295–299, 1998.

Hogancamp, WE, Rodriguez, M, and Weinshenker, BG: The epidemiology of multiple sclerosis. Mayo Clin Proc 72:871–878, 1997.

Hunter, SF, et al: Rational clinical immunotherapy for multiple sclerosis. Mayo Clin Proc 72:765–780, 1997.

Kappos, L, et al: Predictive value of gadolinium-enhanced magnetic resonance imaging for relapse rate and changes in disability or impairment in multiple sclerosis: A meta-analysis. Lancet 353:964–969, 1999.

Krupp, LB: Lyme disease. In Samuels, MA, and Feske, S (eds): Office Practice of Neurology. Churchill Livingstone, New York, 1996, pp 383–387.

Lee, JD, and Reed, K: Approach to the patient with a central nervous system infection. In Samuels, MA, and Feske, S (eds): Office Practice of Neurology. Churchill Livingstone, New York, 1996, pp 363–366.

Lucchinetti, CF, and Rodriguez, M: The controversy surrounding the pathogenesis of the multiple sclerosis lesion. Mayo Clin Proc 72:665–678, 1997.

Metz, L: Multiple sclerosis: Symptomatic therapies. Semin Neurol 18:389–395, 1998.

Miller, A: Diagnosis of multiple sclerosis. Semin Neurol 18:309–316, 1998.

Miller, DH: Multiple sclerosis: Use of MRI in evaluating new therapies. Semin Neurol 18:317–325, 1998.

Navia, BA, Jordan, BD, and Price, RW: The AIDS dementia complex: I. Clinical features. Ann Neurol 19:517–524, 1986.

Newton, HB: Common neurologic complications of HIV-1 infection and AIDS. Am Fam Physician 51:387–398, 1995.

Noseworthy, JH, et al: Demyelinating and immune diseases. Continuum 1994, pp 8–145.

Poser, CM, et al: New diagnostic criteria for multiple sclerosis: Guidelines for research protocols. Ann Neurol 13:227–231, 1983.

Price, RW: Neurological complications of HIV infection. Lancet 348:445–452, 1996.

Rudick, RA: A 29-year-old man with multiple sclerosis. JAMA 280:1432–1439, 1998.

Sellebjerg, F, et al: Double-blind randomized, placebo-controlled study of oral, high-dose methylprednisolone in attacks of MS. Neurology 51:529–534, 1998.

Sorensen, TL, and Ransohoff, RM: Etiology and pathogenesis of multiple sclerosis. Semin Neurol 18:287–294, 1998.

Stolp-Smith, KA, et al: Management of impairment, disability, and handicap due to multiple sclerosis. Mayo Clin Proc 72:1184–1196, 1997.

Tselis, AC, and Lisak, RP: Multiple sclerosis: Therapeutic update. Arch Neurol 56:277–280, 1999.

Weinshenker, BG: The natural history of multiple sclerosis: Update 1998. Semin Neurol 18:301–307, 1998.

Wormser, GP: Treatment and prevention of Lyme disease, with emphasis on antimicrobial therapy for neuroborreliosis and vaccination. Semin Neurol 17:45–52, 1997.

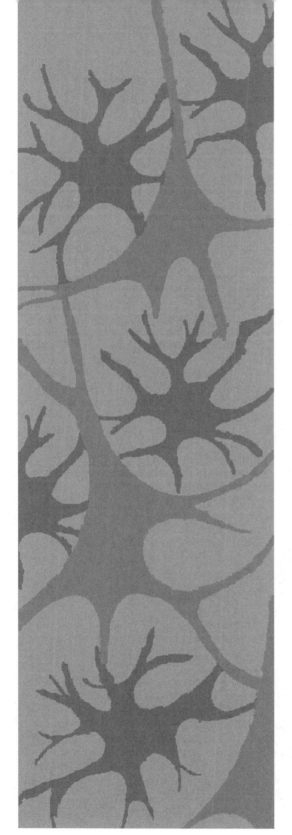

CHAPTER 14

Neuro-oncology

CHAPTER OUTLINE

Primary Brain Tumors
    Diagnostic Approach
    Management
Spinal Cord Tumors
Neurologic Complications of Systemic Disease
    Metastases
        Diagnosis
        Treatment
    Epidural Spinal Cord Compression
    Meningeal Carcinoma
    Neurologic Complications of Therapy
    Paraneoplastic Syndromes
        Definition, Description, and Diagnosis
        Treatment

Neuro-oncology is a rapidly evolving specialty involving the study of cancer and the nervous system. The nervous system can be affected by cancer directly, indirectly, or as a result of treatment-related side effects. The diagnosis and treatment of cancer of the nervous system require the skills of several medical disciplines to help the patient with one of the most frightening medical problems.

PRIMARY BRAIN TUMORS

A 49-year-old man comes for evaluation at the urging of his wife, who is concerned that he is not his "usual self." His wife has noticed a change in his personality, and he admits to being more irritable because of frequent headaches. He has no history of headache, but for the last several months, he has been taking aspirin to treat his frequent headaches. His headache is worse in the morning and gets better as the day progresses. Neurologic examination demonstrates a mild increase in muscle stretch reflexes on the left. Because of the new-onset headache and focal findings on neurologic examination, you obtain a magnetic resonance imaging (MRI) scan of his head, which shows a mass in the right frontal lobe, with mass effect. How do you proceed?

This patient presents with a chronic progressive temporal profile of symptoms. The headache and personality change coupled with focal neurologic signs are consistent with a brain mass, which is confirmed by MRI. The diagnostic possibilities are extensive, with more than 100 types of central nervous system tumors. Tumors of neuroepithelial tissue (glial tumors, or gliomas) include the most common primary brain tumor, astrocytoma. Other major types of tumors are those of cranial and spinal nerves (schwannoma) and the meninges (meningioma),

lymphomas and hematopoietic neoplasms, germ cell tumors, tumors of the sellar region (pituitary), and metastatic tumors.

You need to classify the tumor to determine prognosis and the most appropriate treatment. Certain types of tumors have a predilection for specific locations in the brain. Gliomas (astrocytoma, glioblastoma multiforme, oligodendroglioma), meningiomas, and metastatic tumors usually occur in the cerebral hemispheres. Pituitary adenomas and pineal tumors are midline tumors. In adults, the most common infratentorial tumors are acoustic schwannomas, metastases, and meningiomas. Primary brain tumors in children are usually infratentorial and include cerebellar astrocytomas, medulloblastomas, ependymomas, and brainstem gliomas.

The histologic grade of a brain tumor is important for classification. The four astrocytoma grades correlate directly with mortality rate. Grade 1 astrocytomas (pilocytic astrocytoma) can be cured by surgical removal. Grade 2, or low-grade, astrocytoma is an infiltrating lesion with nuclear atypia but little or no mitotic activity. Grade 3, or anaplastic, astrocytoma has mitoses. Grade 4 (glioblastoma multiforme) has nuclear atypia, mitoses, necrosis, and endothelial proliferation.

DIAGNOSTIC APPROACH

In the case above, the man presented with two of the most common symptoms of brain tumors: headache and personality changes. Headache is the initial symptom in more than one-third of patients with brain tumors, and more than two-thirds will experience headache in the course of their illness. The headache can be mild and intermittent and resemble a tension-type headache. Symptoms of increased intracranial pressure and/or focal findings are more indicative of a brain tumor than headache. In this patient, increased intracranial pressure is indicated by a headache that is worse in the morning and improves in the afternoon. Other symptoms suggestive of increased intracranial pressure include a headache that awakens the patient or is worse with a change in position, cough, or exercise.

Seizures, both focal and generalized, can be the first sign of a brain tumor. Slower growing tumors, such as low-grade astrocytomas or oligodendrogliomas, are more likely to cause seizures than rapidly growing ones. Seizures are more likely to occur when the tumor is in the cerebral cortex. Subcortical or infratentorial tumors are rarely epileptogenic.

Changes in mental status may also be the first symptom of a brain tumor. Patients may complain of problems with concentration or memory, and family members may note a change in personality. In a study of patients older than 65 years who had brain tumors, the most frequent presenting symptoms were confusion, aphasia, and memory loss.

You should focus the neurologic examination on the presence of focal findings that suggest localization of the problem (Table 14–1). All tumors can cause an increase in intracranial pressure. Infratentorial tumors and tumors of the third ventricle frequently obstruct the ventricular system and cause hydrocephalus. Papilledema is a nonlocalizing sign of increased intracranial pressure

TABLE 14–1. CLINICAL FEATURES BASED ON LOCATION OF BRAIN TUMOR

Location	Clinical Features
Frontal cortex	Personality change: disinhibition, irritability, abulia Seizures Hemiparesis Urinary urgency and frequency Gait ataxia Aphasia* Gaze preference
Temporal cortex	Seizures Memory disturbance Superior quadrantanopia
Parietal cortex	Hemianesthesia Aphasia* Neglect† Constructional apraxia Seizures
Occipital cortex	Hemianopia Visual agnosia Seizures
Thalamus	Hemianesthesia Cognitive impairment
Brainstem	Cranial neuropathies Ataxia Limb weakness Nystagmus
Pineal region	Parinaud syndrome (impairment of upward gaze and dissociation of the pupillary light reflex and the near reflex)
Third ventricle	Hydrocephalus Hypothalamic dysfunction Autonomic dysfunction
Cerebellum	Headache Ataxia Hydrocephalus

*If dominant hemisphere is involved.
†If nondominant hemisphere is involved.

and is a late finding. It is important to remember two false-localizing features of increased intracranial pressure: compression of the abducens (CN VI) nerve where it passes over the petrous ligament and compression of the cerebral peduncle by the free edge of the tentorium cerebelli that causes ipsilateral hemiparesis.

Computed tomography (CT) and MRI have been indispensable in evaluating intracranial neoplasms, because they provide information about size, location, midline shift, mass effect, ventricular compression, and obstructive hydrocephalus (Fig. 14–1). The imaging characteristics of the lesion such as location, amount of edema, and type of contrast enhancement can suggest the diagnosis (Table 14–2). The sensitivity of CT in detecting brain tumors is improved by using an intravenous contrast agent. MRI is more sensitive than CT except for detecting calcification and bony involvement. MRI is the preferred imaging technique for evaluation of the posterior fossa, isodense infiltrating gliomas, and leptomeningeal metastases (meningeal carcinoma). Contrast enhancement also increases the sensitivity of MRI. Neuroimaging techniques are rapidly evolving, and radiologic consultation may help you select the most appropriate imaging technique.

Several other diagnostic tests may aid in the diagnosis and management of brain tumors. Audiometry and brainstem evoked potentials are useful in the evaluation of acoustic neuromas by indicating the extent of auditory involvement. Visual field testing is valuable for indicating the presence of tumors in the sellar region (pituitary adenomas) (see Fig. 1–5). The presence of bitemporal hemianopia indicates that a tumor is present in the sellar region and is affecting the optic chiasm. Determining hormonal levels in the blood and urine is helpful in identifying pituitary and hypothalamic tumors. Electroencephalography (EEG) should be performed if the patient has seizures. Focal tumors can cause focal slowing or epileptogenic activity (spikes) seen on EEG. Cerebrospinal fluid (CSF) abnormalities (e.g., pleocytosis) may provide important diagnostic information about leptomeningeal disease. CSF cytology is useful in the diagnosis of pineal tumors and leptomeningeal metastases (meningeal carcinoma). Biologic mark-

ers of germ cell tumors (alpha-fetoprotein, β-subunit of human chorionic gonadotropin, and placental alkaline phosphatase) can be found in the CSF. Remember, lumbar puncture should not be performed in a patient with increased intracranial pressure who is at risk for herniation.

MANAGEMENT

The management of a brain tumor is facilitated by the involvement of several medical specialties, including primary care, neurology, neurosurgery, oncology, radiation oncology, and psychiatry. Most brain tumors require the combination of surgery, radiation therapy, and chemotherapy. Some slow-growing tumors may require only continued neurologic surveillance and serial imaging studies. An example is a small convexity meningioma that is often asymptomatic and requires only observation and reassurance of the patient.

For most brain tumors, surgery is the first step in management. It is curative for many tumors, including meningiomas, pituitary adenomas, pilocytic astrocytomas, and acoustic neuromas. The additional advantages of surgery are that it provides a histologic diagnosis and improves the effectiveness of radiation therapy and chemotherapy.

Radiation therapy is essential in the treatment of all malignant gliomas, low-grade gliomas, and inoperable or recurrent benign tumors. Radiation of the whole brain, stereotactic placement of radioactive isotopes directly into the tumor (brachytherapy), stereotactic radiosurgery (gamma knife), and stereotactic radiotherapy are techniques used to deliver cytotoxic ionizing radiation to tumor cells.

Many chemotherapeutic agents are used to treat brain tumors. Chemotherapy is complicated by the blood-brain barrier, which limits the distribution of water-soluble drugs into the brain. Various strategies have been used to bypass the blood-brain barrier to deliver the medication to the intended target, for example, intrathecal administration and implantation of chemotherapy-impregnated polymer wafers in the surgical cavity after resection.

TABLE 14–2. IMAGING CHARACTERISTICS OF INTRACRANIAL TUMORS

Tumor	Location	NECT	MRI	Enhancement*	Edema	Hemorrhage	Calcification
Low-grade astrocytoma	Cerebral hemisphere	Hypodense	Hyperintense	0/+ Inhomogeneous	Rare	Rare	10%–20%
Anaplastic astrocytoma	Cerebral white matter	Inhomogeneous	Heterogeneous signal	++ Inhomogeneous	Common	Occasional	Uncommon
Glioblastoma multiforme	Cerebral hemisphere	Heterogeneous	Heterogeneous	+++ Inhomogeneous	Common	Common	Rare
Meningioma	Extra-axial dural-based	Hyperdense	Isodense	+++ Homogeneous, on CT, heterogeneous	Present	Rare	20%–25%
Oligodendroglioma	Frontal lobe, cortex	Calcified mixed density	Mixed hypo- and isodense	+/++ Inhomogeneous	Rare	Rare	70%–90%
Ependymoma	Fourth ventricle	Isodense	Hypo-/isodense on T_1, Hyperdense on T_2	+/++ Variable	Hydrocephalus	Can occur	50%
Acoustic neuroma (Schwannoma)	Cerebellopontine angle	Hypo-/isodense	Hypodense on T_1, Hyperdense on T_2	+++ Homogeneous, inhomogeneous, heterogeneous	Rare	Can occur	Rare
Pituitary adenoma	Sellar region	Isodense	Hypodense, mixed intensity	+++	Can occur	Can occur	1%–8%
Craniopharyngioma	Sellar region	Calcification	Hyperdense on T_2, heterogeneous	++ Heterogeneous	Rare	Rare	90%
Metastasis	All cortico-medullary-junction	Iso-/hyperdense	Hypodense on T_1, Hyperdense on T_2	+++ Ring	Present	Common	Rare

*0, absent; +, mild; ++, moderate; +++, extensive.
CT, computed tomography; MRI, magnetic resonance imaging; NECT, non-contrast-enhanced computed tomography; T_1 and T_2, T_1- and T_2-weighted image, respectively.

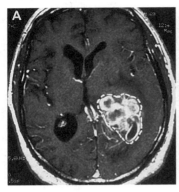
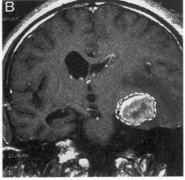

FIG. 14–1. Magnetic resonance imaging of a left posterior temporal glioblastoma multiforme. This mixed-density lesion demonstrates surrounding edema, mass effect, and midline shift. **(A)** Axial section; **(B)** coronal section.

Novel treatment strategies being developed for brain tumors include gene therapy, antiangiogenesis, immunotherapy, and targeting tumor cells. Specialty consultation will provide the most up-to-date treatment recommendations.

Several medications warrant special comment with regard to the treatment of brain tumors. Treatment of seizures is common in these patients, and the usual antiepileptic medications are prescribed (see Table 9–4). It is important to be aware of certain drug interactions, such as the relationship between phenytoin (Dilantin) and dexamethasone (Decadron). Phenytoin induces the liver metabolism of dexamethasone and reduces its half-life and bioavailability. Dexamethasone may also reduce phenytoin levels. Many chemotherapeutic agents, for example, carmustine (BCNU), can affect anticonvulsant levels. In addition to drug interactions, there is an increased incidence of certain anticonvulsant-induced side effects in patients with gliomas, including rash with phenytoin, Stevens-Johnson syndrome with carbamazepine, and shoulder-hand syndrome with phenobarbital. The mechanism for the increased incidence of these effects is not known.

The role of prophylactic anticonvulsant therapy for patients with brain tumors has not been defined and is controversial. The increased risk of allergic reactions and the lack of convincing evidence that such treatment decreases the incidence of seizures argue against it. However, patients with highly epileptogenic tumors like melanoma or those who need to drive a motor vehicle may be reasonable candidates for prophylactic anticonvulsant therapy.

Edema associated with a brain tumor is treated with corticosteroids. The dose of dexamethasone often ranges from 16 mg/day to 100 mg/day, is effective in reducing the headache, and may lessen the neurologic deficits. Common complications of corticosteroid therapy include behavioral changes, fragile skin, osteoporosis, gastrointestinal tract bleeding, visual blurring, hypertension, hyperglycemia, and opportunistic infections. Steroid myopathy occurs after prolonged treatment, in the 9th to 12th week of treatment. The patient develops proximal muscle weakness and wasting. The medication should be discontinued, if possible, or given at the lowest possible dose.

Venous thromboembolic disease is a frequent complication of intracranial malignancy. Inferior vena cava filtration devices have been used to avoid anticoagulation and the risk of hemorrhage into the brain. One study has demonstrated that the complications related to these filtration devices far outweigh the risk of anticoagulation. The risk of brain hemorrhage from anticoagulation may not be significantly increased outside the immediate postoperative period.

SPINAL CORD TUMORS

A 57-year-old man is evaluated because of back pain. For years, he has intermittently experienced low back pain related to excessive lifting and bending. During the last several months, he has had constant back pain that, unlike the previous back pain, is relieved with standing. He reports that both legs feel weak and numb. He has lost control of his urine on several occasions. Neurologic examination shows weakness in both distal lower extremities, sensory loss in the same distribution, absence of the anal reflex, decreased muscle stretch reflexes in the lower extremities, and equivocal plantar reflexes. An MRI scan of the spine is shown in Figure 14–2.

Spinal cord tumors can cause myelopathy, with bilateral lower extremity weakness, spasticity, sensory level, spastic bladder, and extensor plantar reflexes. Involvement of the cauda equina causes lower motor neuron weakness, sensory loss, flaccid bladder, and decreased muscle stretch reflexes (see Fig. 4–3). This patient has a tumor that affects the conus medullaris, with predominant cauda equina symptoms.

The three types of spinal cord tumor are distinguished by their anatomical location. Extradural tumors are outside the dura mater and are discussed below. The other two types of spinal cord tumors, extramedullary (meningiomas and neurofibromas) and intramedullary, are located intradurally. Intramedullary tumors include ependymomas, astrocytomas, oligodendrogliomas, hemangioblastomas, and metastatic tumors.

The treatment of choice for spinal cord tumors is surgical removal. Radiation therapy is used if surgical excision is incomplete. Specialty consultation is recommended for further management advice.

NEUROLOGIC COMPLICATIONS OF SYSTEMIC DISEASE

METASTASES

A 59-year-old woman with a long history of cigarette smoking presents with gait difficulty. For the last several months, she has been "walking like she is drunk." Neurologic examination reveals an ataxic gait, limb ataxia and dysmetria, nystagmus, and poorly performed rapid alternating movements of all extremities. An MRI scan of this patient is shown in Figure 14–3. How do you manage this patient?

Brain metastases are neoplasms that originate outside the nervous system. The incidence is not known precisely, but evidence suggests that intracranial metastases equal—if not exceed—the incidence of primary brain tumors. Brain metastases occur in 20% to 40% of cancer patients, and an increased incidence is anticipated with improved neuroimaging techniques and the extended survival of cancer patients.

Metastases can occur in the parenchyma of the brain, in the leptomeninges, or in the dura mater. The most common source of brain metastases is lung cancer. On autopsy, the majority of "brain metastases of unknown

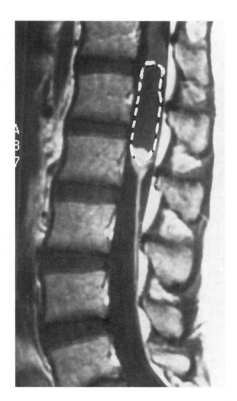

FIG. 14–2. Magnetic resonance imaging of the lumbar spine, showing an ependymoma of the conus medullaris and cauda equina.

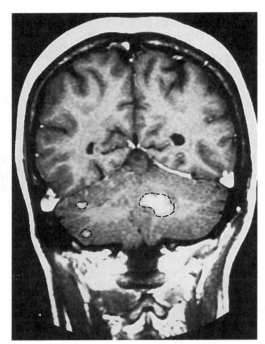

FIG. 14–3. Magnetic resonance imaging of three metastases (encircled) in the cerebellar hemispheres. The primary tumor was small cell carcinoma of the lung.

primary" are found to be the lung. The second leading source is breast cancer. Melanoma, colon cancer, and renal cell carcinoma can also cause brain metastases. Patients younger than 21 years develop metastases from sarcomas and germ cell tumors.

Tumor cells spread to the brain hematogenously. Metastases are usually located at the junction between the gray matter and white matter (the "corticomedullary junction"). The reduced size of blood vessels at this junction is thought to serve as a trap, as for emboli. Metastases are also located at the border zones of the major blood vessels (the "watershed areas"). They can occur anywhere intracranially related to the relative volume of blood flow: 80% cerebral hemispheres, 15% cerebellum, and 5% brainstem.

Diagnosis

Most brain metastases are diagnosed after the systemic cancer has been identified. The

neurologic symptoms reflect the location of the tumors. Contrast-enhanced MRI is the preferred diagnostic test. Metastases are round, well-circumscribed lesions that may be surrounded by edema and enhance with contrast agent. The number of metastases— whether single or multiple—has significant treatment implications. In addition, a single metastasis needs to be distinguished from a primary brain tumor, abscess, cerebral infarct, and hemorrhage. Surgical resection or biopsy may be needed to establish the diagnosis.

Treatment

Treatment options for brain metastases include corticosteroids, radiotherapy, surgery, stereotactic radiosurgery, interstitial brachytherapy, and chemotherapy. Whole brain radiation is used for disseminated or uncontrolled systemic cancer and multiple metastases. If there is a single, surgically accessible metastasis in a patient with limited or no systemic cancer, surgical removal followed by radiation therapy is recommended. In a patient with multiple metastases and a single, surgically accessible, life-threatening lesion, the single lesion should be removed surgically, followed by radiation therapy.

EPIDURAL SPINAL CORD COMPRESSION

A 72-year-old man with known prostate cancer is evaluated because of recent trouble urinating. He also mentions progressive back pain in the thoracic area. Neurologic examination reveals tenderness of the thoracic spine to percussion, lower extremity weakness, decreased vibratory sensation, and hyperactive stretch reflexes with extensor plantar reflexes (Babinski sign). What do you do?

This case is a medical emergency and requires immediate treatment if the patient is to maintain neurologic function. The patient's symptoms and examination findings are consistent with spinal cord compression that is likely metastatic disease from his prostate cancer. Emergency MRI of the spine should be performed to confirm the diagnosis. Give a high dose of corticosteroids (intravenous administration of 100 mg of dexamethasone, followed by 24 mg four times daily) to reduce spinal cord edema. Initiate radiation therapy immediately. Surgical evaluation should be considered for spinal instability, for known radioresistant tumors like renal carcinoma, or for acute deterioration of neurologic function.

MENINGEAL CARCINOMA

Meningeal carcinoma, also known as "leptomeningeal metastases," "neoplastic meningitis," or "carcinomatous meningitis," is the result of disseminated and multifocal seeding of the leptomeninges by malignant cells in the subarachnoid space. The tumors that most commonly metastasize to the meninges are breast and lung tumors and melanoma. It is important that you recognize meningeal carcinoma because of the associated high morbidity and mortality.

The clinical features of meningeal carcinoma are numerous because the disorder can involve all or several levels of the neuraxis. Leptomeningeal metastases can invade the brain and spinal cord parenchyma, cranial nerves, nerve roots, and blood vessels supplying the nervous system. Neck or back pain is a common initial complaint, and lower motor neuron weakness and hyporeflexia are the most common signs. Headache, cognitive changes, gait difficulty, cranial nerve palsies, and radicular symptoms are all possible clinical features. Meningeal carcinoma should be considered in a cancer patient who has evidence of multifocal neurologic involvement. However, single-level neurologic involvement occurs in a large percentage of patients. Like other neurologic complications of systemic cancer, meningeal carcinoma can be the initial presentation of the cancer.

The diagnosis of meningeal carcinoma is made on the basis of positive cytologic findings on CSF analysis. MRI identifies most intraparenchymal lesions and provides information about the risk of herniation with lumbar puncture. Multiple subarachnoid mass lesions and hydrocephalus without an identifiable mass lesion are consistent with the diagnosis. Meningeal enhancement, beading, and root clumping are also suggestive findings.

CSF findings include an increased opening pressure, increased protein concentration, decreased glucose level, and positive cytologic findings. Repeated lumbar punctures may be needed to demonstrate malignant cells in the CSF. Biochemical markers such as carcinoembryonic antigen (CEA) and β-glucuronidase have been used to aid in diagnosis but are limited by poor sensitivity and specificity.

Treatment for meningeal carcinoma includes radiation therapy to symptomatic sites of the neuraxis and intrathecal chemotherapy. Without treatment, the median survival of patients is 4 to 6 weeks.

NEUROLOGIC COMPLICATIONS OF THERAPY

The neurologic complications of cancer therapy are extensive. Chemotherapeutic agents can affect any level of the central or peripheral nervous system (Table 14–3). It is important to recognize these complications in order to modify treatment and to avoid confusion with the direct and indirect effects of the cancer.

Radiation therapy can also damage the central and peripheral nervous systems. Brain injury from radiation is classified by time of onset. An acute encephalopathy can occur during the first few days of therapy. "Early delayed encephalopathy," including headache and somnolence, can occur from 1 to 4 months after the completion of therapy, and "delayed radiotherapy neurotoxicity" can occur from several months to 10 or more years after therapy. Other adverse effects of radiation include cranial neuropathy, myelopathy, peripheral neuropathy, cerebrovascular damage, and radiation-induced tumors. A multidisciplinary approach may be needed to distinguish recurrent cancer from the complications of treatment.

TABLE 14–3. NEUROLOGIC COMPLICATIONS OF CHEMOTHERAPY

Neurologic Complication	Agents
Acute cerebellar syndrome	High-dose cytarabine, 5-fluorouracil, procarbazine, vincristine
Acute encephalopathy	Altretamine, asparaginase, 5-azacitidine, carmustine, cisplatin, high-dose cytarabine, 5-fluorouracil, glucocorticoids, ifosfamide, interferons, interleukin-2, methotrexate, misonidazole, procarbazine, tamoxifen
Aseptic meningitis	Cytarabine, methotrexate, levamisole
Cranial neuropathies	Intra-arterial carmustine (ototoxicity), cisplatin (ototoxicity, vestibulopathy), vincristine (extraocular palsies)
Dementia	Carmofur, carmustine, cytarabine, alpha-interferon, fludarabine, methotrexate
Headache	Glucocorticoids, retinoic acid, tamoxifen
Myelopathy	Intrathecal cytarabine, intrathecal methotrexate, intrathecal thiotepa
Neuropathy	Altretamine, 5-azacitidine, cisplatin, cytarabine, misonidazole, paclitaxel, procarbazine, suramin, teniposide, vinca alkaloids
Seizures	Asparaginase, high-dose busulfan, carmustine, cisplatin, dacarbazine, etoposide, methotrexate, vincristine
Vasculopathy and stroke	Asparaginase, intra-arterial carmustine, intra-arterial cisplatin, methotrexate
Visual loss	Intra-arterial carmustine, cisplatin, tamoxifen

From Wen, PY: Neurologic complications of chemotherapy. In Samuels, MA, and Feske, S (eds): Office Practice of Neurology. Churchill Livingstone, New York, 1996, pp 914–919. By permission of the publisher.

PARANEOPLASTIC SYNDROMES

A 67-year-old man with a long history of smoking is evaluated for weakness and fatigue. His symptoms developed over a few weeks and have been getting progressively worse. Other symptoms include dry mouth, sexual impotence, and blurred vision. Neurologic examination demonstrates mild proximal muscle weakness of the lower extremities with diminished muscle stretch reflexes. What are the diagnostic considerations? How do you proceed to evaluate this patient?

This patient was found to have Lambert-Eaton myasthenic syndrome, a rare syndrome affecting neuromuscular transmission. It is a paraneoplastic syndrome associated with small cell carcinoma of the lung. The term *paraneoplastic syndrome* is used to describe the clinical features of the remote effects of cancer on the nervous system.

Definition, Description, and Diagnosis

Paraneoplastic syndromes are rare disorders that can affect both the central and peripheral nervous systems (Table 14–4). They can be specific for one cell type (e.g., cholinergic synapse in Lambert-Eaton syndrome and Purkinje cells in paraneoplastic cerebellar degeneration). Multiple levels of the nervous system may be affected, as in encephalomyelitis, a paraneoplastic syndrome that affects the brain, brainstem, spinal cord, dorsal root ganglia, and nerve roots.

The serum and CSF of patients with a paraneoplastic syndrome contain antibodies that are directed to neuron proteins expressed by the associated tumor. The immune system recognizes these proteins as foreign and mounts an immune attack. This immune response partially controls tumor growth but also attacks the portion of the nervous system that expresses the antigen. The identification of these antibodies confirms the paraneoplastic origin of the neurologic dysfunction and helps direct the search for the underlying cancer. Several of the anti-

TABLE 14–4. PARANEOPLASTIC SYNDROMES AND CLINICAL FEATURES

Syndrome	Clinical Features
Central Nervous System Syndromes	
Paraneoplastic encephalomyelitis	Combination of clinical features of limbic encephalitis, brainstem encephalitis, cerebellar degeneration, myelopathy, autonomic dysfunction
Limbic encephalitis	Behavioral and psychiatric symptoms, complex partial seizures, dementia
Brainstem encephalitis	Diplopia, dysarthria, dysphagia, spastic quadriparesis, ataxia, gaze palsies
Subacute cerebellar degeneration	Ataxia, dysarthria, limb ataxia, nystagmus
Opsoclonus-myoclonus	Abnormal ocular motility, quick muscle jerks
Retinopathy	Scotomas, blindness, visual hallucinations
Peripheral Nervous System Syndromes	
Motor neuronopathy	Predominant motor weakness
Sensory neuronopathy	Large-fiber sensory loss (joint position and vibration more than pain and temperature), sensory ataxia, dysesthesias, motor involvement (absent or mild)
Autonomic neuronopathy	Gastroparesis, orthostatic hypotension, impotence, reduced sweating, dry eyes and mouth
Length-dependent sensorimotor neuronopathy	Distal sensory loss, muscle weakness
Polyradiculoneuropathy	Proximal sensory loss and motor weakness, pain
Mononeuritis multiplex	Multiple mononeuropathies
Stiff-person syndrome	Stiffness of axial muscles, painful tonic spasms, fixed lumbar lordosis
Neuromyotonia (Isaac syndrome)	Muscle stiffness, myalgias, fasciculations, cramps, hyperhidrosis, tachycardia
Cramp-fasciculation syndrome	Cramps
Neuromuscular Junction and Muscle Syndromes	
Myasthenia gravis	Fatigable weakness
Lambert-Eaton myasthenic syndrome	Fatigue, proximal muscle weakness, reduced or absent muscle stretch reflexes, dry mouth, impotence
Dermatomyositis	Proximal muscle weakness associated with rash
Necrotizing myopathy	Muscle weakness

body-associated paraneoplastic disorders and their related cancers are summarized in Table 14–5.

Paraneoplastic syndromes are difficult to diagnose. The neurologic syndrome often occurs before the discovery of the cancer. In addition, many other inflammatory conditions can mimic these syndromes. Paraneoplastic syndromes have a subacute progressive temporal profile and should be suspected in a patient who has cancer or risk factors for cancer. This diagnosis should also be considered if the patient's clinical features are consistent with one of the characteristic syndromes (see Table 14–4) and no other cause is found on standard evaluation.

The diagnostic approach to the patient depends on whether the patient has a known cancer. If cancer has not been diagnosed, focus the evaluation on detecting the cancer. Some of the tests that may need to be performed are MRI or CT of the chest or abdo-

TABLE 14-5. ANTIBODIES FOUND IN PARANEOPLASTIC SYNDROMES

Antibody	Associated Tumor	Clinical Syndrome
Anti-Yo (PCA)	Gynecologic, breast	Cerebellar degeneration
Anti-Ri (ANNA II)	Breast, gynecologic, SCLC	Opsoclonus, cerebellar ataxia
Anti-Hu (ANNA I)	SCLC, neuroblastoma	Sensory neuronopathy, encephalomyelitis
Anti-voltage-gated calcium channel	SCLC	Lambert-Eaton syndrome
Anti-acetylcholine receptor antibody	Thymoma, SCLC	Myasthenia gravis
Anti-Tr	Hodgkin lymphoma	Cerebellar degeneration
Anti-testicular	Germ cell	Brainstem encephalitis
Antiamphiphysin	Breast, lung	Stiff-person syndrome
Anti-retinal	SCLC, melanoma, gynecologic	Cancer-associated retinopathy

ANNA, antinuclear neuronal antibody; PCA, Purkinje cell antibody; SCLC, small cell carcinoma of the lung.

men, mammography and pelvic ultrasonography in women, testicular ultrasonography in men, lymph node examination, and serum tumor markers. If the patient has a peripheral neuropathy, include a bone survey and serum protein electrophoresis in the evaluation. Tests for paraneoplastic antibodies and CSF analysis are also performed in this clinical situation. The diagnostic evaluation should include CSF analysis for cells, immunoglobulin G (IgG), oligoclonal bands, and cytology. Evaluate the CSF and serum for the presence of paraneoplastic antibodies. If no cancer is detected, follow the patient's condition. If paraneoplastic antibodies are present or CSF analysis results are positive for an immune reaction, repeat the diagnostic evaluation. If a paraneoplastic syndrome occurs in a patient with a known cancer, direct the evaluation at excluding metastatic complications, complications of therapy, or problems related to systemic disease.

Treatment

The first line of treatment for paraneoplastic syndromes is to treat the underlying cancer. However, many of the syndromes do not respond to treatment. Treatment with plasma exchange, intravenous IgG, and other immunosuppressive agents is being investigated.

SUGGESTED READING

Balm, M, and Hammack, J: Leptomeningeal carcinomatosis. Presenting features and prognostic factors. Arch Neurol 53:626–632, 1996.

Black, PMcL: Meningiomas. In Samuels, MA, and Feske, S (eds): Office Practice of Neurology. Churchill Livingstone, New York, 1996, pp 849–854.

Clouston PD, DeAngelis, LM, and Posner, JB: The spectrum of neurological disease in patients with systemic cancer. Ann Neurol 31:268–273, 1992.

Dalmau, J, and Graus, F: Paraneoplastic syndromes. In Samuels, MA, and Feske, S (eds): Office Practice of Neurology. Churchill Livingstone, New York, 1996, pp 925–934.

Dalmau, JO, and Posner, JB: Paraneoplastic syndromes. Arch Neurol 56:405–408, 1999.

Dropcho, EJ: Neurologic complications of radiotherapy. In Samuels, MA, and Feske, S (eds): Office Practice of Neurology. Churchill Livingstone, New York, 1996, pp 919–924.

Fathallah-Shaykh, H: New molecular strategies to cure brain tumors. Arch Neurol 56:449–453, 1999.

Foley, KM: Advances in cancer pain. Arch Neurol 56: 413–417, 1999.

Forsyth, PA, and Posner, JB: Headaches in patients with brain tumors: A study of 111 patients. Neurology 43: 1678–1683, 1993.

Fueyo, J, et al: Targeting in gene therapy for gliomas. Arch Neurol 56:445–448, 1999.

Grossman, SA: Neoplastic meningitis. In Samuels, MA, and Feske, S (eds): Office Practice of Neurology. Churchill Livingstone, New York, 1996, pp 909–914.

Hill, JR, et al: Molecular genetics of brain tumors. Arch Neurol 56:439–441, 1999.

Levin, JM, et al: Complications of therapy for venous thromboembolic disease in patients with brain tumors. Neurology 43:1111–1114, 1993.

Levin, VA: Neuro-oncology: An overview. Arch Neurol 56:401–404, 1999.

Newton, HB: Neurologic complications of systemic cancer. Am Fam Physician 59:878–886, 1999.

Packer, RJ: Brain tumors in children. Arch Neurol 56:421–425, 1999.

Patchell, RA: Metastatic brain tumors. Neurol Clin 13:915–925, 1995.

Patchell, RA, et al: A randomized trial of surgery in the treatment of single metastases to the brain. N Engl J Med 322:494–500, 1990.

Patchell, RA, et al: Postoperative radiotherapy in the treatment of single metastases to the brain: A randomized trial. JAMA 280:1485–1489, 1998.

Perry, JR, Louis, DN, and Cairncross, JG: Current treatment of oligodendrogliomas. Arch Neurol 56:434–436, 1999.

Posner, JB, and Dalmau, JO: Paraneoplastic syndromes affecting the central nervous system. Annu Rev Med 48:157–166, 1997.

Richardson, GS: Pituitary tumors. In Samuels, MA, and Feske, S (eds): Office Practice of Neurology. Churchill Livingstone, New York, 1996, pp 854–861.

Schiff, D: Classification, epidemiology, and etiology of brain tumors. In Samuels, MA, and Feske, S (eds): Office Practice of Neurology. Churchill Livingstone, New York, 1996, pp 808–813.

Schwartz, RB: Neuroradiology of brain tumors. Neurol Clin 13:723–756, 1995.

Shapiro, WR: Current therapy for brain tumors: Back to the future. Arch Neurol 56:429–432, 1999.

Wen, PY: Clinical presentation and diagnosis of brain tumors. In Samuels, MA, and Feske, S (eds): Office Practice of Neurology. Churchill Livingstone, New York, 1996, pp 813–817.

Wen, PY: General principles of management of patients with brain tumors. In Samuels, MA, and Feske, S (eds): Office Practice of Neurology. Churchill Livingstone, New York, 1996, pp 817–824.

Wen, PY: Neurologic complications of chemotherapy. In Samuels, MA, and Feske, S (eds): Office Practice of Neurology. Churchill Livingstone, New York, 1996, pp 914–919.

Index

An *f* following a page number indicates a figure; a *t* indicates a table.

Abdominal reflex, 22
Abducens nerve (CN VI), evaluation of, 12
Abelcet. *See* Amphotericin B
Absence seizure, 154, 155*t*, 156*t*, 161
Acalculia, 7*t*
Acephalic migraine, 50
Acetaminophen (Tylenol)
   for headache, 49*t*
   headache caused by, 52
   for migraine, 51*t*
   for pain, 175*t*, 181
Acetylcholine receptor, antibodies to, 130, 256*t*
Acoustic neuroma, 32, 96, 246, 248, 249*t*
Acromegaly, 113, 118, 129
Acrylamide intoxication, 115*t*
Actigraphy, 166
Action tremor, 206, 208, 216, 217*t*
Acupuncture, 178
Acute cerebellar syndrome, 254*t*
Acute confusional state, 7*t*, 136, 138, 140
Acute disseminated encephalomyelitis, 226*t*, 227*t*, 228
Acute inflammatory demyelinating
      polyradiculoneuropathy (AIDP), 31*t*, 107, 107*t*,
      109*t*, 116–117, 226*t*
Acute symptomatic seizure, 156
Acyclovir
   for facial palsy, 13
   for herpes zoster, 66
   for postherpetic neuralgia, 180
Addison disease, 129, 137*t*
Adies pupil, 8*f*
Adrenal insufficiency, 134
Adrenergic receptor blockers, for pain, 176*t*, 178
Adrenoleukodystrophy, 137*t*, 145*t*
Affective disorders, dizziness in, 91*t*
AIDP. *See* Acute inflammatory demyelinating
      polyradiculoneuropathy
AIDS. *See* Human immunodeficiency virus infection
Akathisia, 167, 205*t*, 206, 222
Akinesia, 204, 205*t*
Alcohol consumption/alcoholism
   dementia in, 139
   disequilibrium in, 101, 101*t*
   dizziness related to, 91*t*
   gait in, 5*t*
   myopathy in, 128, 129*t*
   neuropathy in, 107–108, 113
   pain in, 178
   parkinsonism in, 210
   stroke and, 195
Aldomet. *See* Methyldopa
Allodynia, 106, 174
Allyl chloride, 115*t*
Alprazolam, for tardive syndromes, 222
ALS. *See* Amyotrophic lateral sclerosis
Altitudinal visual field defect, 9

Altretamine, side effects of, 254*t*
Alzheimer disease, 136, 138–139, 143
   clinical features of, 149*t*
   cognitive function in, 7*t*
   dementia in, 137*t*, 143–147
   diagnosis of, 143, 146
   early-onset, 143
   factors that prevent or delay, 145
   genetic factors in, 143–144
   hyposmia in, 7
   late-onset, 143
   magnetic resonance imaging in, 150*f*, 231*f*
   risk factors for, 145
   seizures in, 157*t*
   treatment of, 146
Amantadine (Symmetrel)
   for multiple sclerosis, 236*t*, 237
   for Parkinson disease, 212*t*, 213, 214*t*
Amaurosis fugax, 188, 190
Amicar. *See* Aminocaproic acid
Amikacin, side effects of, 101*t*
Aminocaproic acid (Amicar), side effects of, 129*t*
Aminoglycosides, side effects of, 91*t*
Amiodarone (Cordarone), side effects of, 108, 108*t*,
      129*t*, 211*t*
Amitriptyline (Elavil, Endep)
   for diabetic neuropathy, 112*t*
   for headache prophylaxis, 50*t*
   for migraine, 51*t*
   for migraine prophylaxis, 56
   for multiple sclerosis, 236*t*, 237
   neuropathy related to, 108*t*
   for pain, 175*t*, 177
   for sleep disturbance, 215
Amoxapine (Asendin), side effects of, 211*t*, 222*t*
Amphetamines/amphetamine abuse, 226*t*
   myotoxicity of, 128
   seizures related to, 158
   stroke related to, 199
Amphotericin B (Abelcet)
   for CNS infections, 240*t*
   side effects of, 129*t*
Ampicillin, for CNS infections, 240*t*
Amyloid dementia, 137*t*
Amyloid protein, 144
Amyloidosis, 107, 110*t*, 116, 117*t*, 119
Amyotrophic lateral sclerosis (ALS), 6*t*, 17*t*, 82,
      124–125, 133, 133*t*
Anal reflex, 22–23, 73, 75*t*
Aneurysm, headache in, 45
Angiitis, as cause of dementia, 137*t*
Angiography, 37, 38*f*
   in carotid artery stenosis, 198*f*
   cerebral, 196
   magnetic resonance. *See* Magnetic resonance
      angiography

Angiopathy, 193*t*
Anhidrosis, 7, 100*t*, 106
Anisocoria, 7, 8*f*
Ankle reflex (ankle jerk), 21–22, 73, 80*f*, 101, 106
Ankylosing spondylitis, 70*t*
Anosmia, 7
Antabuse. *See* Disulfiram
Antalgic gait, 5*t*, 73
Anterior cerebral artery, 186*f*, 187*f*
    infarct, 189*f*
    ischemia, 155*t*
Anterior communicating artery, 186*f*
Anterior inferior cerebellar artery, 186*f*
    thrombosis of, 96
Anterior spinal artery, 186*f*
Anti-amphiphilic antibody, 256*t*
Anticholinergics
    for dystonia, 220
    for Parkinson disease, 213
    for tardive syndromes, 222
    for vertigo, 99*t*
Anticoagulants
    as contraindication to lumbar puncture, 28
    dizziness related to, 91*t*
Anticoagulation, 192
Antidepressants
    for pain, 175*t*, 177, 180
    for post-traumatic syndrome, 62
Antiepileptic drugs, 159–164, 160*t*, 162*t*, 163*t*, 164*t*
    for brain tumor, 250
    dizziness related to, 91*t*
    drug interactions, 163, 164*t*
    for headache prophylaxis, 50*t*
    for pain, 176*t*, 177, 180
    for postherpetic neuralgia, 180
    side effects of, 161, 162–163*t*
Antiestrogens, for migraine, 51*t*
Anti-ganglioside antibody, 109
Antihistamines
    dizziness related to, 91*t*
    for vertigo, 99*t*
Anti-Hu antibody, 109, 256*t*
Antihypertensives, dizziness related to, 91*t*
Antineuronal nuclear antibody, 109
Antinuclear antibody, 131
Antioxidants, for Alzheimer disease, 146
Antiphospholipid antibody, 191*f*, 195
Anti-retinal antibody, 256*t*
Anti-Ri antibody, 256*t*
Anti-striated muscle antibody, 131
Anti-testicular antibody, 256*t*
Antithrombin III deficiency, 191*f*
Anti-Tr antibody, 256*t*
Antivert. *See* Meclizine
Anti-Yo antibody, 256*t*
Anxiety disorder, 137*t*
    dizziness in, 91*t*
    pupillary abnormalities with, 8*f*
    spells in, 155*t*
Aortic aneurysm, abdominal, 70*t*
Aortic stenosis, 191*f*
Aphasia, 7*t*, 18*t*, 136, 141, 196
Apolipoprotein E-4, 143–145
Apractic syndromes, 101*t*

Apraxia, 7*t*, 23, 136, 205*t*
Apresoline. *See* Hydralazine
Aralen. *See* Chloroquine
Argyll-Robertson pupil, 8*f*
Aricept. *See* Donepezil
Arm pain, 75, 82
Arnold-Chiari malformation, 18*t*, 98
Arousal difficulty, 168
Arrhythmia, 91*t*, 191*f*, 193*t*
Arsenic intoxication, 107*t*, 109*t*, 110*t*, 115*t*, 145*t*, 178
Artane. *See* Trihexylphenidyl
Arterial dissection, 193*t*, 199
Arterial occlusive disease, 193*t*
Arteriopathy, stroke and, 190
Arteriovenous malformation
    back pain in, 70*t*
    hemorrhage from, headache in, 42–43, 43*t*, 45
    neuroimaging of, 44*t*
    pulmonary, 191*f*
Arteritis (*See also* Temporal arteritis)
    diagnosis of, 193*t*
    types of, and stroke, 190, 191*f*
Arthritis. *See also* Rheumatoid arthritis
    back pain in, 70*t*
    gait in, 5*t*
    geriatric neurologic examination, 25*t*
    pain in, 172*t*
Asendin. *See* Amoxapine
Aseptic meningitis, chemotherapy-related, 254*t*
Asparaginase, side effects of, 254*t*
Aspirin
    for headache, 49*t*
    for migraine, 51*t*
    for pain, 175*t*, 181
    for postherpetic neuralgia, 180
    side effects of, 52, 101*t*
    after stroke, 188
    for stroke prevention, 190–192, 194
Astasia-abasia, 5*t*
Asterixis, 206*t*
Astrocytoma, 246, 248, 249*t*, 251
Asynergia, 204, 205*t*
Ataxia, 101, 204, 205*t*
Ataxic gait, 92
Atenolol (Tenormin)
    for migraine prophylaxis, 55
    side effects of, 52*t*
    for tremor, 218
Atherosclerosis, 11, 190, 191*f*, 194
Athetosis, 204, 205*t*
Ativan. *See* Lorazepam
Atrial fibrillation, as risk factor for stroke, 190, 191*f*, 193–194
Atrial myxoma, 191*f*
Atrial septal defect, 191*f*
Atromid-S. *See* Clofibrate
Attention, tests of, 7*t*, 140
Attention deficit with hyperactivity, 221
Audiometry
    in brain tumor, 248
    in diagnosis of dizziness, 92–93
    diagnosis of hearing loss by, 94*f*
Auditory acuity, 13

Auditory evoked potentials. *See* Brainstem auditory evoked responses
Aura, migraine, 49–50
Automatic movements, 204
Autonomic neuronopathy, 255t
Autonomic neuropathy, 210
    diabetic, 111–112, 111t, 112t
    treatment of, 111
Avlosulfon. *See* Dapsone
Avonex. *See* Interferon beta-1a
Axillary nerve, 21f, 87f
Axonal degeneration, 104
Axonal myopathy, 108
5-Azacitidine, side effects of, 254t
Azathioprine
    for myasthenia gravis, 131
    for myopathy, 128

Babinski sign, 17t, 18t, 21, 23
Back pain. *See also* Spine pain
    causes of, 70t
    complicated, signs of, 71, 74t
    electromyography in, 33
    gait in, 5t
    types, 74t
Baclofen (Lioresal)
    for dystonia, 220
    for multiple sclerosis, 236t, 237
    for neuralgic pain, 64, 64t
    for pain, 176t, 178
    for restless legs syndrome, 168t
    for tardive syndromes, 222
Bacterial meningitis, 31t, 96, 240t
BAER. *See* Brainstem auditory evoked responses
Balance, 13
Ballism, 204, 205t
Baló concentric sclerosis, 227t, 228
Barbiturates, for seizures, 161
Basal ganglion, 206f
Basilar artery, 186f
Basilar migraine, 49
Basilar skull fracture, 96
BCNU. *See* Carmustine
Beesix. *See* Pyridoxine
Behçet disease, 191f, 226t, 232t
Bell palsy, 12–13
Benedryl. *See* Diphenhydramine
Benign childhood epilepsy with centrotemporal spikes, 158
Benign multiple sclerosis, 227t
Benign positional vertigo, 5t, 91t, 92, 92t, 96–98, 98f
Benign rolandic epilepsy, 158
Benzodiazepines
    for dystonia, 220
    for pain, 176t
    for restless legs syndrome, 168, 168t
    for vertigo, 99t
Benztropine (Cogentin)
    for dystonic reactions to medications, 54
    for Parkinson disease, 213
Beta-blockers
    headache related to, 46t
    for headache prophylaxis, 50t

    for migraine prophylaxis, 55–57
Betaseron. *See* Interferon beta-1b
Biceps muscle, evaluation of, 14
Biceps reflex, 21–22, 22t, 80f
Binswanger encephalopathy, 137t, 149
Bitemporal hemianopia, 10f
Bladder
    disturbances in multiple sclerosis, 229, 237
    flaccid, 75t
    loss of control of, 73
    neurogenic, 73, 74t, 237
    spastic, 75t
    uninhibited, 75t
Blepharospasm, 209
Blocadren. *See* Timolol
Blocking tics, 205t
Bone scan, for diagnosis of spine pain, 76, 78t
Bone tumor, back pain in, 70t
Botox. *See* Botulinum toxin
Botulinum toxin (Botox)
    for dystonia, 220
    for tremor, 219, 220t
Botulism, 132
Bowel control, loss of, 73
Brachial artery, compression of, 86
Brachial neuritis, 86
Brachial plexus
    anatomy of, 85, 85f
    compression of, 86
    effect of neoplasms on, 86
    inflammatory condition of, 86
    injury to, 85–86
Brachioradialis reflex, 21–22, 22t, 80f
Bradykinesia, 204, 205t, 207–208
Bradyphrenia, 209
Brain abscess, 43t, 157t, 240–241
Brain attack. *See* Stroke
Brain death, 193t
Brain metastasis, 249t, 251–253
    diagnosis of, 252, 252f
    treatment of, 252, 253
Brain tumor, 98, 246–250, 251–253
    clinical features based on location, 247t
    dementia in, 137t
    diagnostic approach to, 246–248, 247t
    headache in, 246
    histologic grade of, 246
    management of, 248–250
    mental status changes in, 247
    neuroimaging in, 248, 249t, 250f
    personality changes in, 246
    primary, 246–250
    seizures in, 247, 250
    vertigo in, 96t, 98
Brainstem auditory evoked responses (BAERs), 32, 92–93
Brainstem encephalitis, 255t, 256t
Brainstem infarction, 20f
Brainstem tumor, 98
    glioma, 17t, 246
Breast cancer
    brain metastasis in, 252
    meningeal carcinoma in, 253
Brethine. *See* Terbutaline

Broca's area, 142*f*
Bromocriptine (Parlodel)
    for migraine, 51*t*
    for Parkinson disease, 212*t*
    for restless legs syndrome, 168*t*
    side effects of, 217*t*
Brown-Séquard syndrome, 18*t*, 20*f*
Bruns-Garland syndrome. *See* Diabetic
        polyradiculoneuropathy
Bulbocavernosus reflex, 22
Burning feet syndrome, 114
BuSpar. *See* Buspirone
Buspirone (BuSpar), for tremor, 219, 220*t*
Busulfan, side effects of, 254*t*
Butalbital combination (Fiorinal)
    for headache, 49*t*
    headache caused by, 52
Butorphanol
    for migraine, 55
    nasal spray for headache, 49*t*
Buttock pain, 75, 78, 81*t*

Cacosmia, 7
CADASIL, 137*t*
Caffeine
    for headache, 49*t*
    for orthostatic hypotension, 100*t*
    side effects of, 217*t*
Calan. *See* Verapamil
Calcium channel, antibodies to, 132, 256*t*
Calcium channel blockers
    for headache prophylaxis, 50*t*
    for migraine prophylaxis, 56–57
Calculation, tests of, 7*t*
Caloric testing, 13
Canalith repositioning procedure, 98, 98*f*
Cancer, 245–256
    neurologic complications of treatment of, 253, 254*t*
    neuropathic pain in, 180–181
Capsaicin (Zostrix)
    for diabetic neuropathy, 112*t*
    for pain, 176*t*, 178
Captopril, side effects of, 52*t*
Carbamazepine (Tegretol)
    for diabetic neuropathy, 112*t*
    drug interactions, 163–165, 164*t*
    for dystonia, 220
    for multiple sclerosis, 236*t*
    for muscle cramps, 134
    for neuralgic pain, 64, 64*t*
    for pain, 176*t*, 177
    for post-traumatic headache, 62
    for restless legs syndrome, 168*t*
    for seizures, 160*t*, 161
    side effects of, 161, 162*t*
Carbidopa (Lodosyn), for Parkinson disease, 212
Carbidopa/levodopa (Sinemet)
    liquefied, 214, 214*t*
    for Parkinson disease, 211–212, 212*t*, 214*t*
    for restless legs syndrome, 168*t*
    side effects of, 217*t*
    for tremor, 220*t*
Carbon disulfide poisoning, 115*t*

Carbon monoxide poisoning, 210
Carcinomatous meningitis. *See* Meningeal carcinoma
Cardiac disorders, stroke and, 190, 191*f*, 200
Cardiac embolism, 190, 191*f*, 193*t*, 200
Cardiac evaluation, 190
Cardiac fibroelastoma, 191*f*
Cardiomyopathy, 191*f*
Carmofur, side effects of, 254*t*
Carmustine (BCNU), 250
    side effects of, 254*t*
Carotid artery, imaging of, 196, 197*f*
Carotid artery disease, facial pain in, 63
Carotid artery dissection, 191*f*
Carotid artery embolus, 190
Carotid artery stenosis, 189–190
    stroke and, 186, 194–195
    symptomatic, 196–198
Carotid bruit, 196
Carotid endarterectomy, 196–198
Carpal tunnel syndrome, 113, 118–119, 118*f*
    in diabetes, 113
    nerve conduction studies in, 34, 34*t*
    sensory deficit in, 18*t*, 20*f*
Cataplexy, 155*t*, 156*t*, 166–167
Catapres. *See* Clonidine
Catatonia, 205*t*
Catechol-O-methyltransferase inhibitors, for Parkinson
        disease, 212*t*, 213
Cauda equina syndrome, 71, 73*f*, 74*t*, 83–84
Caudate, 204, 206*f*
Causalgia. *See* Complex regional pain syndromes,
        CRPS II
Cefotaxime, for CNS infections, 240*t*
Ceftazidime, for CNS infections, 240*t*
Ceftriaxone
    for CNS infections, 240*t*
    for Lyme disease, 242
Central pain, 180
Central pain syndrome, 172*t*
Central vertigo, 94, 95*t*, 96*t*, 97–99, 98*f*
Cerebellar ataxia, 5*t*, 256*t*
Cerebellar disease/dysfunction, 6*t*, 256*t*
    coordination in, 23
    disequilibrium in, 101, 101*t*
    dizziness in, 92*t*
    gait in, 20, 92
    movement disorders in, 205*t*
    paraneoplastic, 254
    reflexes in, 21
    vertigo in, 95, 98
Cerebellar tumor, 98, 247*t*
Cerebral angiography, 196, 201
Cerebral artery(ies), 186*f*, 187*f*
Cerebral cortex, functional areas of, 142*f*
Cerebral infarct, 210
Cerebral palsy, 5*t*
Cerebral vasculature, 186*f*
    anterior and posterior circulation, 189–190, 190*f*
Cerebrospinal fluid (CSF) analysis, 28–30, 31*t*
    in brain tumor, 248
    in dementia, 142–143
    indications for, 28
    in meningeal carcinoma, 253
    in multiple sclerosis, 231–232

in nervous system infections, 238
in paraneoplastic syndromes, 254
Cerebrovascular disease, 186–201. *See also* Stroke
　angiography in, 37
　dementia in, 148
　diagnostic approach to, 186–192, 193*t*
　　anterior versus posterior circulatory event,
　　　189–190, 189*f*
　　distinguishing hemorrhagic and ischemic events,
　　　188–189
　　hospitalization of patient, 188
　　identifying vascular event, 187–188
　　mechanism of cerebrovascular event, 190–192,
　　　191*f*
Cerebrovascular risk factors, 192–196, 194*t*
Ceroid lipofuscinosis, 217*t*
Cervical dystonia, 219
Cervical myelopathy, 5*t*
Cervical nerves, 71
Cervical radiculopathy, 83*t*
Cervical spondylosis, 80–82
　clinical features of, 232*t*
　diagnosis of, 133
　disequilibrium in, 101*t*
　geriatric neurologic examination, 25*t*
　reflexes in, 22
　weakness in, 17*t*
Chaddock test, 23
Charcot joint, 111
Chemotherapy
　for brain tumor, 248
　neurologic complications of, 253, 254*t*
Chloral hydrate (Noctec), for dementia, 148*t*
Chloroquine (Aralen), side effects of, 108, 108*t*, 129*t*
Chlorpromazine (Thorazine)
　for migraine, 54
　for migraine prophylaxis, 55*t*
　side effects of, 211*t*, 222*t*
Cholinesterase inhibitors
　for Alzheimer disease, 146
　for dementia, 148*t*
Chorea, 204, 205*t*
Chronic daily headache, 58
Chronic hepatic encephalopathy, 137*t*
Chronic hypoglycemic encephalopathy, 137*t*
Chronic inflammatory demyelinating polyneuropathy
　　(CIDP), 34*t*, 107, 107*t*, 109*t*, 110*t*, 118, 226*t*
Chronic pain, 172. *See also* Pain
Churg-Strauss syndrome, 226*t*
Cigarette smoking, stroke and, 195
Cimetidine (Tagamet), side effects of, 52*t*, 108*t*, 129*t*
CIPD. *See* Chronic inflammatory demyelinating
　　polyneuropathy
Cisapride (Propulsid), to increase gastrointestinal
　　motility, 111, 214, 214*t*
Cisplatin (Platinol), side effects of, 91*t*, 101*t*, 108, 108*t*,
　　114, 254*t*
Claudication
　neurogenic, 78–80, 84*t*
　vascular, 84*t*
Clindamycin, for CNS infections, 240*t*
Clioquinol (Vioform), side effects of, 108*t*
Clofibrate (Atromid-S), side effects of, 129*t*
Clonazepam (Klonopin)

for multiple sclerosis, 236*t*
for neuralgic pain, 64, 64*t*
for parasomnias, 168
for pain, 176*t*, 177
for restless legs syndrome, 168*t*
for seizures, 160*t*, 161
side effects of, 162*t*
for sleep disturbance, 215
for tardive syndromes, 222
for tremor, 219, 220*t*
for vertigo, 99*t*
Clonidine (Catapres)
　for orthostatic hypotension, 100*t*
　for pain, 176*t*, 178–180
　for restless legs syndrome, 168*t*
Clopidogrel (Plavix)
　after stroke, 188
　for stroke prevention, 191–192
Clozapine (Clozaril)
　for levodopa-induced psychosis, 212–213
　side effects of, 222*t*
Clumsy hand syndrome, 190
Cluster headache, 58–59, 65*f*
　migraine–cluster headache syndrome, 59
　prophylactic medication for, 50*t*, 60*t*
　treatment of, 59, 60*t*
Coagulation disorder, 190, 193*t*
Cocaine
　myotoxicity of, 128
　seizures related to, 158
　stroke related to, 199
　vasculitis related to, 226*t*
Codeine
　for headache, 49*t*
　for migraine, 51*t*
　for pain, 175*t*, 181
　for restless legs syndrome, 168*t*
Cogan syndrome, 97, 226*t*
Cogentin. *See* Benztropine
Cognex. *See* Tacrine
Cognitive function
　loss of. *See* Memory loss
　in Parkinson disease, 215
　tests of, 6, 7*t*
Cog-wheel rigidity, 208–209
Coital headache, 59, 61*t*
ColBENEMID, side effects of, 108*t*, 129*t*
Collagen-vascular disorder. *See* Connective tissue
　　disease
Collateral circulation, 196, 197*f*
Color vision, 230
Coma, 32, 193*t*
Commissural syndrome, 18*t*, 20*f*
Common peroneal nerve, 87*f*
Compazine. *See* Prochlorperazine
Complex partial seizure, 154, 155*t*
Complex regional pain syndromes, 172*t*, 174, 179
　CRPS I, 179
　CRPS II, 179
Compression neuropathy, 119–120, 119–120*f*
Computed tomography (CT), 34–35, 36*f*
　in brain tumor, 248, 249*t*
　in cerebrovascular event, 188–189, 189*f*
　in dementia, 142–143

Computed tomography (CT)—*Continued*
  in dizziness, 94
  in headache, 44, 44t
  indications for, 37t
  in myasthenia gravis, 131
  in nervous system infections, 238
  in spine pain, 77, 78t
  in stroke, 190
Confusional spells, 156t
Confusional states, 154, 155t
Congestive heart failure, 4, 190, 191f
Connective tissue disease, 226t, 237–238
  with dermatomyositis, 127
  diagnostic features of, 239t
  headache in, 43, 43t, 46t
  neuropathy in, 108, 110t, 114–115, 116t, 118
  stroke and, 200
  weakness in, 125
Conus medullaris, 71
Conversion disorder, 5t, 19, 102, 181–182
  resemblance to peripheral nerve disease, 106t
Coordination
  impaired, 204
  tests of, 19, 23
Copaxone. *See* Glatiramer acetate
Coprolalia, 221
Cordarone. *See* Amiodarone
Corgard. *See* Nadolol
Corneal reflex, 12, 22
Cortical lesion
  sensory deficit in, 18, 18t, 20f
  weakness in, 17t
Cortical-basal ganglionic degeneration, 137t, 210t, 217t
Corticospinal tract, 15, 15f
  abnormalities of, 22–23, 230
  pyramidal decussation, 15
Corticosteroids
  for brain tumor, 250
  for cluster headache, 59
  for cluster headache prophylaxis, 60t
  for facial palsy, 13
  for multiple sclerosis, 236
  for myasthenia gravis, 131
  for myopathy, 128
  for postherpetic neuralgia, 180
  side effects of, 52t, 129
  for spinal cord compression, 253
Cough headache, 59, 61t
Cramps, 134
Cramp-fasciculation syndrome, 255t
Cranial arteritis. *See* Temporal arteritis
Cranial nerves. *See also specific nerves*
  in diabetes mellitus, 113
  examination of, 6–14, 8–13f, 25t
Cranial neuropathy, 111t
  chemotherapy-related, 254t
Craniopharyngioma, 25, 249t
Craniovertebral junction anomaly, 92
Creatine kinase, plasma, 125, 128–129
Cremasteric reflex, 22–23
Creutzfeldt-Jakob disease, 137t, 143, 145t, 210
Critical illness neuropathy, 107t, 114
Crossed straight leg raising test, 75
CRPS. *See* Complex regional pain syndrome

Cryoglobulinemia, 110t, 116, 117t, 226t
Cryptococcus neoformans infection, 137t, 237–239
Cryptogenic seizure, 156–157
CSF analysis. *See* Cerebrospinal fluid analysis
CT. *See* Computed tomography
Cubital tunnel syndrome, 113
Cuprimine. *See* Penicillamine
Cupulolithiasis, 25t
Cushing disease, 137t
Cushing syndrome, 129
Cyanide poisoning, 115t, 210
Cyclophosphamide, for myopathy, 128
Cyclosporine (Neoral), side effects of, 129t, 217t
Cylert. *See* Pemoline
Cyproheptadine (Periactin)
  for migraine, 57
  for multiple sclerosis, 236t
Cystic fibrosis, 128
Cysticercosis, 25, 137t
Cytarabine, side effects of, 254t
Cytomegalovirus infection, 241
Cytosine arabinoside, side effects of, 211t

Dacarbazine, side effects of, 254t
Danazol
  headache caused by, 52t
  for migraine, 51t
Dantrium. *See* Dantrolene
Dantrolene (Dantrium), for multiple sclerosis, 236t, 237
Dapsone (Avlosulfon), side effects of, 108t
Darvocet. *See* Propoxyphene
Decadron. *See* Dexamethasone
Decerebrate posturing, 209
Declarative memory, 141
Decorticate posturing, 209
Deep brain stimulation
  for Parkinson disease, 215–216
  for tremor, 220t
Deep tendon reflex(es), 21, 22t, 76
Deep vein thrombophlebitis, 190
Delirium, 136
  dementia versus, 143, 144t
Deltasone. *See* Prednisone
Deltoid muscle, evaluation of, 14
Dementia, 136
  causes of, 137t
  chemotherapy-related, 254t
  delirium versus, 143, 144t
  depression versus, 137t, 138, 139t, 141, 143, 144t
  differential diagnosis of, 145t
  family history of, 138
  forms of, 143–150
  geriatric neurologic examination, 25t
  laboratory tests in, 141–143, 144t, 145t
  mental status examination in, 139–141, 140–141t
  neuroimaging in, 37t
  neurologic examination in, 139
  parasomnias in, 168
  screening for, 6
  symptomatic treatment of, 148t
Dementia pugilistica, 137t
Dementia with Lewy bodies, 147, 149t, 208, 210t
Demyelinating neuropathy, 108–109, 109t, 118

Demyelinating syndromes, 145t, 227
Depakote. *See* Valproate
Depression, 136
  dementia versus, 137t, 138, 139t, 141, 143, 144t
  dizziness in, 102
  geriatric neurologic examination, 25t
  mental status examination in, 138
  in multiple sclerosis, 236–237
Dermatomes, 19, 20, 21f
Dermatomyositis, 127–128, 226t, 255t
Desyrel. *See* Trazodone
Devic syndrome, 227t, 228
Dexamethasone (Decadron)
  for brain tumor, 250
  for CNS infections, 240t
  drug interactions of, 250
  for spinal cord compression, 253
Dextroamphetamine, for orthostatic hypotension, 100t
Dextromethorphan, for pain, 176t, 178
Diabetes mellitus
  geriatric neurologic examination, 25t
  oculomotor nerve dysfunction in, 11
  radiculopathy in, 77
  stroke and, 190, 194
Diabetic amyotrophy, 112
Diabetic neuropathy, 107–113, 118
  autonomic neuropathy, 111–112, 111t
  carpal tunnel syndrome in, 118
  cranial neuropathy, 111t
  disequilibrium in, 101t
  generalized sensorimotor neuropathy, 110–111, 111t
  laboratory tests in, 110t
  mononeuropathy, 111t, 112–113
  mononeuropathy multiplex, 111t
  nerve conduction studies in, 34t
  pain in, 178–179
  polyradiculoneuropathy, 111t, 112
  reflexes in, 21
  sensory deficit in, 18t
  temporal profile of, 107t
  treatment of, 111, 112t
  truncal neuropathy, 112
Dialysis dementia, 137t
3,4-Diaminopyridine, for Lambert-Eaton syndrome, 132
Diazepam (Valium)
  for multiple sclerosis, 236t
  for restless legs syndrome, 168t
  for vertigo, 99t
Dibenzyline. *See* Phenoxybenzamine
Diclofenac, side effects of, 52t
Didanosine (Videx), side effects of, 108t, 242
Diet, stroke and, 195
Digit span test, 7t
Dihydroergotamine
  for chronic daily headache, 58
  for cluster headache, 60t
  for headache, 49t
  for migraine, 51t, 53, 54t
  for migraine prophylaxis, 55t
  for status migrainosus, 54, 55t
Dilantin. *See* Phenytoin
Dilaudid. *See* Hydromorphone
Dimenhydrinate (Dramamine), for vertigo, 99t
Diphasic dyskinesia, 215

Diphenhydramine (Benadryl), for sleep disturbance, 215
Diphtheria, 107t, 109t
Diplegic gait, 5t
Diplopia, 11–12, 17t
Disequilibrium, 90, 100–102, 100t. *See also* Orthostatic hypotension
  causes of, 91t, 101t
  clinical features of, 92t
  diagnosis of, 92t
  drug-related, 101t
  mechanisms of, 91t
  multisensory, 100
Diskitis, 70t
Disseminated intravascular coagulation, 191f
Disulfiram (Antabuse), side effects of, 108t
Ditropan. *See* Oxybutynin
Diuretics, side effects of, 91t, 128
Divalproex sodium (Depakote). *See also* Valproate
  for cluster headache, 59
  for cluster headache prophylaxis, 60t
  for migraine prophylaxis, 56–57
  for neuralgic pain, 64, 64t
Dix-Hallpike test, 92, 93f
Dizziness. *See also* Disequilibrium; Presyncope; Vertigo
  causes of, 91t
  diagnostic approach to, 90–94, 93–94f, 155t, 156t
  drug-related, 90, 91t
  ill-defined, 90, 91t, 92t, 102
  mechanisms of, 91t
  patient history in, 90
  types of, 91t
Donepezil (Aricept)
  for Alzheimer disease, 146
  for dementia, 148t
Dopamine agonists
  for Parkinson disease, 211, 212t
  for restless legs syndrome, 168, 168t
Dopamine receptor blockers
  for tardive syndromes, 222, 222t
  parkinsonism related to, 207
Dorsal column disease, resemblance to peripheral nerve disease, 106t
Dorsal column-lemniscal pathway, 16–17
Dorsal cord syndrome, 18t
Double vision, 229
Doxycycline, for Lyme disease, 242
Dramamine. *See* Dimenhydrinate
Drop attack, 154–155, 155t, 156t
Droperidol (Inapsine), for vertigo, 99
Drug abuse. *See also specific drugs*
  headache in, 46t
  seizure in, 158
  stroke and, 199
Drugs
  dementia related to, 137t, 139
  dizziness related to, 90, 91t
  headache related to, 43t, 52t
  myopathy related to, 128, 129t
  neuropathy related to, 108t
  ototoxic. *See* Ototoxic drugs
  parkinsonism related to, 211t
  tardive syndromes related to, 222t
  that exacerbate myasthenia gravis, 131–132

Drugs—*Continued*
  tremor related to, 217*t*
Duchenne muscular dystrophy, 125–126, 126*t*
Duragesic. *See* Fentanyl
Dynamic tremor, 216
Dysarthria, 5–6, 6*t*, 14
Dyskinesia, 204, 215
Dysmetria, 204, 205*t*
Dyssynergia, 205*t*
Dystonia, 205*t*, 209, 222
  definition of, 219–220
Dystonia—*Continued*
  in Parkinson disease, 215
  treatment of, 220
  types of, 219–220

Echolalia, 221
Echopraxia, 221
EEG. *See* Electroencephalography
Effexor. *See* Venlafaxine
Ehlers-Danlos syndrome, 199
Elavil. *See* Amitriptyline
Eldepryl. *See* Selegiline
Elderly. *See* Geriatric patient
Electrocardiography, in headache, 46*t*
Electrodiagnostic tests, in neuropathy, 33–34, 108–109
Electroencephalography (EEG), 30–32, 32*t*
  in brain tumor, 248
  in dementia, 142–143
  in headache, 45
  in seizures, 158
Electromyography (EMG), 33–34
  insertional activity, 34, 35*f*
  interference pattern, 34, 35*f*
  motor unit action potential, 34, 35*f*
  in neuropathy, 108–109
  spontaneous activity, 34, 35*f*
  in weakness, 125
Electronystagmography (ENG), 92–93
Emboli, cardiac, as cause of stroke, 191*f*
EMG. *See* Electromyography
EMLA, for pain, 176*t*
Encephalitis, 238
  dystonia in, 219
  encephalography in, 32*t*
  headache in, 43, 43*t*
  parkinsonism in, 210
  seizures in, 157*t*
Encephalomyelitis, paraneoplastic, 254, 255*t*, 256*t*
Encephalopathy
  chemotherapy-related, 254*t*
  electroencephalography in, 32, 32*t*
Endep. *See* Amitriptyline
Endocrine myopathy, 128–130
Endocrine neuropathy, 113
Endometriosis, 70*t*
ENG. *See* Electronystagmography
Entacapone, for Parkinson disease, 212*t*, 213
Ependymoma, 246, 249*t*, 251
Ephedrine, for orthostatic hypotension, 100*t*
Epidural abscess, 70*t*, 157*t*
Epidural hematoma, 157*t*
Epidural spinal cord compression, 252–253

Epilepsy. *See* Seizures
Episodic dyscontrol, 155*t*, 156*t*
Equilibrium, 4
Erb palsy, 85
Erectile dysfunction, 132
Ergot derivatives, for orthostatic hypotension, 100*t*
Ergotamine
  for cluster headache, 59, 60*t*
  for cluster headache prophylaxis, 60*t*
  headache caused by, 52
  for migraine, 51*t*, 53, 54*t*
  for migraine prophylaxis, 55*t*
Erythema migrans, 242
Eskalith. *See* Lithium
Essential tremor, 206, 206*t*, 217–218, 217*t*
  familial, 204
  Parkinson disease versus, 218, 218*t*
Estradiol, for migraine, 51*t*
Estrogen
  for Alzheimer disease, 146
  headache caused by, 51, 52*t*
  migraine and, 50, 51*t*
Estrogen replacement therapy, 145
  neuroprotective effect of, 213
Ethambutol (Myambutol), side effects of, 108*t*
Ethosuximide (Zarontin)
  for seizures, 160*t*, 161
  side effects of, 162*t*
Ethylene oxide intoxication, 115*t*
Etoposide, side effects of, 254*t*
Etrafon. *See* Perphenazine/amitriptyline
Evoked potentials, 32–33
  in brain tumor, 248
  in multiple sclerosis, 231
Executive functioning
  disturbances in, 136
  tests of, 7*t*
Exertional headache, 59
Extensor digitorum brevis muscle, of foot, 106*f*
Extraocular muscles
  assessment of, 125
  dysfunction of, 10–11, 11*f*
Extrapyramidal syndrome, 91*t*, 92, 101*t*
Eye movements, 10–12, 11*f*. *See also* Nystagmus, Ophthalmoplegia.

Fabry disease, 178, 191*f*
Facial expression
  muscles of, 12
  in Parkinson disease, 206, 208
Facial nerve (CN VII), 5
  compression of, 206*t*
  evaluation of, 12–13
  peripheral distribution of, 12, 13*f*
Facial nerve palsy, 12–13, 242
Facial pain, 63–66
  atypical, 65
  glossopharyngeal neuralgia, 64
  herpes zoster, 65–66
  occipital neuralgia, 64–65
  postherpetic neuralgia, 65–66
  temporomandibular joint dysfunction, 66
  trigeminal neuralgia, 63–64

Facial paralysis, evaluation of, 13
Facial sensation, evaluation of, 12
Facial spasm, 206t
Facioscapulohumeral dystrophy, 126, 126t
Factitious disorder, 181–182
Falling, in Parkinson disease, 209, 215
Famciclovir
    for herpes zoster, 66
    for postherpetic neuralgia, 180
Familial amyloid polyneuropathy, 110t
Familial tremor, 204, 218
Fasciculations, 14, 17t, 124–125, 134
Felbamate (Felbatol)
    for seizures, 160t, 161
    side effects of, 162t
Felbatol. *See* Felbamate
Femoral nerve, 22t, 87f
Femoral neuropathy, 86
Fentanyl (Duragesic), for pain, 175t, 181
Festination, 209
Fetal nigral transplantation, for Parkinson disease,
        215–216
Fibromuscular dysplasia, 191f, 199
Final common pathway. *See* Lower motor neuron
Finger flexor reflex, 22
Finger-to-nose test, 19, 23
Fiorinal. *See* Butalbital combination
Flagyl. *See* Metronidazole
Florinef. *See* Fludrocortisone
Fluconazole, for CNS infections, 240t
Fludarabine, side effects of, 254t
Fludrocortisone (Florinef), for orthostatic hypotension,
        100t, 212
5-Fluorouracil, side effects of, 254t
Fluoxetine (Prozac)
    for multiple sclerosis, 236t, 237
    for pain, 175t
    side effects of, 217t
Fluphenazine (Prolixin)
    side effects of, 211t, 222t
    for tics, 221
Focal cortical degeneration, 137t, 145t
Focal dystonia, 205t, 219
Focal neuropathy, 118–120, 118–120f
Foot ulcer, 111
Footdrop, 106, 120, 125, 132–133
Foramen magnum lesion, 155t, 156t
Freezing phenomenon, 205t, 209
Frontal cortex, tumor of, 247t
Frontal gait, 5t, 102
Frontal lobe lesion, 101t, 102
Frontotemporal dementia, 137t, 139–140, 145t, 150
Fugue state, 155t, 156t
Funduscopic examination, 7, 9f
    of optic nerve, 228, 228f, 230
Fungal meningitides, 45
Furadantin. *See* Nitrofurantoin
Furosemide, side effects of, 101t

Gabapentin (Neurontin)
    for diabetic neuropathy, 112t
    for multiple sclerosis, 236t
    for neuralgic pain, 64, 64t
    for pain, 176t, 177, 179
    for postherpetic neuralgia, 180
    for post-traumatic headache, 62
    for restless legs syndrome, 168t
    for seizures, 160t, 161, 163
    side effects of, 162t
    for tremor, 219, 220t
Gabitril. *See* Tiagabine
Gag reflex, 14
Gait abnormality, 4, 5t, 205t
    in geriatric patients, 24
    in Parkinson disease, 209, 215
    in spine pain, 73
Gait apraxia, 5t, 102
Gait examination, 4–5, 5t, 20, 25t
    in dizziness, 90–91
Gamma-aminobutyric acid (GABA) derivatives, for
        neuralgic pain, 63–64
Ganciclovir, for cytomegalovirus infection, 241
Gastrocnemius-soleus reflex, 21, 22t
Gastroparesis, 111
Gemfibrozil (Lopid), side effects of, 129t
Genetic factors
    in Alzheimer disease, 143–144
    in multiple sclerosis, 234
    in neuropathy, 107–108
Gentamicin, side effects of, 101t
Geriatric patient, neurologic examination of, 24–25,
        25t
Germ cell tumor, 248
Geste antagoniste, 220
Giant cell arteritis. *See* Temporal arteritis
Ginkgo biloba, 146–147
Glatiramer acetate (Copaxone), for multiple sclerosis,
        235, 235t
Glial tumor. *See* Glioma
Glioblastoma multiforme, 246, 249t, 250f
Glioma, 17t, 246, 248, 250
Globus pallidus, 204, 206f
Glossopharyngeal nerve (CN IX), 5
    evaluation of, 14
Glossopharyngeal neuralgia, 14, 64
Gold (Myochrysine), side effects of, 108, 108t
Granulomatous angiitis, 191f
Graphesthesia, 18
Greater occipital nerve, 21f
Grip strength, 14, 125
Guillain-Barré syndrome. *See* Acute inflammatory
        demyelinating polyradiculoneuropathy

Halcion. *See* Triazolam
Haldol. *See* Haloperidol
Hallervorden-Spatz disease, 137t
Hallucinations
    hypnagogic, 166–167
    levodopa-related, 212–213
    olfactory, 7
Haloperidol (Haldol)
    for dementia, 148t
    side effects of, 211t, 217t, 222t
    for tics, 221
Handwriting, effect of tremor on, 218, 219f
Hartnup disease, 137t

Headache. *See also specific types.*
chemotherapy-related, 254*t*
chronic daily, 58
classification of, 45–46
cluster. *See* Cluster headache
diagnostic testing in, 44–45, 46*t*
doctor-patient relationship and, 46–47
electroencephalography in, 45
laboratory tests in, 46*t*
lumbar puncture in, 45
migraine. *See* Migraine headache
new daily persistent, 58
post-lumbar puncture, 30
post-traumatic, 61–62
postural, 45
primary, 42
psychologic issues in, 47
rebound, 48
red flags, 42–44, 43*t*
secondary, 42
of short duration, 59–61, 61*t*
in temporal arteritis. *See* Temporal arteritis
temporal profile of, 42–43, 43*t*
tension-type. *See* Tension-type headache
treatment of
abortive, 47–48, 49*t*
goals of, 47
medication, 47
with over-the-counter analgesics, 47
pitfalls of, 48*t*
principles of, 46–48
prophylactic, 47–48, 50*t*
Headache log, 47, 55
Hearing loss
conductive, 13, 92–93, 94*f*
evoked potentials in, 32
sensorineural, 13, 92–93, 94*f*
Hearing test, 13, 25*t*, 92–93
Hemangioblastoma, 251
Hematologic disorders, stroke and, 190, 191*f*, 199–200
Hemianesthesia, 196
Hemianopia, 196
bitemporal, 10*f*
homonymous, 9–10, 10*f*
Hemicrania continua, 58
Hemiparesis, 18*t*, 196
Hemorrhage, into neoplasm, 188
Hemorrhagic stroke, 188–189, 201, 201*f*
Heparin therapy, 192
Hepatitis, confusion with CIDP, 118
Hereditary peripheral neuropathy, 34*t*, 107–108, 109*t*, 110*t*
Hereditary spastic paraplegia, 232*t*
Heredodegenerative disorders, 207, 217*t*
Herniated disk, 71, 72*f*, 82
back pain in, 72, 75
diagnosis of, 78*t*
myelography in, 37, 38*f*
radiculopathy in, 77–78
reflexes in, 21
Heroin, 226*t*
myotoxicity of, 128
stroke related to, 199
Herpes zoster, 65–66, 77, 116

Hexacarbon poisoning, 115*t*
Hexosaminidase A deficiency, 133*t*
Hip, referred pain from, 75
Hip pain, 78
Histoplasmosis, 237
HIV infection. *See* Human immunodeficiency virus infection
HMG-CoA reductase inhibitors, 194
Hollenhorst plaque, 196
Homocysteine, 195
Homocystinuria, 191*f*
Homonymous hemianopia, 9–10, 10*f*
Horner syndrome, 8, 8*f*, 199
5-HT₁ receptor agonists, for migraine, 53, 54*t*
Human immunodeficiency virus (HIV) infection, 238–242, 239*t*, 240*t*, 241*t*
AIDS dementia complex, 241
clinical features of, 232*t*
dementia in, 137*t*, 145*t*
headache in, 46*t*, 241
HIV encephalopathy, 241
HIV headache, 241
hyposmia in, 7
neuropathy in, 107, 107*t*, 110*t*, 116–117
pain in, 178
parkinsonism in, 210
Human T-cell lymphotrophic virus infection, 232, 232*t*
Huntington disease, 6*t*, 137*t*, 139, 204, 205*t*, 207, 217*t*
Hydralazine (Apresoline), side effects of, 108*t*
Hydrocarbon solvent poisoning, 101*t*
Hydrocephalus, 247–248
dementia in, 145*t*
disequilibrium in, 101*t*
movement disorders in, 205*t*
normal-pressure, 5*t*, 144*t*
dementia in, 137*t*, 139, 143, 149–150, 150*f*
disequilibrium in, 102
gait disorder in, 150
parkinsonism in, 210
removal of CSF in, 30
obstructive, 137*t*
Hydromorphone (Dilaudid), for pain, 175*t*
Hyperaldosteronism, 129
Hyperalgesia, 174
Hypercalcemia, 46*t*, 137*t*
Hypercapnia, 46*t*, 137*t*
Hypercoagulable state, 200
Hyperkinesia, 204, 205*t*
Hypernatremia, 46*t*
Hyperparathyroidism, 113, 129, 133, 133*t*
Hyperpathia, 179
Hyperreflexia, 22, 73
Hypertension, 193
oculomotor nerve dysfunction in, 11
stroke and, 190, 191*f*
Hypertensive hemorrhage, 36*f*, 201, 201*f*
Hyperthyroidism, 21, 113, 129, 133, 133*t*
Hypnagogic hallucination, 166–167
Hypnic headache, 59, 61*t*
Hypocalcemia, 129, 134, 157*t*
Hypochondriasis, 181–182
Hypoglossal nerve (CN XII), 5
evaluation of, 14
Hypoglycemia, 46*t*, 134, 137*t*, 157*t*, 217

Hypokinesia, 204, 205*t*
Hypomagnesemia, 134, 157*t*
Hyponatremia, 134, 157*t*
Hypoparathyroidism, 129
Hypophosphatemia, 114
Hyporeflexia, 21–22
Hypotension, orthostatic. *See* Orthostatic hypotension
Hypothalamic tumor, 248
Hypothyroidism
    dementia in, 138–139
    disequilibrium in, 101*t*
    neuropathy in, 113, 118
    parkinsonism in, 210
    reflexes in, 21
    weakness in, 129
Hypoxemia, 137*t*
Hypoxia, 46*t*, 137*t*, 157*t*

Ibuprofen (Motrin)
    for headache, 49*t*
    headache caused by, 52
    for migraine, 51*t*, 53
    for migraine prophylaxis, 55*t*
    for orthostatic hypotension, 100*t*
    for pain, 175*t*
Ice pick headache, 59, 61*t*
Idiopathic central nervous system hypersomnia, 166–167
Idiopathic pain, 172*t*
Idiopathic seizure, 156–157
Ifosfamide, side effects of, 254*t*
Illness-affirming behavior, 181–182
Immune-mediated disorders, 226, 226*t*
Immunoglobulin, for myasthenia gravis, 131
Impotence, 132
Inapsine. *See* Droperidol
Inclusion body myositis, 127, 133, 133*t*, 226*t*
Incontinence, 73, 75*t*
Inderal. *See* Propranolol
Indomethacin
    for cluster headache, 59
    for cluster headache prophylaxis, 60*t*
    for headache, 49*t*, 59, 61*t*
    headache caused by, 52*t*
    for migraine prophylaxis, 55*t*, 56
    for orthostatic hypotension, 100*t*
Infectious diseases, of nervous system, 238–242
    causing polyneuropathy, 116
    treatment of, 240*t*
Inferior oblique muscle, 10, 11*f*
Inferior rectus muscle, 10, 11*f*
Inflammatory bowel disease, confusion with CIDP, 118
Inflammatory neuropathy
    acute inflammatory demyelinating polyneuropathy (AIDP), 31*t*, 107, 107*t*, 109*t*, 116, 226*t*
    chronic inflammatory demyelinating polyradiculoneuropathy (CIDP), 34*t*, 107, 107*t*, 109*t*, 118, 226*t*
Inflammatory spondyloarthropathy, 72, 74*t*
Initial tremor, 216
Inner ear disease, autoimmune, 97
Insomnia, 166–168
Intention tremor, 204

Interferon, side effects of, 254*t*
Interferon beta-1a (Avonex), for multiple sclerosis, 235, 235*t*
Interferon beta-1b (Betaseron), for multiple sclerosis, 235, 235*t*
Interleukin-2, side effects of, 254*t*
Internal carotid artery, 186*f*, 196
Internal hamstring reflex, 22
Interosseous muscles, of hand, 106*f*
Intervertebral disk disease, 70*t*. *See also* Herniated disk
Intracerebral hemorrhage, 149, 188, 201
Intracranial pressure, increased, 246–248
Isaac syndrome, 255*t*
Ischemic stroke, 188–190, 191*f*
Ishihara plates, 230
Isolated brainstem syndrome, 227*t*, 228
Isometheptene-dichloralphenazone-acetaminophen, for migraine prophylaxis, 55*t*
Isometric tremor, 217, 217*t*
Isoniazid (Nydrazid), side effects of, 108*t*
Isosorbide, side effects of, 52*t*

Jaw reflex, 22
Jendrassik method, 22

Kawasaki disease, 226*t*
Ketalar. *See* Ketamine
Ketamine (Ketalar), for pain, 176*t*
Ketorolac
    for migraine, 52–53
    for migraine prophylaxis, 55*t*
Kinetic tremor, 216–217, 217*t*
Klonopin. *See* Clonazepam
Klumpke's paralysis, 85
Knee jerk, 80*f*

Labetalol (Normodyne), side effects of, 129*t*
Laboratory tests
    in dementia, 141–143, 144*t*, 145*t*
    in diabetic neuropathy, 110*t*
    in headache, 46*t*
    in Lyme disease, 242
    in multiple sclerosis, 230–232
    in neuropathy, 109, 110*t*
Labyrinthine ischemia, 96
Labyrinthitis, 91*t*, 96, 188
Lacunar infarct, 190, 192*f*, 231*f*
Lambert-Eaton myasthenic syndrome, 132, 226*t*, 254, 255*t*, 256*t*
Lamictal. *See* Lamotrigine
Lamotrigine (Lamictal)
    for neuralgic pain, 64, 64*t*
    for pain, 176*t*, 177
    for seizures, 160*t*, 161
    side effects of, 162*t*
Language
    normal development of, 24*t*
    tests of, 7*t*
Language problem, 141
Lateral femoral cutaneous nerve, 21*f*, 87*f*
    compression of, 120

Lateral femoral cutaneous nerve—*Continued*
    injury to, 86
Lateral medullary syndrome, 8
Laxatives, in muscle weakness, 128
Lead intoxication, 110t, 115t, 137t, 145t
Leg pain, 75, 81t
Leprosy, 107, 116
Leptomeningeal metastasis. *See* Meningeal carcinoma
Lesser occipital nerve, 21f
Leucovorin, for CNS infections, 240t
Leukemia, 110t, 157t, 191f, 226t
Leukoaraiosis, 143, 149, 149f, 231f
Leukodystrophy, 232t
Levamisole, side effects of, 254t
Levodopa, for Parkinson disease, 214, 214t
Lewy bodies, dementia with, 137t, 147
Lhermitte sign, 229
Lidocaine, for pain, 176t, 177–178
Limb pain
    plexopathy, 70, 85–86, 85f, 87f
    radiculopathy, 77–78, 79f
    from spinal disease, 70
Limb-girdle dystrophy, 126t
Limbic encephalitis, 255t
Lioresal. *See* Baclofen
Lithium (Eskalith, Lithobid)
    for cluster headache, 59
    for cluster headache prophylaxis, 60t
    for headache of short duration, 61t
    side effects of, 108t, 217t
Lithobid. *See* Lithium
Locomotion, defined, 4
Lodosyn. *See* Carbidopa
Lopid. *See* Gemfibrozil
Lopressor. *See* Metoprolol
Lorazepam (Ativan)
    for dementia, 148t
    for vertigo, 99t
Lou Gehrig disease. *See* Amyotrophic lateral sclerosis
Lovastatin (Mevacor), side effects of, 129t, 211t
Lower body parkinsonism, 5t, 102
Lower extremity, nerves of, 87f
Lower motor neuron, 15, 15f
Lower motor neuron lesion, 6t, 15, 16t, 17t
Loxapine (Loxitane), side effects of, 222t
Loxitane. *See* Loxapine
LSD, stroke related to, 199
Lumbar puncture, 28–30
    complications of, 30
    contraindications to, 28
    for headache, 45, 61t
    procedure for, 28–30, 29f
Lumbar radiculopathy, 81–82t
Lumbosacral plexopathy, 86
Lumbosacral polyradiculoneuropathy, 112
Lung cancer, 109
    brain metastasis in, 251–252, 252f
    meningeal carcinoma in, 253
    paraneoplastic syndrome in, 254
Lyme disease, 231–232, 242
    clinical features of, 232t, 242
    dementia in, 137t
    headache in, 43, 43t, 45, 46t
    laboratory testing in, 242

    neuropathy in, 110t
    optic neuritis in, 237
    stroke and, 200
Lymphoma, 226t
    dementia in, 137t
    diagnosis of, 133, 133t
    neuropathy in, 110t, 118
    primary CNS, 232t, 240, 241t
    seizures in, 157t

Macrodantin. *See* Nitrofurantoin
Magnetic resonance angiography (MRA), 36–37, 37f,
        44t, 196
Magnetic resonance imaging (MRI), 35–37, 37f
    of brain metastasis, 252f
    in brain tumor, 248, 249t, 250f
    of cerebrovascular event, 189
    contraindications to, 36
    in dementia, 142–143, 149f, 150f
    in dizziness, 94
    in headache, 44t
    indications for, 37f
    in lacunar infarct, 192f
    in multiple sclerosis, 230–231, 231f, 233f, 234
    in myasthenia gravis, 131
    in nervous system infections, 238
    in seizures, 158–159
    in spine pain, 77, 78t
Maintenance of wakefulness test, 166
Malingering
    dizziness in, 102
    pain in, 181–182
    resemblance to peripheral nerve disease, 106t
Manganese intoxication, 210
Marburg variant, 227t, 228
Marcus Gunn pupil, 230
Marfan syndrome, 199
Mass lesion, 241
    dementia in, 145t
    headache in, 43, 43t
    neuroimaging in, 44t
    seizures in, 158
Mastectomy, pain after, 181
Mastication, muscles of, 11–12
Meclizine (Antivert), for vertigo, 99t
Median nerve, 21f, 87f
    compression of. *See* Carpal tunnel syndrome
    nerve conduction studies using, 33, 33f
Medulla, 15, 15f
Medulloblastoma, 246
Melanoma, meningeal carcinoma in, 253
Mellaril. *See* Thioridazine
Memory, tests of, 7t, 141
Memory loss. *See also* Dementia
    diagnostic approach to, 136–143
    patient history in, 136–139
Ménière disease, 91t, 92t, 96–97, 101t, 156t
Meningeal carcinoma, 31t, 45, 145t, 248, 253
Meningioma, 25, 96, 246, 248, 249t, 251
Meningitis. *See also specific types*
    acute, 238
    chronic, 238
    CSF analysis in, 28, 232

diagnosis of, 193*t*
disequilibrium in, 101*t*
headache in, 43, 43*t*
in HIV-infected patient, 238
seizures in, 157*t*
treatment of, 240*t*
Menopause, migraine after, 51
Menstrual dysfunction, seizures and, 165
Menstrual migraine, 50, 51*t*
Mental disorders, pain and, 181–182
Mental status changes
in brain tumor, 247
neuroimaging in, 37*t*
testing for, 6, 7*t*
Mental status examination, 6, 7*t*, 25*t*
in dementia, 139–141, 140–141*t*
Meperidine
for headache, 49*t*
for migraine, 51*t*, 55
for migraine prophylaxis, 55*t*
Meralgia paresthetica, 86, 120
Mercury intoxication, 110*t*, 115*t*, 137*t*, 145*t*, 210
Mesoridazine (Serentil), side effects of, 222*t*
Mestinon. *See* Pyridostigmine
Metabolic neuropathy, 113–114
Metachromatic leukodystrophy, 137*t*, 145*t*
Metastasis. *See* Brain metastasis
Methanol intoxication, 210
Methazolamide (Neptazane), for tremor, 219,
    220*t*
Methotrexate
for myopathy, 128
side effects of, 91*t*, 254*t*
Methyldopa (Aldomet), side effects of, 52*t*, 211*t*
Methylphenidate (Ritalin)
for orthostatic hypotension, 100*t*
side effects of, 217*t*
Methylprednisolone (Solu-Medrol)
for multiple sclerosis, 236
for optic neuritis, 237
Methysergide
for cluster headache, 59
for cluster headache prophylaxis, 60*t*
for headache prophylaxis, 50*t*
for migraine prophylaxis, 57
Metoclopramide (Reglan)
for gastroparesis, 111
for orthostatic hypotension, 100*t*
side effects of, 211*t*, 212, 217*t*, 222*t*
Metoprolol (Lopressor)
headache caused by, 52*t*
for migraine prophylaxis, 55
for tremor, 218
Metronidazole (Flagyl), side effects of, 52*t*, 108*t*
Mevacor. *See* Lovastatin
Mexiletine (Mexitil)
for diabetic neuropathy, 112*t*
for pain, 176*t*, 177, 179, 180
Mexitil. *See* Mexiletine
MGUS. *See* Monoclonal gammopathy of undetermined
    significance
Micrographia, 207–208
Midbrain (rubral) tremor, 217*t*
Middle cerebral artery, 186*f*, 187*f*

Middle cerebral artery infarct, 10*f*, 18*t*, 189*f*, 190
Midodrine (ProAmatine), for orthostatic hypotension,
    100*t*, 212
Midrin
for headache, 49*t*
for migraine, 53
Migraine equivalent, 50
Migraine headache, 48–57
associations of, 50–52, 65*f*
basilar, 49
dizziness in, 91*t*
frequency of, 50
hyperosmia in, 7
menstrual, 50, 51*t*
neuroimaging in, 44–45
ophthalmoplegic, 49
pathogenesis of, 48
in pediatric patient, 57
phases of, 48–49
prophylaxis for, 50*t*
quality and duration of pain in, 65*f*
retinal, 49
with seizure disorder, 45
spells in, 154, 155*t*, 156*t*
stroke and, 52
tension-type headache and, 57–58
transformed, 52–53, 58
transient ischemic attack versus, 187
treatment of, 52–57, 54–56*t*
types of, 48, 49–50
vertigo in, 96–97
Migraine mimic, 199
Migraine-cluster headache syndrome, 59
Migrainous stroke, 199
Mini-Mental State Examination (MMSE), 6, 140–141,
    140*t*
Miosis, 7
Mirapex. *See* Pramipexole
Misonidazole, side effects of, 254*t*
Mitochondrial disease, 137*t*
Mitral valve prolapse, 191*f*
MMSE. *See* Mini-Mental State Examination
Moban. *See* Molindone
Modafinil, for narcolepsy, 167
Molindone (Moban), side effects of, 222*t*
Monoamine oxidase inhibitors
for migraine prophylaxis, 57
for narcolepsy, 167
for Parkinson disease, 212*t*
Monoclonal gammopathy, 118
Monoclonal gammopathy of undetermined significance
    (MGUS), 109*t*, 116, 117*t*, 226*t*
Mononeuritis multiplex, 113, 242, 255*t*
Mononeuropathy multiplex, 107, 111*t*
Morphine, for pain, 175*t*, 181
Motion sickness, 92*t*
Motor examination, 14–16, 16*f*, 16*t*, 25*t*, 125
Motor fluctuations, in Parkinson disease, 213–215, 214*t*
Motor neuron disease, 132–134
electromyography in, 33
multifocal, 110*t*, 133, 133*t*
resemblance to peripheral nerve disease, 106*t*
weakness in, 17*t*, 125
Motor system, anatomy of, 15, 15*f*

Motor tic, 221
Motrin. See Ibuprofen
Movement disorders, 155t, 204–222
    classification of, 204
    clinical examples of, 205t
    definitions used to describe, 205t
    diagnostic approach to, 204–206, 205–206t
Moyamoya disease, 191f
MPTP overdose, 210
MRA. See Magnetic resonance angiography
MRI. See Magnetic resonance imaging
Multifocal dystonia, 219
Multi-infarct dementia, 137t, 138, 147–148
Multi-infarct state, disequilibrium in, 101t
Multimodal association cortex, 142f
Multiple myeloma, 70t, 110t, 116, 117t
Multiple sclerosis, 206t, 226–237, 226t
    CSF analysis in, 31t, 231–232, 229t
    dementia in, 137t
    diagnostic approach to, 188, 228–230, 229t, 232t, 233
    disease-modifying therapy in, 235–236, 235t
    dizziness in, 91t
    epidemiology of, 233–234
    evoked potentials in, 32
    gait in, 5t
    genetic factors in, 234
    laboratory tests in, 230–232
    magnetic resonance imaging in, 230–231, 231f, 233f, 234
    ocular problems in, 230
    optic neuritis in, 227–228, 227t, 228f, 237
    pain in, 180
    pregnancy in, 234–235
    prognosis in, 234
    reflexes in, 22
    resemblance to peripheral nerve disease, 106t
    speech problems in, 6t
    spells in, 155t
    symptomatic therapy in, 236–237, 236t
    types of, 227–228, 227t
    vertigo in, 96–98
    visual field defect in, 10f
Multiple sleep latency test, 166–167
Multisensory disequilibrium, 100
Multisystem degenerative disorders, 137t, 207–208, 217t
Muscle biopsy, 125–126
Muscle cramps. See Cramps
Muscle strain, 70t
Muscle strength, evaluation of, 75–76
Muscle stretch reflexes. See Deep tendon reflexes
Muscle tone, tests of, 208. See also Dystonia.
Muscular dystrophy, 125–126, 126t
Musculocutaneous nerve, 21f, 22t
Myambutol. See Ethambutol
Myasthenia gravis, 226t, 255t, 256t
    diagnosis of, 130–131, 133t
    factors that exacerbate, 131–132
    resemblance to peripheral nerve disease, 106t
    treatment of, 131
    weakness in, 15, 17t, 124, 130–132
Myelography, 37–38, 38f
    for diagnosis of spine pain, 77, 78t
Myelopathy

    back pain in, 74t
    cervical spondylotic, 82
    chemotherapy-related, 254t
    CSF analysis in, 232
    deficits associated with, 73f
    diagnosis of, 78t
    disequilibrium in, 101t
    resemblance to peripheral nerve disease, 106t
    with spinal cord tumor, 251
    weakness in, 17t
Myocardial infarction, stroke risk after, 191f, 193–194
Myochrysine. See Gold
Myoclonic seizure, 161
Myoclonus, 204, 206t
Myofascial pain syndrome, 172t
Myopathy. See also specific types
    associated with drugs and toxins, 128, 129t
    axonal, 108
    electromyography in, 35f
    endocrine, 128–130
    inflammatory, 127–128
        associated conditions and findings, 127–128
        treatment of, 128
    inherited, 126–127, 126t
    resemblance to peripheral nerve disease, 106t
    weakness in, 15, 17t, 124
Myositis, 242. See also specific types
Myotonic dystrophy, 126–127

Nadolol (Corgard)
    for migraine prophylaxis, 55
    for tremor, 218
Naprosyn. See Naproxen
Naproxen (Naprosyn)
    for headache, 49t
    for headache prophylaxis, 50t
    for migraine, 51t, 53
    for migraine prophylaxis, 55t, 56
    for orthostatic hypotension, 100t
    for pain, 175t
Naratriptan
    for migraine, 53, 54t
    for migraine prophylaxis, 55t
Narcolepsy, 155t, 156t, 166–167
Narcotics
    headache caused by, 52
    for migraine, 54–55
    for migraine prophylaxis, 55t
    for pain, 174–178
Navane. See Thiothixene
Neck flexion, 15, 229
    assessment of, 125
Neck pain, 75, 82
Neck stiffness, 238
Nefazodone (Serzone), for pain, 175t, 178
Neglect, 7t, 196
Neoplastic meningitis. See Meningeal carcinoma
Neoral. See Cyclosporine
Nephrotic syndrome, 118
Neptazane. See Methazolamide
Nerve conduction studies, 33–34, 33f, 34t
    conduction time, 34, 34t
    conduction velocity, 34, 34t

distal latency, 34, 34t
  in neuropathy, 108–109
  proximal latency, 34
Nerve root syndromes, 80f
Neuralgia. *See also specific types*
  medications for neuralgic pain, 64t
Neuralgic amyotrophy, 86
Neuroacanthocytosis, 217t
Neurofibroma, 251
Neurofibromatosis, 157t, 158
Neuroimaging, 34–38. *See also specific modalities*
  in dementia, 142–143
  in dizziness, 92–94
  in headache, 44–45, 44t
  in multiple sclerosis, 227, 230–231, 231f, 232t, 233f,
    234
Neuroleptic malignant syndrome, 209
Neurologic complications
  of cancer therapy, 253, 254t
  of systemic disease, 251–256
Neurologic examination
  coordination examination, 23
  cranial nerve examination, 6–14, 8–13f
  in dementia, 139
  gait examination, 4–5, 5t, 25t
  in geriatric patient, 24–25, 25t
  mental status examination, 6, 7t, 25t
  motor examination, 14–16, 16f, 16t, 25t
  in pediatric patient, 24, 24t
  reflex examination, 19–23, 22t, 25t
  sensory examination, 16–19, 18t, 20–21f, 25t
  speech evaluation, 5–6, 6t
Neurologic history, 4
Neuromuscular junction, disorders of, 124, 130–132
Neuromyotonia, 255t
Neuronal migration, disorders of, 158
Neurontin. *See* Gabapentin
Neuro-oncology, 245–256
Neuropathic pain, 172t
Neuropathy, 103–120. *See also specific types*
  acquired vs. hereditary, 107–108
  asymmetric, 107
  chemotherapy-related, 254t
  demyelinating, 108–109, 109t
  diagnostic approach to, 104–109
  drug-related, 108t
  electrodiagnostic tests in, 108–109
  gait in, 5t
  laboratory tests in, 109, 110t
  localization of, 104
  painful, 178–179
  paraneoplastic, 255t
  temporal pattern of, 107, 107t
  weakness in, 124
Neuropsychiatric tests, 141–142
Niacin deficiency, 113
Nifedipine
  for migraine prophylaxis, 56
  side effects of, 52t
Nightmares, 168
Nimodipine, for migraine prophylaxis, 56
Nitrofurantoin (Furadantin, Macrodantin), side effects
    of, 108t
Nitroglycerin, side effects of, 52t

Nitrous oxide, side effects of, 108t
NMDA antagonists, for pain, 176t, 178
Nociceptive pain, 172t
Noctec. *See* Chloral hydrate
Nonsteroidal anti-inflammatory drugs (NSAIDs)
  for Alzheimer disease, 145–146
  for headache prophylaxis, 50t
  for migraine, 52–53
  for migraine prophylaxis, 55t, 56
  for orthostatic hypotension, 212
  for pain, 175t, 179, 181
  for postherpetic neuralgia, 180
Normodyne. *See* Labetalol
Nortriptyline (Pamelor)
  for diabetic neuropathy, 112t
  for migraine prophylaxis, 56
  for pain, 175t, 177
NSAIDs. *See* Nonsteroidal anti-inflammatory drugs
Nutritional deficiency/disorder
  myopathy in, 128
  neuropathy in, 107t, 113–114
  weakness in, 125
Nydrazid. *See* Isoniazid
Nylen-Bárány test. *See* Dix-Hallpike test
Nystagmus, 230
  positional, 93
  vertigo and, 94–95, 95t

Obsessive-compulsive disorder, 206t, 221
Obturator nerve, 21f, 87f
Occipital cortex, tumor of, 247t
Occipital neuralgia, 64–65
Occlusive disease, stroke and, 190, 191f
Oculogyric crisis, 222
Oculomotor nerve (CN III)
  evaluation of, 10–11, 11f
  palsy, 11, 113
Olanzapine (Zyprexa)
  for psychosis in Parkinson disease, 213
  for tardive syndromes, 222
  tardive syndromes related to, 222t
Olfactory nerve (CN I), evaluation of, 7
Oligodendroglioma, 246, 249t, 251
Olivopontocerebellar degeneration, 137t, 207, 210t,
    232t
Oncovin. *See* Vincristine
Ophthalmoplegia, 49, 130, 230
Opiates
  for pain, 175t, 180–181
  pupillary abnormalities and, 8f
  for restless legs syndrome, 168, 168t
Opsoclonus, 256t
Opsoclonus-myoclonus, 255t
Optic atrophy, 9f
Optic chiasm lesion, 9, 32
Optic nerve (CN II), evaluation of, 7–10, 8–10f
Optic neuritis, 9, 226t, 232t, 237
  evoked potentials in, 32
  in multiple sclerosis, 227–228, 227t, 228f, 237
  visual field defect in, 10f
Oral contraceptives
  drug interactions, 164–165
  migraine and, 51

Oral-buccal-lingual dyskinesia, 221–222
Orap. *See* Pimozide
Organ transplantation, 118
Organophosphate intoxication, 115t, 129t
Orthostatic hypotension, 92t
  levodopa-related, 212
  medications for, 100t
  treatment of, 111
Orthostatic tremor, 217t
Oscillopsia, 101
Osteosclerotic myeloma, 109t, 110t, 116, 117t
Otolithiasis, 96
Otolithic catastrophe, 97
Otomastoiditis, 96
Ototoxic drugs, 5t, 13–14, 91t, 92t, 101, 101t
Oxybutynin (Ditropan), for multiple sclerosis,
  236t
Oxycodone (Percocet)
  for pain, 175t, 181
  for restless legs syndrome, 168t
Oxygen therapy, for cluster headache, 59, 60t

Paclitaxel (Taxol), side effects of, 108t, 114, 254t
Pain, 172–182. *See also specific sites*
  categories of, 172t
  diagnostic approach to, 173–174
  evaluation of chronic pain, 172–173
  how patient copes with, 174
  idiopathic, 172t
  management principles, 173
  mental disorders and, 181–182
  motivational-affective aspect of, 173
  neuropathic, 172t
  nociceptive, 172t
  rescue medication, 181
  sensory-discriminative aspect of, 173
  treatment of, 174–178, 175–176t
Pain history, 173–174
Pain sensation, 16–18, 18t
  tests of, 20–21
Pallidotomy
  for Parkinson disease, 215–216
  for tremor, 220t
Pamelor. *See* Nortriptyline
Pancoast tumor, 8
Panic attack, 155t, 156t
Panic disorder, 91t, 92t, 102
Papilledema, 9f, 43, 247–248
Papillitis, 228
Paraneoplastic syndromes, 137t, 226t, 254–256
  antibodies found in, 256, 256t
  clinical features of, 232t, 254–256, 255t
  definition of, 254–256
  diagnosis of, 254–256
  disequilibrium in, 101, 101t
  neuropathy in, 107t
  pain in, 178, 180
  parkinsonism in, 210
  treatment of, 256
Parasomnias, 155t, 156t, 166, 168
Parathyroid disease, 210
Paresthesia, 81t, 103–120. *See also* Neuropathy
  diagnostic approach to, 104–109

Parietal cortex, tumor of, 247t
Parietal lobe function, tests of, 140–141
Parietal lobe lesion, 10, 10f, 205t
Parkinson disease, 147, 204, 207–216. *See also*
  Parkinsonism
  behavioral signs of, 209
  bradykinesia in, 208
  clinical features of, 149t, 205t, 210t
  coordination in, 23
  dementia in, 137t, 139, 209, 215
  differential diagnosis of, 210, 210f
  disequilibrium in, 101t, 102
  dyskinesia in, 215
  essential tremor versus, 218, 218t
  facial expression in, 206, 208
  falls in, 209, 215
  gait in, 5t, 209, 215
  hyposmia in, 7
  managing late complications of, 213–215
  medical treatment of, 210–213, 212t
  motor fluctuations in, 213–215, 214t
  parasomnias in, 168
  parkinsonism versus, 207
  postural instability in, 209
  psychiatric complications in, 215
  rigidity in, 208–209
  sleep disturbance in, 209, 215
  speech problems in, 6t
  surgical therapy for, 215–216
  tremor in, 208, 216, 217t
  weakness in, 207
Parkinsonism, 206–216. *See also* Parkinson disease
  clinical presentation of, 206
  diagnosis of, 207, 210, 210f
  disequilibrium in, 102
  gait in, 4, 5t
  geriatric neurologic examination, 25t
  Parkinson disease versus, 207
  postural instability in, 24–25
  primary, 207
  secondary, 207, 210, 217t
  vascular, 210t
Parkinsonism plus, 207
Parlodel. *See* Bromocriptine
Paroxetine (Paxil)
  for dementia, 148t
  for pain, 175t
Paroxysmal hemicrania, 59, 61t
Partial seizure, 155t, 158, 160–161, 187–188
Paxil. *See* Paroxetine
Pediatric patient
  developmental landmarks for, 245
  migraine in, 57
  neurologic examination of, 24, 24t
Pemoline (Cylert), for multiple sclerosis, 236t, 237
Penicillamine (Cuprimine), side effects of, 128, 129t
Penicillin
  for CNS infections, 240t
  side effects of, 158
Percocet. *See* Oxycodone
Pergolide (Permax)
  for restless legs syndrome, 168t
  side effects of, 217t
Periactin. *See* Cyproheptadine

Perilymph fistula, 96
Periodic paralysis, 129
Peripheral nerves
    distribution of, 21f
    structure of, 105f
Peripheral nerve disease, 104–116
    clinical features of, 105t
    disequilibrium in, 101, 101t
    disorders that mimic, 106t
    dizziness in, 91t
    gait in, 5t
    geriatric neurologic examination, 25t
    infection, 241
    muscle cramps in, 134
    muscle studies in, 34
    nerve conduction studies in, 34
    reflexes in, 22
    sensory deficit in, 18t, 20f
    weakness in, 15, 17t
Permax. *See* Pergolide
Pernicious anemia, 113
Peroneal nerve, 21f
    compression of, 120, 120f
    nerve conduction studies using, 33
Peroneal palsy, 5t, 17t
Perphenazine (Trilafon), side effects of, 211t, 222t
Perphenazine/amitriptyline (Etrafon, Triavil), side
        effects of, 211t, 222t
Personality change, 138
Personality disorder, 137t
Pes cavus, 108, 108f
PET. *See* Positron emission tomography
Phalen maneuver, 119
Pharyngeal reflex, 22
Phencyclidine
    myotoxicity of, 128
    seizures related to, 158
    stroke related to, 199
Phenelzine sulfate, for migraine prophylaxis, 57
Phenergan. *See* Promethazine
Phenobarbital
    drug interactions, 163, 165
    for seizures, 160t, 161
    side effects of, 161, 163t
    for tremor, 220t
Phenothiazines, for migraine, 54
Phenoxybenzamine (Dibenzyline), for restless legs
        syndrome, 168t
Phentolamine, for pain, 178
Phenylpropanolamine
    for orthostatic hypotension, 100t
    side effects of, 199, 217t
Phenytoin (Dilantin)
    for diabetic neuropathy, 112t
    drug interactions, 163–165, 164t, 250
    for multiple sclerosis, 236t
    for muscle cramps, 134
    for neuralgic pain, 64, 64t
    for pain, 176t, 177
    for seizures, 160t, 161
    side effects of, 5t, 108t, 161, 163t
Pheochromocytoma, 217
Phonic tic, 221
Phrenic nerve, 5

Physical activity, stroke and, 195
Physiologic tremor, 217, 217t
Pick disease, 137t, 139, 145t, 150
Pill-rolling tremor, 208
Pilocytic astrocytoma, 248
Pimozide (Orap)
    side effects of, 222t
    for tics, 221
Pineal tumor, 246, 247t, 248
"Pins and needles." *See* Paresthesia
Piroxicam, side effects of, 52t
Pituitary adenoma, 246, 248, 249t
Pituitary apoplexy, 42, 43t
Pituitary disease, 9, 10f
Plain radiographs, for diagnosis of spine pain, 76, 78t
Plantar reflex, 23, 73
Plasmapheresis, for myasthenia gravis, 131
Platinol. *See* Cisplatin
Plavix. *See* Clopidogrel
Plexopathy, 70, 85–86, 85f, 87f
Poliomyelitis, 134
Polyarteritis nodosa, 97, 115, 115t, 137t, 191f, 226t, 239t
Polychlorinated biphenyl intoxication, 115t
Polymyositis, 17t, 35f, 127–128, 226t
Polyneuropathy
    nerve conduction studies in, 34
    pain in, 172t
Polysomnography, 166–168
Pontine lesion, 206t
Porphyria, 107t, 110t, 114
Position sense, 16–18, 18t
    tests of, 21
Position-specific tremor, 217, 217t
Positron emission tomography (PET), 142–143
Postcentral gyrus, lesions of, 18
Postconcussion syndrome, 137t
Post-endarterectomy syndrome, 63
Posterior cerebral artery, 186f, 187f
Posterior cerebral artery infarct, 189f
Posterior communicating artery, 186f
Posterior fossa infarct, 193t
Posterior fossa surgery, monitoring evoked potentials
        during, 32
Posterior fossa tumor, 91t
Posterior inferior cerebellar artery, 186f
    thrombosis of, 96
Posterior tibial nerve, nerve conduction studies using,
        33
Post-herpes simplex encephalitis, 137t
Postherpetic neuralgia, 65–66, 172t, 179–180
Postoperative pain, 172t, 180–181
Postpolio syndrome, 134
Postradiation pain, 180
Post-traumatic headache, 61–62
Post-traumatic pain, 172t
Postural balance, 100–102
Postural headache, 45
Postural instability
    in Parkinson disease, 209
    tests for, 209
Postural tremor, 216, 217t, 218
Posture, in geriatric patient, 25t
Posturography, 92–93
Pramipexole (Mirapex)

Pramipexole—*Continued*
  for Parkinson disease, 212*t*
  for restless legs syndrome, 168*t*
  side effects of, 217*t*
Pravachol. *See* Pravastatin
Pravastatin (Pravachol)
  indications for, 194
  myotoxicity of, 129*t*
Praxis, tests of, 7*t*
Prazosin, for pain, 178
Precentral gyrus, 15, 15*f*
Prednisone (Deltasone)
  for cluster headache prophylaxis, 60*t*
  for myopathy, 128
  side effects of, 129*t*
  for temporal arteritis, 63
Prefrontal cortex, 142*f*
Pregnancy
  antiepileptic drugs and, 165
  migraine during, 50–51, 51*t*
  in multiple sclerosis, 234–235
  neuropathy in, 118
Presbycusis, 13, 25*t*
Presbyopia, 25*t*
Presyncope, 90, 99–100
  causes of, 91*t*
  clinical features of, 92*t*
  diagnosis of, 92*t*
  management of, 100, 100*t*
  mechanisms of, 91*t*
Prilocaine, for pain, 176*t*, 178
Primary lateral sclerosis, 133
Primidone (Mysoline)
  drug interactions, 163
  for seizures, 160*t*
  side effects of, 161, 163*t*
  for tremor, 219, 220*t*
Prion disease, 143, 210
ProAmatine. *See* Midodrine
Procainamide (Pronestyl), side effects of, 128, 129*t*
Procarbazine, side effects of, 254*t*
Prochlorperazine (Compazine)
  for migraine, 51*t*, 54
  for migraine prophylaxis, 55*t*
  side effects of, 211*t*, 212, 222*t*
Progressive bulbar palsy, 133
Progressive multifocal leukoencephalopathy, 137*t*, 240, 241*t*
Progressive supranuclear palsy, 101*t*, 137*t*, 207–209, 210*t*
Prolixin. *See* Fluphenazine
Promethazine (Phenergan)
  side effects of, 211*t*, 222*t*
  for vertigo, 99*t*
Pronestyl. *See* Procainamide
Propoxyphene (Darvocet), for restless legs syndrome, 168*t*
Propranolol (Inderal)
  headache caused by, 52*t*
  for headache of short duration, 61*t*
  for headache prophylaxis, 50*t*
  for migraine, 51*t*
  for migraine prophylaxis, 55
  for orthostatic hypotension, 100*t*

  for tremor, 218–219, 220*t*
Proprioception, 16
  tests of, 19, 33
Propulsid. *See* Cisapride
Prozac. *See* Fluoxetine
Pseudobulbar palsy, 6*t*, 148–149
Pseudoephedrine (Sudafed)
  for orthostatic hypotension, 100*t*
  side effects of, 217*t*
Pseudoseizure, 155*t*, 156*t*
Pseudotumor cerebri, 30, 31*t*, 43–44, 43*t*
Pseudoxanthoma elasticum, 191*f*
Psychiatric illness
  in Parkinson disease, 215
  spells in, 154, 155*t*, 156*t*
Psychogenic gait, 5*t*
Psychogenic overlay, 102
Psychogenic pain, 182
Psychologic issues
  headache and, 47
  spine pain and, 76
Ptosis, 7, 17*t*
Pull test, 24–25, 206, 209
Pupil
  abnormalities of, 7, 8*f*
  sympathetic control of, 8*f*
Pupillary light reflex, 7, 8*f*
Pupillography, 166
Putamen, 204, 206*f*
Pyramidal decussation, 15
Pyridostigmine (Mestinon)
  for Lambert-Eaton syndrome, 132
  for myasthenia gravis, 131
Pyridoxine, side effects of, 108, 108*t*
Pyridoxine deficiency, 113–114
Pyrimethamine, for CNS infections, 240*t*

Quadrantanopia, 10*f*
Quadriceps reflex, 21, 22*t*
Quetiapine (Seroquel)
  for psychosis in Parkinson disease, 213
  for tardive syndromes, 222
  tardive syndromes related to, 222*t*
Quinine sulfate, for muscle cramps, 134

Radial nerve, 21*f*, 22*t*, 87*f*
  compression of, 119–120
Radiation therapy
  for brain tumor, 248
  neurologic complications of, 86, 253
  postradiation pain, 180
Radiculopathy, 77–78, 79*f*
  algorithm for evaluation and treatment of, 79*f*
  back pain in, 75
  cervical, 83*t*
  lumbar, 81–82*t*
  sensory deficit in, 18*t*, 20*f*
  spinal mobility in, 75
  spinal surgery for, 83–84
  weakness in, 17*t*
Ramsay Hunt syndrome, 13, 66
Ranitidine, side effects of, 52*t*

Rebound headache, 48
Recall, tests of, 7t
Reflex arc, 21
Reflex examination, 19–23, 22t, 25t
Reflex sympathetic dystrophy. See Complex regional
    pain syndromes
Refsum disease, 110t
Reglan. See Metoclopramide
Relapsing-remitting multiple sclerosis, 227–228, 227t,
    234
REM sleep behavior disorder, 168
Remote symptomatic seizure, 156
Renal failure, headache in, 46t
Repose tremor, 218
Requip. See Ropinirole
Rescue medication, 181
Reserpine (Serpasil)
    side effects of, 211t
    for tardive syndromes, 222
Resistance to activated protein C, 191f
Rest tremor, 207–208, 216, 217t
Restless legs syndrome, 167–168, 168t, 204, 206
Retinal embolus, 196
Retinal ischemia, 196
Retinal migraine, 49
Retinoic acid, side effects of, 254t
Retinopathy, paraneoplastic, 255t, 256t
Retrovir. See Zidovudine
Reversible ischemic neurologic deficit (RIND), 186
Rheumatoid arthritis, 226t, 239t
    back pain in, 70t
    neuropathy in, 115, 116t, 118
    vertigo in, 97
Rigidity, 205t, 208–209
Riluzole, for amyotrophic lateral sclerosis, 133
RIND. See Reversible ischemic neurologic deficit
Rinne test, 13, 92–93
Risperdal. See Risperidone
Risperidone (Risperdal)
    for dementia, 148t
    for psychosis in Parkinson disease, 213
    side effects of, 211t, 222t
Ritalin. See Methylphenidate
Rizatriptan, for migraine, 53
Romberg sign, 101, 106, 113
Romberg test, 19
Ropinirole (Requip)
    for Parkinson disease, 212t
    for restless legs syndrome, 168t
    side effects of, 217t

Saddle anesthesia, 74t
Sarcoidosis, 107, 110t, 137t, 191f, 200, 226t, 232, 232t,
    237
Saturday night palsy, 120
Schilling test, 113
Schizophrenia, 205t
Schwannoma, 246
Sciatic nerve, 87f
Sciatic stretch test, 75
Sciatica, 18t, 78
Scleroderma, 127, 226t
Scoliosis, in history of neuropathy, 107–108

Scopolamine (Transderm-Scop), for vertigo, 99t
Secondary progressive multiple sclerosis, 227t, 228, 234
Segmental dystonia, 219
Seizures, 155–165, 187–188. See also specific types
    algorithm for evaluation of, 159f
    in brain tumor, 247, 250
    causes, 156, 157t
    chemotherapy-related, 254t
    electroencephalography in, 30, 32t, 158
    first, diagnostic approach to, 155–160
    magnetic resonance imaging in, 158–159
    migraine with seizure disorder, 45
    neuroimaging in, 37t
    prognosis in, 158
    provoked, 156, 157t, 159
    risk for recurrence of, 159
    syncope versus, 156
    treatment of, 159–164, 160t, 162t, 163t, 164t
    unprovoked, 156–157
    in women, 164–165
Selective serotonin reuptake inhibitors (SSRI)
    for dementia, 148t
    for pain, 175t, 177
Selegiline (Eldepryl)
    for Alzheimer disease, 146
    for Parkinson disease, 212t, 213, 214t
Semivoluntary movements, 204
Sensory ataxia, 5t
Sensory examination, 16–21, 18t, 20–21f, 25t
Sensory loss, 103–120. See also Neuropathy
    diagnostic approach to, 104–109
Sensory trick, 220
Serentil. See Mesoridazine
Seroquel. See Quetiapine
Serpasil. See Reserpine
Sertraline (Zoloft), for dementia, 148t
Serum sickness, 226t
Serzone. See Nefazodone
Short Test of Mental Status, 140–141
Shoulder pain, 82, 86
Shoulder-hand syndrome, 250
Shy-Drager syndrome, 207, 210t
Sick sinus syndrome, 191f
Sickle cell anemia, 191f, 199–200
Simvastatin (Zocor)
    indications for, 194
    side effects of, 129t
Sinemet. See Carbidopa/levodopa
Single-photon emission computed tomography
    (SPECT), 142
Sjögren syndrome, 115, 116t, 226t, 232t, 239t
Sleep apnea, 166–167
    diary, 166
    disorders, 155t, 156t, 165–168
        in Parkinson disease, 209, 215
        dyskinesias during, 204
        paralysis, 166–167
        periodic movements of, 167, 204
        terror, 168
Sleep/wake cycle disorders, 166
Sleep-walking, 168
Small-vessel disease
    dementia in, 148–149
    gait in, 5t

Small-vessel disease—*Continued*
  stroke and, 190, 191*f*
Smell, sense of, 7
Snout reflex, 24
Social skills, normal development of, 24*t*
Sodium channel antagonists, for pain, 63–64, 64*t*, 176*t*,
  177
Sodium intake, 195
Solu-Medrol. *See* Methylprednisolone
Somatization disorder, 181
Somatoform disorder, resemblance to peripheral nerve
  disease, 106*t*
Somatoform pain, 172*t*, 182
Somatosensory evoked potentials, 32–33
Somesthetic cortex, lesions of, 18
Somnolence, daytime, 166–167
Spastic dysarthria, 6*t*
Spastic gait, 5*t*
Spasticity, 208, 237
SPECT. *See* Single-photon emission computed
  tomography
Speech, evaluation of, 5–6, 6*t*, 14
Spells, 154–155
  algorithm for evaluation of, 159*f*
  differential diagnosis of, 154–155, 155*t*
  electroencephalography in, 30–31
  focal, 154, 155*t*
  with memory loss, 156*t*
  without focal symptoms, 155*t*, 156*t*
  generalized, 154
Sphenoid wing meningioma, 232*t*
Spina bifida, 70*t*
Spinal accessory nerve (CN XI), 5
  evaluation of, 14
Spinal cord, 15, 15*f*, 71
Spinal cord compression, 38, 78*t*
  epidural, 252–253
Spinal cord injury, 23, 180
Spinal cord lesion, sensory deficit in, 18*t*
Spinal cord tumor, 250–251
  back pain in, 70*t*
  types of, 251
Spinal dural arteriovenous fistula, 70*t*
Spinal mobility, 75
Spinal muscular atrophy, 133
Spinal nerves, 71, 71*f*
  nerve root syndromes, 80*f*
Spinal stability, 78*t*
  surgery for instability, 83–84
Spinal stenosis
  back pain in, 72, 74*t*, 75, 78–80
  diagnosis of, 78*t*
  myelography in, 37
Spinal surgery, 83–85
  complications of, 84–85
  indications for, 83–84
Spine
  anatomy of, 71, 71*f*
  congenital defects of, 75
Spine pain. *See also* Back pain
  algorithm for evaluation and treatment of, 79*f*
  associated clinical conditions, 74*t*
  cervical spondylosis, 80–82
  diagnostic tests for, 76–77

evaluation of, 71–76
  provocative tests, 75
  quality and location of, 71
  radiculopathy, 77–78, 79*f*
  red flags of, 74*t*
  sensory loss with, 76
  spinal stenosis, 37, 78–80
  temporal profile of, 72
  types of, 74*t*
  from whiplash, 82–83
Spinocerebellar degeneration, 232*t*
Spinothalamic tract, 16–17
  tests of, 19
Spondylolisthesis, 76, 77*f*
Spondylolysis, 76, 77*f*, 78*t*
Spondylosis, 70*t*, 72
SSRIs. *See* Selective serotonin reuptake inhibitors
Status migrainosus, 53–54, 55*t*
Stavudine, side effects of, 242
Stelazine. *See* Trifluoperazine
Steppage gait, 125
Stereognosis, 18
Stereotypy, 206*t*
Sternocleidomastoid muscle, evaluation of, 14
Steroid myopathy, 250
Stevens-Johnson syndrome, 250
Stiff muscles, 205*t*
Stiff-person syndrome, 205*t*, 255*t*, 256*t*
Stinger, 85
Straight leg raising test, 75
Strategic infarct, 147–148
Striatonigral degeneration, 101*t*, 207, 210*t*
Stroke. *See also* Cerebrovascular disease
  arterial dissection, 199
  cardiac causes of, 190, 191*f*, 200
  in carotid artery stenosis, 186
  chemotherapy-related, 254*t*
  computed tomography in, 34
  disequilibrium in, 102
  dystonia in, 219
  gait in, 5*t*
  geriatric neurologic examination, 25*t*
  headache in, 43
  hematologic disorders and, 200–201
  hemorrhagic, 188–189, 201, 201*f*
  illicit drug use and, 199
  ischemic, 188–190, 191*f*
  mechanism of, 190–192, 191*f*
  migraine and, 52
  migrainous, 199
  minor, 186
  neuroimaging in, 37*t*
  pain in, 180
  parasomnias in, 168
  prevention of first, 192–196, 194*t*
  seizures in, 157*t*
  speech problems in, 6*t*
  thrombolytic therapy for, 200–201
  after transient ischemic attack, 186
  in young adults, 198–200
Sturge-Weber syndrome, 157*t*
Subacute bacterial endocarditis, 74*t*
Subacute cerebellar degeneration, 255*t*
Subacute combined degeneration, 101*t*

Subacute sclerosing panencephalitis, 137t
Subarachnoid hemorrhage, 201
    computed tomography in, 36f, 188
    CSF analysis in, 31t
    dementia in, 149
    diagnosis of, 193t
    headache in, 42–43, 43t
Subcortical arteriosclerotic encephalopathy, 149
Subdural abscess, 157t
Subdural hematoma
    computed tomography in, 36f, 188
    dementia in, 137t, 149
    headache in, 43, 43t
    seizures in, 157t
Substantia nigra, 204, 206f
Subthalamic nucleus, 204, 206f
Suck reflex, 24
Sudafed. *See* Pseudoephedrine
Sulfadiazine, for CNS infections, 240t
Sumatriptan
    for cluster headache, 60t
    for headache, 49t
    for migraine, 51t, 53, 54t
    for migraine prophylaxis, 55t
Superficial reflexes, 21
Superior cerebellar artery, 186f
    thrombosis of, 96
Superior oblique muscle, 10–11, 11f
Sural nerve, 21f
Suramin, side effects of, 254t
Swallowing, and vagus nerve, 14
Sweating, 100t
    with pain, 179
Swinging-flashlight test, 230
Symmetrel. *See* Amantadine
Syncope
    causes of, 154
    seizure versus, 156
Synovir. *See* Thalidomide
Syphilis
    clinical features of, 232t
    CSF analysis in, 232
    dementia in, 137t, 145t
    diagnosis of, 193t
    disequilibrium in, 101t
    headache in, 46t
    neuropathy in, 110t, 116
    optic neuritis in, 237
    stroke and, 200
    vertigo in, 96–97
Syringomyelia, 18t, 20f, 23, 106t
Systemic disease, neurologic complications of,
        251–256
Systemic lupus erythematosus, 116t, 137t, 191f, 226t,
        232t, 237, 239t
Systemic sclerosis, 115, 116t

Tabes dorsalis, 106t
Tacrine (Cognex)
    for Alzheimer disease, 146
    for dementia, 148t
Tagamet. *See* Cimetidine
Tamoxifen
    for migraine, 51t
    side effects of, 254t
Tardive syndromes
    diagnosis of, 221–222
    treatment of, 222
Tardive tremor, 217t
Task-specific tremor, 217, 217t
Tasmar. *See* Tolcapone
Taxol. *See* Paclitaxel
TEE. *See* Transesophageal echocardiography
Tegretol. *See* Carbamazepine
Temperature sensation, 16–18, 18t
    tests of, 19
Temporal arteritis, 65f, 226t, 239t
    dementia in, 137t
    headache in, 43t, 46t, 62–63
    polymyalgia rheumatica and, 63
Temporal cortex, tumor of, 247t
Temporal lobe
    lesions, 10, 10f
    role in learning, 7, 141, 142f
    seizures, aura in, 7
Temporomandibular joint dysfunction, 66
Teniposide, side effects of, 254t
Tenormin. *See* Atenolol
TENS. *See* Transcutaneous electrical nerve stimulation.
Tensilon test, 130–131
Tension-type headache, 45, 49t, 57–58, 65f
    chronic, 57–58
    episodic, 57–58
    migraine and, 57–58
    prophylaxis for, 50t
    treatment of, 58
Terbutaline (Brethine), side effects of, 217t
Terminal tremor, 216–217
Tetanus, 209
Tethered cord, 70t
Tetrabenazine, for tardive syndromes, 222
Thalamic infarct, 18t, 20f, 149
Thalamic pain syndrome, 18t
Thalamic syndrome, 17–18
Thalamic tumor, 247t
Thalamotomy
    for Parkinson disease, 215–216
    for tremor, 220t
Thalidomide (Synovir), side effects of, 108, 108t
Thallium intoxication, 107t, 115t, 178
Theo-Dur. *See* Theophylline
Theophylline (Theo-Dur), side effects of, 158, 217t
Thioridazine (Mellaril)
    for dementia, 148t
    side effects of, 211t, 222t
Thiotepa, side effects of, 254t
Thiothixene (Navane), side effects of, 211t, 222t
Third ventricle, tumor of, 247t
Thoracic outlet syndrome, 86, 119
Thorazine. *See* Chlorpromazine
Thrombocythemia, 191f
Thrombocytosis, 193t
Thrombolytic therapy
    complications of, 200–201
    exclusion criteria for, 200
    for stroke, 200–201
Thrombophlebitis, 191f

Thrombosis, 191*f*
Thrombotic thrombocytopenic purpura, 191*f*
Thymectomy, 131
Thyroid disease, 8, 134, 137*t*
Thyrotoxicosis, 46*t*, 118, 217
TIA. *See* Transient ischemic attack
Tiagabine (Gabitril), for seizures, 161
Tibial nerve, 21*f*, 22*t*, 87*f*
Tics, 204, 206*t*, 220–221
    definition of, 221
    treatment of, 221
    types of, 221
Tick paralysis, 107*t*
Ticlid. *See* Ticlopidine
Ticlopidine (Ticlid)
    after stroke, 188
    for stroke prevention, 191–192
Tigan. *See* Trimethobenzamide
Timolol (Blocadren)
    for migraine prophylaxis, 55
    for tremor, 218
Tinel sign, 119
Tinnitus, 13
Tissue plasminogen activator (t-PA), thrombolytic
    therapy with, 200
Tizanidine (Zanaflex), for multiple sclerosis, 236*t*
Tobramycin, side effects of, 101*t*
Tocainide, for muscle cramps, 134
Todd paralysis, 158
Tolcapone (Tasmar), for Parkinson disease, 212*t*,
    213
Tonic-clonic seizure, generalized, 32*t*, 161
Topamax. *See* Topiramate
Topiramate (Topamax)
    for seizures, 160*t*, 161
    side effects of, 163*t*
Top-shelf syndrome, 98
Torticollis, 204, 205*t*, 219
Tourette syndrome, 205*t*, 220–221
Toxins, myopathy related to, 128, 129*t*
    dementia related to, 138–139
    neuropathy related to, 107*t*, 108, 114, 115*t*
    spells related to, 156*t*
Toxoplasmosis, 240, 241*t*
t-PA. *See* Tissue plasminogen activator
Traction/inflammatory headache, 45
Tramadol (Ultram)
    for diabetic neuropathy, 112*t*
    for pain, 175*t*
    for restless legs syndrome, 168*t*
Transcutaneous electrical nerve stimulation, 178
Transderm-Scop. *See* Scopolamine
Transesophageal echocardiography (TEE), 200
Transformed migraine, 52–53, 58
Transient global amnesia, 154, 155*t*, 156*t*
Transient ischemic attack (TIA), 155*t*, 186
    differential diagnosis of, 187–188
    treatment of, 190–192
    vertigo in, 96–97
Transverse myelitis, 226*t*, 227*t*, 228
Trapezius muscle, evaluation of, 14
Trauma
    neuropathy related to, 107*t*
    postconcussion syndrome, 137*t*

    post-traumatic headache, 61–62
    post-traumatic pain, 172*t*
    seizures after head injury, 157*t*, 158
Traumatic dementia, 138
Traumatic tap, 30
Trazodone (Desyrel)
    for dementia, 148*t*
    for sleep disturbance, 215
Tremor, 204, 206*t*. *See also specific types*
    definition of, 216, 217*t*
    drug-related, 217*t*
    in Parkinson disease, 208, 216, 217*t*
    treatment of, 218–219, 220*t*
    types of, 216–219, 217*t*, 218*t*
Trendelenburg gait, 73
Triavil. *See* Perphenazine/amitriptyline
Triazolam (Halcion), for restless legs syndrome,
    168*t*
Triceps muscle, evaluation of, 14
Triceps reflex, 21, 22*t*, 80*f*
Trichloroethylene intoxication, 115*t*
Tricyclic antidepressants
    for headache, 58
    for headache prophylaxis, 50*t*
    for migraine prophylaxis, 56–57
    for narcolepsy, 167
    for pain, 175*t*, 177–178
    for postherpetic neuralgia, 180
    side effects of, 91*t*, 158
Trifluoperazine (Stelazine), side effects of, 211*t*, 222*t*
Trigeminal nerve (CN V), 5
    evaluation of, 11–12
    sensory distribution of branches of, 12, 12*f*
Trigeminal neuralgia, 12, 63–64, 65*f*, 229
Trihexyphenidyl (Artane)
    for Parkinson disease, 213
    for tremor, 220*t*
Trilafon. *See* Perphenazine
Trimethobenzamide (Tigan), for nausea, 212
Trimethoprim-sulfamethoxazole, side effects of, 52*t*
Trochlear nerve (CN IV), evaluation of, 11, 11*f*
Truncal neuropathy, 112
Tuberculosis, 137*t*, 200, 237, 240
Tuberous sclerosis, 157*t*, 158
Tumors, and seizures, 158, 157*t*. *See also* Neuro-
    oncology.
Two-point discrimination test, 18, 18*t*
Tylenol. *See* Acetaminophen

Uhthoff sign, 229
Ulnar nerve, 21*f*, 87*f*
    compression of, 119, 119*f*
    nerve conduction studies using, 33
Ultram. *See* Tramadol
Ultrasonography, carotid, 196
Upper cord lesions, 155*t*
Upper extremity, nerves of, 87*f*
Upper motor neuron, 15, 15*f*
Upper motor neuron lesion, 15, 16*t*, 17*t*, 21–23
Uremia, 137*t*, 157*t*
Urinary retention, 75*t*, 229
Urinary tract infection, 70*t*, 74*t*, 229
"Useless hand," 229

Vagus nerve (CN X), 5
  evaluation of, 14
Valacyclovir, for postherpetic neuralgia, 180
Valium. *See* Diazepam
Valproate (Depakote). *See also* Divalproex sodium.
  drug interactions, 164, 164*t*
  for headache prophylaxis, 50*t*
  for migraine, 51*t*
  for pain, 176*t*, 177
  for seizures, 160–161, 160*t*
  side effects of, 161, 163*t*, 217*t*
Valsalva maneuver, 92
Vancomycin, for CNS infections, 240*t*
Vascular claudication, 84*t*
Vascular dementia, 138–139, 145*t*, 147–149
Vascular headache, 45, 49*t*, 50*t*
Vascular malformation, seizures in, 158
Vascular parkinsonism, 210*t*
Vasculitis, 237–238
  angiography in, 37
  CNS, 226*t*
  CSF analysis in, 232
  dementia in, 137*t*, 145*t*
  diagnostic features of, 239*t*
  headache in, 45
  neuropathy in, 107, 107*t*, 110*t*, 114–115
  pain in, 178
Vasculopathy, chemotherapy-related, 254*t*
Vasospasm, 191*f*
Venlafaxine (Effexor), for pain, 175*t*, 178
Venous thromboembolic disease, with brain tumor,
    250
Verapamil (Calan)
  for cluster headache, 59
  for headache prophylaxis, 50*t*, 60*t*
  for migraine, 51*t*
  for migraine prophylaxis, 56
  for muscle cramps, 134
  side effects of, 211*t*
Vertebral artery, 186*f*
Vertebrobasilar artery, 187*f*
Vertebrobasilar artery disease, 96–97
Vertebrobasilar ischemia, 10*f*, 91*t*, 156*t*
Vertigo, 90, 94–99, 95*f*, 95*t*, 96*t*
  causes of, 91*t*
  central, 94, 95*t*, 96*t*, 97–99, 98*f*
  clinical features of, 92*t*
  diagnosis of, 92*t*, 155*t*, 156*t*
  mechanisms of, 91*t*
  medications for, 99*t*
  nystagmus and, 94–95, 95*t*
  peripheral, 94, 95*t*, 96–97, 96*t*
  positional, 90–91
Vestibular ataxia, 5*t*
Vestibular dysfunction, bilateral, 100–101, 101*t*
Vestibular lesion, 93–94
Vestibular neuritis, 101*t*
Vestibular neuronitis, 91*t*, 92*t*, 96
Vestibular nucleus, 94
Vestibular pathway, anatomy of, 95*f*
Vestibular receptors, 94
Vestibulocochlear nerve (CN VIII), 90
  evaluation of, 13–14
Vestibulopathy, 155*t*, 188

Vibratory sensation, 16–18, 18*t*
  tests of, 19, 33
Videx. *See* Didanosine
Vigabatrin, for pain, 177
Vinblastine, side effects of, 114
Vincasar PFS. *See* Vincristine
Vincristine (Oncovin, Vincasar PFS), side effects of,
    108*t*, 114, 129*t*, 254*t*
Vioform. *See* Clioquinol
Viral meningitis, CSF analysis in, 31*t*
Viral neuronitis, 96
Visual acuity, 7
Visual evoked potentials, 32
Visual field, 7
  tests of, 9, 248
Visual field defects, 9–10, 10*f*
  in carotid artery disease, 196
Visual loss
  acute, 9
  chemotherapy-related, 254*t*
Visual testing, 7
Visual-spatial ability, tests of, 7*t*
Vitamin B$_1$ deficiency, 113, 137*t*
Vitamin B$_2$ deficiency, 113–114
Vitamin B$_{12}$ deficiency, 82
  clinical features of, 232*t*
  dementia in, 137*t*, 138–139
  disequilibrium in, 101*t*
  gait in, 5*t*
  neuropathy in, 110*t*, 113
  sensory deficit in, 18*t*
Vitamin C, neuroprotective effect of, 213
Vitamin D deficiency, 128
Vitamin E
  for Alzheimer disease, 146
  deficiency, 113, 128
  excess, 128, 129*t*
  neuroprotective effect of, 213
Voluntary movements, 204

Waddling gait, 125
Waldenström macroglobulinemia, 110*t*, 116, 117*t*
Wallenberg syndrome. *See* Lateral medullary syndrome
Warfarin, 192
Weakness
  diagnostic approach to, 124–126
  electromyography in, 125
  family history in, 124–125
  motor examination in, 15, 125
  motor neuron disease, 132–134
  muscle biopsy in, 125–126
  in myopathy
    associated with drugs and toxins, 128
    endocrine, 128–130
    inflammatory, 127–128
    inherited, 126–127, 126*t*
  neuromuscular junction disorders, 130–132
  patterns by anatomical division, 16, 17*t*
Weber test, 13, 93
Wegener granulomatosis, 137*t*, 191*f*, 226*t*, 239*t*
Wernicke's area, 142*f*
Whiplash injury, 62, 82–83
Whipple disease of the brain, 137*t*

Wilson disease, 137*t*, 145*t*, 204, 207, 217*t*
Withdrawal emergent syndrome, 222
Working memory, 141
Writer's cramp, 204
Writing
   small (micrographia), 207–208
   to assess therapy for tremor, 218
Wry neck, 219

X-rays. *See* Plain radiographs.

Zalcitabine, side effects of, 242

Zanaflex. *See* Tizanidine
Zarontin. *See* Ethosuximide
Zidovudine (Retrovir)
   for HIV infection, 241
   side effects of, 129*t*, 242
Zocor. *See* Simvastatin
Zolmitriptan
   for migraine, 53, 54*t*
   for migraine prophylaxis, 55*t*
Zoloft. *See* Sertraline
Zostrix. *See* Capsaicin
Zyprexa. *See* Olanzapine